INSTRUCTOR'S MANUAL WITH TEST BANK

for

UNDERSTANDING NORMAL AND CLINICAL NUTRITION

SIXTH EDITION

Eleanor Noss Whitney
Corrine Balog Cataldo
Sharon Rady Rolfes

Mary Rhiner, MA, RD, LD
Kirkwood Community College

Melaney Jones, MS

Lori Turner, PhD., RD
University of Arkansas, Fayetteville

Margaret Hedley, MSc, RD
University of Guelph

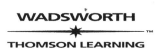

WADSWORTH

THOMSON LEARNING ™

Australia • Canada • Mexico • Singapore • Spain • United Kingdom • United States

Table of Contents

Lecture Outlines Keyed to Media Resources

Prepared by

MARY RHINER, MA, RD, LD
Kirkwood Community College

and

Melaney Jones

CONTENTS

An Overview of Nutrition
Chapter 1

Chapter Summary

Food choices are often based on behavioral or social motives. Nutrition awareness can help people make healthy food choices.

The nutrient classes include carbohydrate, fat, protein, vitamins, minerals and water. Essential nutrients, those that the body cannot make or cannot make in sufficient quantities, must be obtained from food. Nutrients are classified as elements or compounds, organic or inorganic.

Protein, fat, and carbohydrate are energy-yielding nutrients. When metabolized their chemical bonds are broken and energy is released. This energy is measured in kCalories. Alcohol, though not a nutrient, also contributes to food energy. Energy is used in the body to fuel metabolic and physical activities. Excess energy is stored, mostly as fat.

Vitamins and minerals play a different role from the energy-yielding nutrients. They are consumed in much smaller quantities. They function structurally or as chemical helpers. Water, the often forgotten and ignored nutrient, is needed in the most abundant quantity and is indispensable to body activities.

The science of nutrition studies the nutrients in food and the body's handling of those nutrients. Nutrition research using epidemiological studies, case-control studies, animal studies and human intervention trials tries to answer questions about nutrition.

Dietary recommendations reflect collaborative efforts of the United States and Canada. The recommendations are called Dietary Reference Intakes (DRI) and focus on 14 nutrients. The four categories that are used for planning and assessing diets include the Estimated Average Requirements, Recommended Dietary Allowances, Adequate Intakes and Tolerable Upper Intake Levels. Recommendations are based on scientific research.

Recommendations must be used with the following perspectives: that recommendations apply to healthy people, that a large margin of safety is included, that diets contain a variety of foods, that average daily intakes are considered and finally, that each of the four categories serve a unique purpose.

Nutritional assessment evaluates the many factors that influence or reflect nutritional health for individuals and populations. Various methods of data collection are used including collection of the historical information, anthropometric measures, physical examinations, laboratory tests, food consumption surveys and nutrition status surveys.

Nutrition plays a role in many of the leading causes of illness and death in the United States. Government and other agencies have developed diet recommendations to forestall or prevent disease. These include limiting sugar, fat, cholesterol, salt and alcohol, and increasing starch while consuming a variety of foods. Maintaining appropriate body weight and increasing physical activity is also recommended.

Highlight 1 describes the criteria for qualified nutrition experts, identifying valid nutrition information and identifying fake credentials and quacks. It presents ways to identify reliable nutrition information on the Internet. In addition, this Highlight provides lists of reliable sources of nutrition information.

Chapter Outline	**Terms/Overheads/Handouts**
I. Food Choices	**nutrition**
	foods
	chronic
	acute
	diet
A. Personal Preference	
B. Habit	
C. Ethnic Heritage or Tradition	
D. Social Interactions	
E. Availability, Convenience, and Economy	
F. Positive and Negative Associations	
G. Emotional Comfort	
H. Values	
I. Body Weight and Image	
J. Nutrition	**functional foods**
II. The Nutrients	
A. Nutrients in Foods and the Body	**energy**
	nutrients
	O1 Elements in the Six Classes of Nutrients
1. Composition of foods	
2. Composition of the body	
3. Chemical composition of nutrients	**organic**
	inorganic
4. Essential nutrients	**essential**
5. Nonnutrients	**phytochemicals**
	nonnutrients

B. The Energy-Yielding Nutrients   **energy-yielding nutrients**
    1. Energy measured in kCalories   **calories**
    2. Energy from foods
    3. Energy in the body   **metabolism**
    4. Other roles
C. The Vitamins   **vitamins**
D. The Minerals   **minerals**
E. Water
III. The Science of Nutrition
A. Nutrition Research   *02 Research Designs*

    1. Types of studies
        a) Epidemiological studies
        b) Case-control studies
        c) Animal studies
        d) Human intervention trials
    2. Controls   **subjects**
                                                  experimental group
                                                  control group
                                                  randomization

    3. Sample size
    4. Placebos   **placebo**
                                                  placebo effect
                                                  blind experiment
    5. Double Blind   **double-blind experiment**
    6. Correlations and Causes   **variables**
                                                  correlation
                                                  positive correlation
                                                  negative correlation
                                                  replication
                                                  peer review
B. Research versus Rumors   **validity**
IV. Dietary Reference Intakes   **Dietary Reference**
                                                  Intakes (DRI)
A. Establishing Nutrient Recommendations   *O3 Estimated Average*
                                                  Requirements and
                                                  RDA Compared
                                                  O4 The Nutrient RDA and
                                                  the Energy RDA
                                                  Compared
    1. Estimated Average Requirements   **requirement**
                                                  Estimated Average
                                                  Requirement

SUMMARY AND OUTLINE: CHAPTER 1

4

VII. Highlight: Nutrition Information-
Experts and Quacks -On the Net and
In the News

A.   Nutrition on the Net

H1-1 Evaluation of
Published Nutrition
Information
fraud
quackery
Internet (net)
websites
cyberspace
World Wide Web (WWW
The Web)
H1-2 Research Project
Using the Internet
H1-3 Tufts University
Nutrition Navigator

B.   Nutrition in the News
C.   Identifying Nutrition Experts
   1.   Physicians
   2.   Registered dietitians

dietitian

registered dietitian (RD)
registration
American Dietetic
Association (ADA)

   3.   Others

dietetic technician
registered (DTR)
public health dietitians

D.   Identifying Fake Credentials

accredited
correspondence schools
nutritionist
license to practice

E.   Identifying Valid Information

misinformation

SUMMARY AND OUTLINE: CHAPTER 1

6

SUMMARY AND OUTLINE: CHAPTER 1

Planning a Healthy Diet
Chapter 2

Chapter Summary

Basic diet planning principles include choosing an <u>adequate</u> diet that provides enough energy and nutrients to meet the needs of healthy people. The diet must be <u>balanced</u> - using enough but not too much of each type of food. <u>Overeating must be avoided</u>. Foods should be delivering the most nutrients for the least amount of food energy (<u>nutrient dense</u>). <u>Variety</u> and <u>moderation</u> contribute to all of these factors.

The Dietary Guidelines for Americans apply principles of good eating and offer practical advice on healthy habits.

A tool for successful diet planning includes the Daily Food Guide. This familiar plan sorts foods into five major food groups based on nutrient content and origin. It is simple and flexible. Serving sizes and number of servings to consume from each group are recommended for various age groups. Energy intakes are not specified. The USDA's Food Pyramid graphically illustrates the Daily Food Guide.

The Exchange Lists categorize foods by their nutrient and energy content. Portion sizes vary to allow energy amounts to be similar. Lists for starches/breads, vegetables, fruits, meats, milk and milk products and fats are provided. Meat and milk are subdivided by fat content. Exchange lists allow people to more easily control energy and fat intakes.

Using diet planning tools together allows individuals to plan nutrient-dense, well-balanced diets that provide variety and moderation and avoid overeating.

Shopping for nutrient dense foods is a priority. Choose whole grain and enriched breads, cereals and other grains. Fresh green and yellow-orange vegetables are important, as are citrus and yellow-orange fruits. Choose legumes often. Lean meats, fish and poultry with visible fat removed and prepared using low fat cooking methods is preferred. Fortified low-fat milk and milk products are recommended over imitation products.

The Food and Drug Administration (FDA) has revised food labeling regulations to include required labeling on almost all packaged foods. Posters or brochures provide nutrition information for fresh meats, vegetables and fruits.

Requirements for ingredient lists, serving sizes, and nutrition facts are outlined. The Daily Values (DV) are used as standard values for labeling. Percent Daily Values for 2000 kCalorie diets are used for reference. Nutrient claims and health claims on labels must meet specified FDA criteria.

Consumer education is an important component of the FDA labeling plan.

Highlight 2 outlines the college dilemma in preparing nutritious meals when time, groceries and kitchen facilities are limited.

Chapter Outline	**Terms/Overheads/Handouts**
I. Principles and Guidelines	
A. Diet-Planning Principles	
1. Adequacy	**adequacy (dietary)**
2. Balance	**balance (dietary)**
3. kCalorie (energy) control	**kCalories (energy) control**
4. Nutrient density	**nutrient density** **empty-kCalorie foods**
5. Moderation	**moderation (dietary)**
6. Variety	**variety (dietary)**
B. Dietary Guidelines for Americans	
1. Aim for fitness	
a) Aim for a healthy weight	
b) Be physically active each day	
2. Build a healthy base	
a) Use pyramid to guide food choices	
b) Choose variety in grains, especially whole grains	
c) Choose variety in fruits and vegetables	
d) Keep foods safe to eat	
3. Choose sensibly	
a) Choose a diet low in saturated fat and cholesterol and moderate in total fat	
b) Choose beverages and foods that limit your intake of sugar	
c) Choose and prepare foods with less salt	
d) If you drink alcoholic beverages, do so in moderation	
II. Diet-Planning Guides	
A. Food Group Plans	**food group plans**
1. Daily food guide	*H2-1 Compare Your Food Intake to the Daily Food Guide*
2. Notable nutrients	
3. Miscellaneous foods	
4. Mixtures of foods	
5. Nutrient density	
6. Recommended servings	

SUMMARY AND OUTLINE: CHAPTER 2

SUMMARY AND OUTLINE: CHAPTER 2

D. From Guidelines to Groceries
    1. Breads, cereals and other grains

refined
enriched
whole grain
020 Nutrients in Bread

    2. Vegetables
    3. Legumes
    4. Fruit
    5. Meat, fish and poultry

textured vegetable protein

    6. Milk

imitation foods
food substitutes
nonfat milk, fat-free milk, skim, zero-fat, no-fat, low-fat milk
reduced-fat milk

III. Food Labels

O21 Introducing a Food Label

A. The Ingredient List
B. Serving Sizes
C. Nutrition Facts

O22 Introducing a Food Label "Nutrition Facts"

D. The Daily Values
E. Nutrient Claims
F. Health Claims
G. Consumer Education

Daily Values (DV)
nutrient claims
health claims
H2-2 Most Frequently Eaten Raw Fruits, Vegetables, and Seafood

IV. Highlight: College Bound and Hungry
    1. Use the food pyramid
    2. Make shopping list

SUMMARY AND OUTLINE: CHAPTER 2

Digestion, Absorption, and Transport
Chapter 3

Chapter Summary

The gastrointestinal tract is a flexible muscular tube that prepares nutrients for absorption. Food enters the mouth, where it is reduced to a coarse mash. Peristalsis passes the bolus through the esophagus to the stomach. The stomach retains the bolus, adds water, and grinds it to a suspension of small particles. The semiliquid mass (chyme) passes to the small intestine where it is further broken down. Various glands and organs work together to secrete digestive juices containing hormones and enzymes that help in breaking down foods to absorbable units. Undigested and unabsorbed nutrients pass through the large intestine to be eliminated.

Muscular actions of digestion include peristalsis, the motions of the circular and longitudinal muscles of the stomach, segmentation, and sphincter contractions.

Nutrients absorbed through the microvilli of the small intestine travel to one of two systems - the bloodstream directly or the lymphatic system. Once inside the vascular system, nutrients travel freely and can be used by any cells in the body.

Details of the gastrointestinal system are regulated by the endocrine (hormone) and nervous system. PH levels, sphincters, and digestive and enzymatic secretions help in making the digestive tract responsive to conditions in its environment. A healthy digestive tract will help to promote proper functioning of the system. Balance, variety, moderation and adequacy of the diet promotes optimal utilization of foods consumed.

Highlight 3 reviews common digestive problems. Choking may require use of the Heimlich maneuver. Serious vomiting can cause fluid and electrolyte imbalances. Diarrhea, characterized by frequent and loose stools, requires rest and fluid replacement. Constipation, although generally not serious, may reflect a need for lifestyle changes. Belching and gas is more of a complaint than a serious problem. Heartburn and "acid indigestion" is painful and may be caused by different factors, thus the treatments vary. Ulcer treatment includes seeking medical advice and avoiding foods and beverages that cause difficulties. Many of the common digestive problems reflect hurried lifestyles rather than any particular foods eaten.

Chapter Outline	Terms/Overheads/Handouts
I. Digestion	**digestion**
	absorption
A. Anatomy	*O23 The Gastrointestinal Tract*
	gastrointestinal (GI) tract
	lumen
	gastro
	intestinalis
1. Mouth	**mouth**
	mastication
	pharnyx
	digestive system
	epiglottis
	bolus
2. Esophagus/stomach	**esophagus**
	sphincter
	esophageal sphincter
	stomach
	chyme, chymos
	pyloric sphincter, pylorus
3. Small intestine	**gall bladder**
	pancreas
	small intestine
	duodenum, duodecim
	jejunum
	ileum
4. Large intestine (Colon)	**large intestine, colon, sigmoid**
	ileocecal valve
	appendix
	rectum
	anus
B. Muscular Actions	**motility**
1. Peristalsis	**peristalsis, peri, stellien**
2. Stomach action	*O24 Stomach Muscles*
3. Segmentation	**segmentation**
4. Sphincter contractions	**reflux**

SUMMARY AND OUTLINE: CHAPTER 3

C. Secretions of Digestion	*O25 The Salivary Glands*
	O26 The pH Scale
	gland
	exocrine, exo
	endocrine, endo
	krine
	catalyst
	hydrolysis, hydro,
	  lysis
	digestive enzymes
	  -ase
	  carbohydrase
	  lipase
	  protease

1. Saliva	**salivary glands** **saliva**
2. Gastric juice	**gastric glands** **gastric juice** **hydrochloric acid** **mucus** **mucus membrane** **goblet cells** **pH**
3. Pancrestic juice and intestinal enzymes	**pancreatic juice** **bicarbonate**
4. Bile	**liver** **bile** **emulisifier**
5. Protective factors	**intestinal flora, flora**
D. Final Stages	**stools** **feces**
II. Absorption	**absorption**

A. Anatomy	**villi, villus**
	microvilli, microvillus
	O27 The Small Intestinal
	  Villi
	crypts
	O28 Absorption of
	  Nutrients

B. Intestinal Cells
  1. Cell capabilities
  2. Specialization
  3. Food combining "myth"
  4. Nutrient transport preparation

SUMMARY AND OUTLINE: CHAPTER 3

III. The Circulatory Systems
   A. Vascular System

O29 The Vascular System
H3-1 Transport of
   Nutrients into
   Blood
arteries
capillaries
veins
portal vein, portal
hepatic vein, hepatic

   B. Lymphatic System

lymphatic system
lymph
thoracic duct
subclavian vein
lacteals
O30 The Liver

IV. Regulation of Digestion and
    Absorption

homeostasis, homeo,
   stasis

   A. Hormones and Nerve
      Pathways

hormones

     1. pH level of stomach

gastrin

     2. Pyloric sphincter
     3. Alkaline pH

secretin

     4. Pancreatic enzymes
     5. Presence of fat

cholesystokinin (CCK)

     6. Intestinal motility

gastric-inhibitory
   peptide

   B. System at Its Best

V. Highlight: Common Digestive Problems
   A. Choking

trachea
Helmlich maneuver
larnyx

   B. Vomiting

vomiting

   C. Diarrhea

diarrhea
colitus
colonic irrigation
irritable bowel syndrome
indigestion

   D. Constipation

constipation
defecate, defaecare
hemorrhoids
diverticulitis
diverticula

   E. Belching and Gas

belching
hiccups

SUMMARY AND OUTLINE: CHAPTER 3

F. Heartburn and "Acid Indigestion"   **acid controllers**
                                              antacids
                                              heartburn
                                              gastroesophageal reflux
                                              indigestion
G. Ulcers   **ulcer**
                                              peptic ulcer

SUMMARY AND OUTLINE: CHAPTER 3

SUMMARY AND OUTLINE: CHAPTER 3

The Carbohydrates:
Sugars, Starches, and Fibers
Chapter 4

Chapter Summary

The simple carbohydrates include the monosaccharides (glucose, fructose and galactose) and the disaccharides (sucrose, maltose and lactose). The complex carbohydrates include the polysaccharides (glycogen, starch and fiber).

Carbohydrate digestion involves hydrolyzing bonds to absorbable forms. This process begins in the mouth and continues through the stomach and small intestine. Fibers are not digested. Carbohydrates that are absorbed circulate to the liver, where cells convert the compounds to glucose.

Some individuals lack lactase - the enzyme responsible for the digestion of lactose. This is characterized by bloating, gas, abdominal discomfort and diarrhea upon the consumption of lactose-containing foods.

The main function of glucose in the body is to provide energy. Glycogen is the storage form of glucose - found only in the liver and muscle cells. Glucose can be made from protein. Extra glucose can be converted into fat. The homeostasis of blood glucose is important for health. Hormones that help to maintain blood glucose in the normal range include insulin, glucagon and epinephrine.

Sucrose poses no major health concerns except for increased risk of dental caries. It may be associated with nutrient deficiencies. Sugar does not cause obesity, heart disease, misbehavior in children nor criminal behavior in adults. It is recommended that the diet contain no more than 10% of total kCalories from refined sugars.

Health effects of starch and fiber include weight control, low blood pressure, decreased risk of some forms of cancer, better control of diabetes and improved GI functioning. Excessive fiber may result in abdominal discomfort, low nutrient availability and bulk production.

Highlight 6 classifies the list of FDA approved artificial sweeteners, their properties and allowable intakes and uses. Safety aspects and benefits of

18

artificial sweeteners are discussed. Advantages and disadvantages of sugar alcohols are provided.

Chapter Outline	Terms/Overheads/Handouts
I. The Chemist's View	**carbohydrates, carbo, hydrate** **simple carbohydrates** **complex carbohydrates** **hexoses** *O31 Atoms and their Bonds*
II. Simple Carbohydrates	*O32 Simplified Diagrams of Glucose*
A. Monosaccharides	*O33 Chemical Structures of the Monosaccharides* **monosaccharides, mono, saccharide**
1. Glucose	**glucose** **dextrose, ose**
2. Fructose	**fructose, fruct**
3. Galactose	**galactose**
B. Disaccharides	**disaccharides, di**
1. Condensation	**condensation** *O34 Condensation of Two Monosaccharides*
2. Hydrolysis	**hydrolysis** *O35 Hydrolysis of a Disaccharide*
3. Maltose	**maltose**
4. Sucrose	**sucrose, sucro**
5. Lactose	**lactose, lact**
III. Complex Carbohydrates	**polysaccharides, poly, oligosaccharide**
A. Glycogen	**glycogen, glyco, gen**
B. Starches	**starches** **available carbohydrates** *O36 Glycogen and Starch Molecules Compared*
C. Fibers	**fibers** *H4-1 Characteristics of Fiber*
1. Cellulose	
2. Hemicellulose	
3. Pectins	

SUMMARY AND OUTLINE: CHAPTER 4

        4.   Gums and mucilages
        5.   Lignin
        6.   Other classifications   **soluble fibers**
                                                      insoluble fibers
                                                      phytic acid
                                                      phytate

IV. Digestion and Absorption   **dextrins**
    A. Processes
        1.   Mouth
        2.   Stomach   **satiety**
        3.   Small intestine   **maltase**
                                                      sucrase
                                                      lactase
        4.   Large intestine   **resistant starch**
                                                      ferment
        5.   Absorption in bloodstream   *O37 Absorption of*
                                                      Monosaccharides
    B. Lactose Intolerance   **lactose intolerance**
        1.   Symptoms
        2.   Causes   **lactase deficiency**
        3.   Prevalence
        4.   Dietary changes   **acidophilus**
V. Glucose in the Body
    A. Carbohydrate Metabolism   **available carbohydrates**
                                                      unavailable
                                                          carbohydrates

        1.   Storing glucose as glycogen
        2.   Using glucose for energy
        3.   Making glucose from protein   **gluconeogenesis, gluco,**
                                                          neo, genesis
                                                      protein-sparing action
        4.   Making ketone bodies   **ketone bodies**
                                                      ketosis
                                                      acid-base balance

        5.   Converting glucose to fat
    B. Blood Glucose Constancy
        1.   Glucose homeostasis   *O38 Maintaining Blood*
                                                      Glucose Homeostasis
        2.   Regulating hormones   **insulin**
                                                      glucagon
                                                      epinephrine (adrenaline)

        3.   Balancing within normal range
        4.   Outside normal range
        5.   Diabetes   **diabetes**
                                                      type 1 diabetes

SUMMARY AND OUTLINE: CHAPTER 4

type 2 diabetes
juvenile-onset diabetes
noninsulin-dependent
  diabetes mellitus
hypoglycemia
glycemic effect
glycemic index

6. Hypoglycemia
7. Glycemic effect

VI. Health Effects and Recommended
Intakes of Sugars

brown sugar
confectioners' sugar
corn sweeteners
corn syrup
dextrose
granulated sugar
high-fructose corn syrup
honey
invert sugar
levulose
maple sugar
molasses
raw sugar
turbinado sugar
white sugar

A. Health Effects of Sugar
    1. Nutrient deficiencies
    2. Dental caries

dental caries, caries
plaque (dental)

B. Accusations about Sugar
    1. Obesity
    2. Heart disease
    3. Misbehavior and criminal behavior
C. Recommended intakes of sugar
VII. Health Effects and Recommended Intakes
    of Starch and Fibers
    A. Health Effects of Starch and Fiber
        1. Weight control
        2. Heart disease
        3. Cancer
        4. Diabetes
        5. GI health
        6. Harmful effects of excessive fiber

    B. Recommended Intakes of Starch and Fiber
        1. Choose variety
        2. Read food labels

SUMMARY AND OUTLINE: CHAPTER 4

VIII. Highlight: Alternatives to Sugar

    A. Artificial Sugars

        1. Saccharin
        2. Aspartame
        3. Acesulfame-K
        4. Sucralose
        5. Alitame, cyclamate

        6. Acceptable daily intake

        7. Weight control

    B. Sugar Replacers
        1. Sugar alcohols

nutritive sweeteners
stevia
artificial sweeteners
nonnutritive sweeteners
saccharin
aspartame
acesulfame potassium
sucralose
alitame
cyclamate
ADI (Acceptable Daily Intake)

sugar replacers
sugar alcohols
polyols
maltitol
mannitol
sorbitol
xylitol
isomalt
lactitol

SUMMARY AND OUTLINE: CHAPTER 4

SUMMARY AND OUTLINE: CHAPTER 4

The Lipids: Triglycerides, Phospholipids, and Sterols
Chapter 5

Chapter Summary

The lipids include triglycerides (fats and oils), phospholipids, and sterols. In foods fats provide flavor, tenderness and palatability.

Triglycerides are composed of fatty acids and glycerol. The fatty acids can be long, medium or short chained, and saturated, monounsaturated, or polyunsaturated. Omega-3 and omega-6 polyunsaturated fatty acids have special importance in nutrition. Essential fatty acids include linoleic and linolenic acid.

Processed fat in food is often hydrogenated to alter the texture of the food and prolong its shelf life. The cis-fatty acid configuration is found naturally in foods and the trans-fatty acid configuration is found in processed foods. Altered fatty acids may have adverse health effects.

Triglycerides provide energy, insulation, and protection from shock and help the body use protein and carbohydrate. Fatty acid saturation affects cooking qualities, storage and susceptibility to disease. The body can make some fatty acids. Deficiencies do occur in some cases. Triglycerides in the diet provide fat-soluble vitamins, add satiety, and deliver flavor, texture and tenderness to foods.

Phospholipids are used as emulsifiers in foods. They function as part of the cell membrane. Cholesterol is found in animal foods only. Sterols include vital body compounds such as bile, sex hormones and Vitamin D.

Fat is emulsified by bile in the small intestine to make it accessible for lipase to digest it. After absorption, fats are transported in the bloodstream by lipoproteins. These include chylomicrons, very-low-density lipoproteins, low-density lipoproteins, and high-density lipoproteins. The distinction between lipoproteins has important implications for health.

Fat is efficiently stored in fat cells. Fat stores have virtually unlimited capacity. When needed for energy, the enzyme lipase responds and fat is broken down. When fat is metabolized in the absence of carbohydrate, ketone bodies are formed.

Lipid profiles are important to evaluate risk of heart disease. Excess fat contributes to obesity, cancer, hypertension, and diabetes. Current recommendations include reducing fat intake to 30% or less of total energy intake, saturated fat to one-third of total fat or less than 10% of energy intake, and cholesterol to less that 300 milligrams per day.

Highlight 4 describes the use of fat replacements. Some are carbohydrate-based, protein-based and fat-based while some are classified as synthetic. Properties, caloric values and uses of each are outlined. Fat replacements offer low-fat alternatives to high fat foods and provide the desired flavor and texture preferred by many people. There are some side effects.

Chapter Outline	**Terms/Overheads/Handouts**
I. The Chemist's View of Triglycerides and Fatty Acids	lipids
A. The Fatty Acids	**fatty acid**
1. The carbon chain	*O39 A Saturated Fatty Acid* *O40 A Monounsaturated Fatty Acid* *O41 A Polyunsaturated Fatty Acid* *O43 Formation of a Triglyceride* *O44 A Mixed Triglyceride*
2. Degree of unsaturation	**saturated fatty acid** **saturated fat** **unsaturated fatty acid** **unsaturated fat** **monounsaturated fatty acid, mono** **polyunsaturated fatty acid (PUFA), poly** **polyunsaturated fat** **linoleic acid** **linolenic acid**
3. Double bond location	**point of unsaturation** **omega** **omega-3 fatty acid** **omega-6 fatty acid** *O42 Omega-3 and Omega-6 Fatty Acids Compared* *O45 Comparison of Dietary Fats*

B.   Triglycerides

triglycerides, tri, glyceride, acyl
O44 A Mixed Triglyceride

C.   Degree of unsaturation

fats
oils

    1.   Firmness
    2.   Stability

oxidation
antioxidants

    3.   Hydrogenation

hydrogenation
O46 Hydrogenation

    4.   Trans-fatty acids

trans-fatty acids
O47 Cis- and Trans- Fatty Acids Compared

II.   The Chemist' s View of Phospholipids and Sterols

   A.   The Phospholipids

phospholipid
lecithin
O48 Lecithin
choline

    1.   Phospholipids in foods
    2.   Roles of phospholipids

   B.   The Sterols

sterols
cholesterol
endogenous
exogenous
O49 Cholesterol and Vitamin D3

    1.   Sterols in foods
    2.   Roles of sterols

atherosclerosis, athero, scleros, osis

III.   Digestion, Absorption and Transport of Lipids

hydrophobic, hydro, phobia, lipo, phile
hydrophillic

   A.   Lipid Digestion

monoglyceride
diglyceride

    1.   Mouth
    2.   Stomach
    3.   Small intestine

O50 Emulsification of Fat by Bile
O51 Digestion of a Triglyceride

    4.   Route of bile

   B.   Lipid Absorption

micelles
chylomicrons
O52 Absorption of Lipids

SUMMARY AND OUTLINE: CHAPTER 5

C.   Lipid Transport

lipoproteins
*O53 Size Comparisons of
   the Lipoproteins*
O54 A Typical Lipoprotein
*O55 The Lipoproteins
   Compared*

1.   Chylomicrons   **chylomicrons**
2.   Very-low-density lipoporteins   **VLDL**
3.   Low-density lipoproteins   **LDL**
4.   High-density lipoproteins   **HDL**
5.   Health implications

IV.   Lipids in the Body
  A.   Triglycerides
  B.   Essential Fatty Acids   **essential fatty acids**
     1.   Linoleic Acid   **arachidonic acid**
     2.   Linolenic Acid   **eicosapentaenoic acid**
                             docosahexaenoic acid
     3.   Eicosanoids   **eicosaniods**
     4.   Fatty acid deficiencies
  C.   Lipid Metabolism
     1.   Storing fat as fat   **adipose tissue**
                             O56 An Adipose Cell
                             lipoprotein lipase

     2.   Making fat from carbohydrate or protein
     3.   Making fat from fat
     4.   Using fat for energy   **hormone-sensitive
                              lipase**

V.   Health Effects and Recommended Intakes
   of Lipids
  A.   Health Effect of Lipids   **blood lipid profile**
     1.   Heart disease   **cardiovascular disease,
                              cardio, vascular**

     2.   Risks from saturated fats
     3.   Risks from trans-fats
     4.   Benefits of monounsaturated fats
     5.   Benefits from omega-3 polyunsaturated fats
     6.   Cancer
     7.   Obesity
     8.   Fat restrictions

B.   Recommended Intakes of Fat   *H5-1 How to Modify*
                                                                              A Recipe

        1.   Reduce total fat intake
        2.   Reduce saturated fat and trans-fat intake
        3.   Reduce cholesterol intake
        4.   Balance omega-3 and omega-6 intakes
        5.   Select lean meats and nonfat milks
        6.   Eat vegetables, fruits and grains
        7.   Use fats and oils sparingly
        8.   Invisible fat
        9.   Wise choices
        10.   Read food labels

VI.   Highlight: Alternatives to Fat
    A.   Carbohydrate-Based Fat Replacers
    B.   Protein-Based Fat Replacers
    C.   Fat-Based Fat Replacers
    D.   Synthetic Fat Replacers

SUMMARY AND OUTLINE: CHAPTER 5

SUMMARY AND OUTLINE: CHAPTER 5

Protein: Amino Acids
Chapter 6

Chapter Summary

Protein is vital to the structural and working materials of all cells. The structure of protein allows many diverse functions in the body as compared to fat and carbohydrate. Protein carries nitrogen, oxygen, hydrogen and carbon atoms. Twenty different amino acids form the building blocks of protein. Essential amino acids are those the body cannot make in sufficient amounts to meet needs.

Protein is denatured in the stomach so digestive enzymes can attack peptide bonds. Digestive enzymes in the small intestine continue to hydrolyze protein to single amino acids. Carriers transport the amino acids into the cells.

Protein functions in the growth and maintenance of tissue. Enzymes, hormones and antibodies are proteins. Proteins help with fluid and acid-base balance and aid in the transport of nutrients, the clotting of blood, and vision.

Amino acids, the building blocks of protein, are used by the cells to make other compounds. When fat and carbohydrate are limited, amino acids can be deaminated and used for energy. Excess amino acids are stored as fat.

Food proteins can be limiting in essential amino acids or incomplete. Plant proteins may need to be complemented. Proteins of high quality are easily digested and offer the body all the essentials amino acids. Amino acid scoring, biological value, net protein utilization, protein efficiency ratio and PDCAAS are measures used to evaluate protein quality.

Protein-energy malnutrition is classified as kwashiorkor, marasmus or a mix of the diseases. Infections are common and rehabilitation requires careful nutrition therapy. Excessive intake of protein may pose health risks.

Protein recommendations include allowing 15% of total kCalories as protein. Protein recommendations are also expressed in proportion to body weight at 0.8gm/kg of healthy body weight. The use of amino acid supplements is inappropriate.

Highlight 6 reviews vegetarian diets. Benefits of meatless diets include ease of controlling body weight, lowering blood pressure, and fewer incidences of coronary artery disease and cancer. Diet planning includes meeting protein, iron, zinc, calcium, vitamin B12 and vitamin D needs. Special attention to diet during pregnancy, lactation, infancy, childhood and adolescence is recommended.

Chapter Outline	**Terms/Overheads/Handouts**
I. The Chemist's View of Protein	**protein**
A. Amino Acids	**amino acids**
1. Unique side groups	
2. Nonessential amino acids	**nonessential amino acids**
3. Essential amino acids	**essential amino acids** **indispensible** **dispensible**
4. Conditionally essential amino acids	**conditionally essential amino acid**
B. Proteins	
1. Amino acid chains	**peptide bond** **dipeptide, di, peptide** **tripeptide, tri** **polypeptide, poly, oligo** *O57 Amino Acid Structure* *O58 Examples of Amino Acids* *O59 Formation of a Dipeptide*
2. Amino acid sequences	
3. Protein shapes	
4. Protein functions	**hemoglobin, hemo, globin**
5. Protein denaturation	**denaturation**
II. Digestion and Absorption of Protein	
A. Digestion process	
1. Stomach	**pepsin, pepsinogen**
2. Small intestine	**peptidase, tri, di, endo, exo** **proteases**
B. Absorption process	
III. Proteins in the Body	
A. Protein Synthesis	*O60 Protein Synthesis*
1. Delivering instructions	
2. Amino acid line up	

SUMMARY AND OUTLINE: CHAPTER 6

3. Sequencing errors	**sickle-cell anemia**
4. Nutrients and gene expression	

B. Roles of Protein

1. Building materials	**matrix**
	collagen
2. Enzymes	**enzymes**
	O61 Enzyme Action
3. Hormones	
4. Fluid balance	**fluid balance**
	edema
5. Acid-base regulation	**acids**
	bases
	acidosis
	alkalosis
6. Transporters	*O62 A Membrane-Bound Transport Protein*
7. Antibodies	**antigens**
	antibodies
	immunity
8. Energy and glucose source	
9. Other roles	

C. Protein Metabolism

1. Protein turnover and amino acid pool	**protein turnover**
	endogenous protein, endo, gen
	exogenous, exo
	amino acid pool
2. Nitrogen balance	**nitrogen balance**
3. Using amino acids to make proteins or nonessential amino acids	
4. Using amino acids to make other compounds	**neurotransmitters**
5. Using amino acids for energy	
6. Deaminating amino acids	**deamination**
7. Using amino acids to make fat	

IV. Protein in Foods

H6-1 Plant Proteins in Human Nutrition: Myths and Realities

A. Protein Quality

1. Limiting amino acids	**limiting amino acid**
2. Complete protein	**complete protein**
3. Complementary proteins	**mutual supplementation**
	O63 Examples of Mutual Supplementation
	complementary proteins

    4.   Digestibility

    5.   Reference protein
B. Measures of Protein Quality
    1.   Amino acid scoring
    2.   Biological value
    3.   Net protein utilization

    4.   Protein efficiency ratio

    5.   PDCAAS

protein digestibility
high-quality protein
reference protein

amino acid scoring
biological value (BV)
**net protein utilization
(NPU)**
**protein efficiency ratio
(PER)**
**protein digestibility-
corrected amino acid
score (PDCAAS)**

C. Protein Regulation for Food Labels
V. Health Effects and Recommended
     Intakes of Protein
  A. Protein-Energy Malnutrition   **protein-energy
malnutrition (PEM)**
**protein-calorie
malnutrition (PCM)**
acute PEM
chronic PEM

    1.   Classifying PEM   *O64 Features of Maramus
& Kwashiorkor in
Children*

    2.   Marasmus   **marasmus**
    3.   Kwashiorkor   **kwashiorkor**
                                 aflatoxin

    4.   Marasmus-kwashiorkor mix
    5.   Infections   **dysentery**
    6.   Rehabilitation
B. Health Effects of Protein
    1.   Heart disease
    2.   Cancer
    3.   Adult bone loss (osteoporosis)
    4.   Weight control
    5.   Kidney disease
C. Recommended Intakes of Protein
    1.   Protein RDA
    2.   Adequate energy
    3.   Protein in abundance
D. Protein and Amino Acid Supplements

VI. Highlight: Vegetarian Diets

vegans
pure vegetarians
strict vegetarians
total vegetarians
vegetarians

A. Health Benefits
   1. Weight control
   2. Blood pressure
   3. Coronary artery disease   **vegans**
   4. Cancer   **omnivores,omni,vores**
B. Vegetarian Diet Planning   **tofu**
           tempeh
   1. Protein   **lacto-ovo-**
           vegetarians, ovo
           meat replacements
           textured vegetable
           protein

   2. Iron
   3. Zinc
   4. Calcium   **lactovegetarians**
   5. Vitamin B12
   6. Vitamin D
C. Vegetarian Diets through the Life Span
   1. Pregnancy and lactation
   2. Infancy
   3. Childhood and adolescence
D. Closing Thoughts   **macrobiotic diets**

SUMMARY AND OUTLINE: CHAPTER 6

Metabolism:
Transformations and Interactions
Chapter 7

Chapter Summary

After a balanced meal, the energy-yielding nutrients are digested and absorbed. Carbohydrate yields glucose which is used by the brain cells and other cells. It is metabolized to pyruvate and acetyl CoA to provide energy. Some glucose may be stored as glycogen. Fat yields glycerol and fatty acids. These are also metabolized to acetyl CoA, enter the TCA cycle and provide energy. Some are reassembled and stored as fat. Protein yields amino acids that primarily function to build body protein. Amino acids will be metabolized for energy, if needed. Carbohydrate, fat and protein enter the TCA cycle by different routes, but the energy-yielding pathways are the same.

Surplus carbohydrate is stored as glycogen. When glycogen stores are filled, excess is routed to fat. Surplus fat is stored as fat with seemingly unlimited capacity. Surplus protein is deaminated. It can be used for energy. If not needed for energy, it is stored as fat.

Stored energy is drawn upon as the body shifts from a fed state to a fasting state. Fat stores last longer than carbohydrate stores. It is important that the nervous system and brain cells have glucose available to them. Protein may be called upon to meet this need. Ketosis, a condition of high blood and urine ketones, is a danger sign. Ketosis suppresses the appetite and slows metabolism. This adaptation of the body helps to prolong life in life threatening situations or starvation.

Quick weight loss schemes may promote the loss of weight but not the loss of fat.

Highlight 7 describes the relationship between nutrition and alcohol. Ethanol produces a state of euphoria in the human body. It reacts likes a drug, offering some benefits with dangerous short term and long term side effects. Various amounts consumed have different effects on different people.

Alcohol is metabolized by the liver cells at the rate of 1/2 ounce per hour depending on the individual and the circumstances. The pathway for alcohol metabolism is different than that of the other energy-yielding nutrients. Alcohol interferes with a multitude of chemical and hormonal reactions.

Chapter Outline	**Terms/Overheads/Handouts**
I. Chemical Reactions in the Body	**photosynthesis, photo, synthesis** **fuel** **metabolism** **energy metabolism meta, bole**
A. Building Reactions	**anabolism, ana**
B. Breakdown Reactions	**catabolism, kata**
C. Transfer of Energy in Reactions	**coupled reactions** **adenosine triphosphate (ATP)**
D. The Site of Reactions - Cells	*O68 A Typical Cell*
E. Helpers in Reactions 1. Enzymes 2. Coenzymes	**coenzymes, co**
II. Breaking Down Nutrients for Energy	*O69 A Simple Overview of Energy Metabolism* **pyruvate** **acetyl CoA, CoA** **acetate, acetic acid**
A. Glucose	*O65 Anabolic and Catabolic Reactions: Glycogen* **glycolysis, glyco, lysis**
1. Glucose-to-pyruvate and back	
2. Glucose-to-pyruvate, anaerobic pathway	**anaerobic, an** **aerobic** *O70 Glycolysis*
3. Pyruvate-to-acetyl CoA	*O71 Pyruvate-to-Acetyl CoA* *O73 The Breakdown of Acetyl CoA* *O72 The Paths of Pyruvate and Acetyl CoA*
4. Glucose retrieval via Cori cycle	**Cori cycle** **lactic acid**
5. Muscle's need for oxygen	
6. Pyruvate-to-acetyl CoA, irreversible	

SUMMARY AND OUTLINE: CHAPTER 7

7. Acetyl CoA-to-carbon dioxide	**TCA cycle**
	Kreb's cycle
8. Acetyl CoA-to-fat	*O74 In Summary: The Glucose-To-Energy Pathway*
	O66 Anabolic and Catabolic Reactions: Triglycerides
B. Glycerol and Fatty Acids	
	O75 The Fats-to-Energy Pathway
1. Glycerol-to-pyruvate	
2. Fatty acids-to-acetyl CoA	**fatty acid oxidation**
	beta oxidation
3. Glucose not retrievable from fatty acids	
C. Amino Acids	*O67 Anabolic and Catabolic Reactions: Protein*
	O76 Amino Acid-To-Pathway
Energy	
1. Amino acid catabolism	
2. Glucose retrievable from amino acids	
3. Amino acids-to-fat	
4. Deamination	**keto**
	O77 Keto Acids
	ammonia
5. Transamination	**transamination**
	O78 Transamination to Make a Nonessential Amino Acid
6. Ammonia-to-urea in liver	**urea**
	O79 Urea Synthesis
7. Urea excreted via kidneys	*O80 Urea Excretion*
8. Water for urea excretion	
D. The Final Stages of Catabolism	
1. The TCA cycle	**oxaloacetate**
2. The electron transport chain	**electron transport chain (ETC)**
	O81 Electron Transport Chain

3. kCalories/g secret revealed

III. The Body's Energy Budget

    A. Economics of Feasting   *O83 Feasting*

        1. Surplus protein

        2. Surplus carbohydrate

        3. Surplus fat

    B. Transition from Feasting to Fasting

    C. Economics of Fasting   *O84 Fasting*

                                         O85 Continued Fasting

        1. Glucose for the brain

        2. Protein to meet glucose needs

        3. Fat's small glucose contribution
             from glycerol

        4. Ketosis shift   *O86 Ketone Body*
                                              Formation

        5. Appetite suppression

        6. Metabolic slowdown

        7. Starvation symptoms

IV. Highlight: Alcohol and Nutrition

    A. Alcohol in Beverages   **alcohol**
                                               ethyl alcohol, ethanol

beer

wine

distilled liquor

drug

proof

moderation

drink

    B. Alcohol in the Body   *O87 Alcohol Metabolism*

alcohol dehydrogenase

    C. Alcohol Arrives in the Liver   **acetaldehyde**

alcohol abuse

nicotinamide adenine
           dinucleotide (NAD)

    D. Alcohol Disrupts the Liver   **fatty liver**

fibrosis

cirrhosis,cirrhos

microsomal ethanol-
           oxidizing system
           (MEOS),micro,soma

SUMMARY AND OUTLINE: CHAPTER 7

E. Alcohol and the Brain

narcotic
euphoria
antidiuretic hormone (ADH)

F. Alcohol and Malnutrition

H7-1 Alcohol's Effects on Nutrients in the Body
alcoholism

G. Short Term Effects
H. Long Term Effects
I. Personal Strategies

moderation

SUMMARY AND OUTLINE: CHAPTER 7

SUMMARY AND OUTLINE: CHAPTER 7

Energy Balance and Body Composition
Chapter 8

Chapter Summary

Energy balance is a simple yet complex formula. Energy from food and beverages is measured by the use of the bomb calorimeter. Hunger, appetite and satiety resulting from stimuli from nutrients and hormones play a role. Energy expenditure includes basal metabolism, physical activity, thermic effect of food and adaptive thermogenesis. An individual can estimate energy requirements. If the energy consumed equals the energy expended, the individual is in energy balance. If energy consumed is more than energy expended, weight increases. If energy consumed is less that energy expended, weight decreases.

A variety of techniques are used to measure body weight and body composition. Height/weight charts and body mass indexes are used as guidelines for weight. Waist circumference and waist-to-hip measure body fat distribution. Fatfold measures, hydrodensitometry and bioelectrical impedance measure body composition. Body fat distribution and composition may be critical in determining risks to health.

Both overweight and underweight are conditions associated with health risk. There is a strong relationship between obesity and cardiovascular disease, diabetes and cancer.

Highlight 8 discusses guidelines for identifying fad diets and weight loss schemes.

Chapter Outline   Terms/Overheads/Handouts

I. Energy Balance
II. Energy In: The KCalories Food Provide
    A. Food Composition   **bomb calorimeter, calor,**
                                                   metron
                                                 direct calorimetry

42

A. Defining Healthy Body Weight
   1. Body weight and its standards
   2. Body mass index

body mass index (BMI)
overweight
underweight
O90 BMI Values Used to
   Assess Weight
O91 Different Body
   Compositions
   Compared
O94 BMI Silhouettes

B. Body Fat and Its Distribution
   1. Some people need less
   2. Some people need more
   3. The criterion of health

H8-1 Medical Problems
   Associated with Obesity

   4. Fat distribution

intra-abdominal fat
central obesity,
   abdominal fat,
   upper-body fat
O95 Visceral Fat and
   Subcutaneous Fat

   5. Waist circumference
   6. Other measures

waist circumference
O92 Methods Used to
   Assess Body Fat
 fat-fold measure,
   skinfold test
hydrodensitometry
bioelectrical impedance

C. Health Risks Associated with Body
   Weight and Body Fat

O93 Body Mass Index and
   Mortality

   1. Health risks of underweight
   2. Health risks of overweight
   3. Cardiovascular disease
   4. Diabetes

insulin resistance

   5. Cancer

SUMMARY AND OUTLINE: CHAPTER 8

44

V. Highlight: The Latest and Greatest
       Weight-Loss Diet - Again
   A. The Diet's Appeal
   B. The Diet's Achievements
       1. Don't count kCalories
       2. Satisfy hunger
       3. Follow a plan
   C. The Diet's Shortcomings
       1. Too much fat
       2. Unbalanced nutrition
       3. Too little variety
   D. The Body's Perspective

SUMMARY AND OUTLINE: CHAPTER 8

Weight Control:
Overweight and Underweight
Chapter 9

Chapter Summary

Various theories are used to explain obesity. Fat cell development, fat cell metabolism, and set-point theory are theoretical explanations. Genetics and environmental factors have been proposed as causes of obesity. Differences of opinion lead to controversies in weight loss treatment.

Choices for treatment of obesity are many. Aggressive treatments include drugs and surgery. Weight regains are common. Reasonable treatments for obesity involve planning well-balanced eating plans with physical activity. Behavior and attitude are important aspects. Weight maintenance programs are valuable after weight goals are met.

Underweight conditiond pose health problems also. Strategies for weight gain include intake of energy-dense foods, regular meals, large portions, extra snacks and exercise to build muscles.

Anorexia nervosa, bulimia nervosa and binge eating are eating disorders characterized by sociological, neurochemical and psychological problems. The nutritional component of treatment involves dietary intervention and education. Highlight 9 discusses characteristics and treatment plans.

Chapter Outline

	Terms/Overheads/Handouts
I. Overweight	**epidemic,epi,demos** *O96 Prevalence of Obesity among Adults across the U.S.* *O97 Distribution of Body Weights in U.S. Adults* *O98 Weight Gain Patterns during Adulthood*

46

A. Fat Cell Development	**hyperplastic obesity** **hypertrophic obesity** *O99 Fat Cell Development*
B. Fat Cell Metabolism	
C. Set-Point Theory	**set point**
II. Causes of Obesity	
A. Genetics	

1. Leptin	**leptin, leptos**
	*O100 Leptin's Action in the
	    Body: Negative Energy
	    Balance*
	*O101 Leptin's Action in the
	    Body: Positive Energy
	    Balance*
	*O102 Mice With and
	    Without Leptin
	    Compared*

2. Uncoupling proteins	**brown adipose tissue**
B. Environment	
1. Overeating	**toxic food environment**
2. Physical inactivity	
III. Controversies on Obesity Treatment	
A. Elusive Goals	
B. Dangers of Weight Loss	
1. Fad diets	

2. Weight cycling	**weight cycling**
	**rachet effect, yo-yo
	    effect**
	*O103 Weight Cycling
	    Effect of
	    Repeated Dieting*
	*O104 The Psychology of
	    Weight Cycling*

3. Psychological problems	
IV. Aggressive Treatments of Obesity	
A. Drugs	
1. Sibutramine	**sibutramine** **serotonin**
2. Orlistat	**orlistat**
3. Other drugs	
4. Over-the-counter drugs	
5. Herbal products	
6. Other gimmicks	**cellulite**
B. Surgery	**clinical severe obesity**

V. Reasonable Treatments of Obesity

O105 Reasonable Weight Goals and Expectations Compared
H9-1 Evaluation of a Weight-Loss Program

    A. Eating Plans
        1. Realistic energy intake
        2. Nutritional adequacy
        3. Small portions
        4. Complex carbohydrates
        5. Choose fats sensibly
        6. Empty kCalories
        7. Adequate water intake
    B. Physical Activity
        1. Activity and energy expenditure
        2. Activity and basal metabolism
        3. Activity and body composition
        4. Activity and appetite control
        5. Activity and psychological benefits
        6. Choosing activities
        7. Spot reducing
    C. Behavior and Attitude
        1. Behavior modification
        2. Awareness of behaviors

behavior modification
H9-2 Eating Attitudes Test
H9-3 Exploring Eating Habits

        3. Change behaviors
        4. Personal attitude
        5. Support groups
    D. Weight Maintenance
    E. Prevention
    F. Public Health Programs
VI. Underweight
    A. Problems of Underweight
    B. Weight-Gain Strategies
        1. Energy-dense foods
        2. Regular meals daily
        3. Large portions
        4. Extra snacks
        5. Juice and milk
        6. Exercising to build muscles

48

VII. Highlight: Eating Disorders	**eating disorder**
A. The Female Athlete Triad	**female athlete triad**
	O106 The Female Athlete Triad
1. Disordered Eating	
2. Amenorrhea	**amenorrhea**
	primary amenorrhea
	secondary amenorrhea
3. Osteoporosis	**stress fractures**
B. Other Dangerous Practices of Athletes	**muscle dysmorphia**
C. Preventing Eating Disorders in Athletes	
D. Anorexia Nervosa	**anorexia nervosa, an, orex, nervos**
1. Characteristics	**cathartic**
a) Role of the family	
b) Self-starvation	
c) Physical consequences	
2. Treatment	
E. Bulimia Nervosa	**bulimia nervosa**
1. Characteristics	
a) Role of the family	
b) Binge eating	
c) Purging	**cathartic**
	emetic
2. Treatment	**unspecified eating disorders**
F. Binge-Eating Disorder	**binge-eating disorder**
G. Eating Disorders in Society	

The Water-Soluble Vitamins:
B Vitamins and Vitamin C
Chapter 10

Chapter Summary

The structure and function of vitamins differ from the energy-yielding nutrients. Vitamins are individual units. They do not yield energy but assist the enzymes that release energy. The amounts needed by the body are considerably less as compared to the energy-yielding nutrients. Vitamins are essential nutrients with unique characteristics.

The water-soluble vitamins are needed in frequent, small amounts. They are absorbed directly into the blood, and travel freely. They are excreted in the urine, so are unlikely to reach toxic levels.

Thiamin, riboflavin, niacin, pantothenic acid, biotin, vitamin B6, folate, and vitamin C are reviewed. Functions, recommended intakes, deficiency symptoms and diseases, problems with toxicity, and significant food sources are outlined in detail. The unique characteristics of each vitamin are given. Interrelationships are discussed.

Highlight 10 reviews arguments for and against vitamin and mineral supplements. Guidelines for appropriate supplementation are given.

Chapter Outline

	Terms/Overheads/Handouts
I. Overview of Vitamins	**vitamins, vita, amine** *O107 Coenzyme Action*
A. Bioavailability	**bioavailability**
B. Precursors	**precursors, provitamins**
C. Organic Nature	
D. Solubility	**water-soluble vitamins** **fat-soluble vitamins**
E. Toxicity	

50

II. B Vitamins-As Individuals
    A. Thiamin   **thiamin**
        1. Recommendations
        2. Deficiency   **Wernicke-Korsakoff syndrome**
                                                     beriberi, beri, beriberi
        3. Food sources   *O108 Thiamin in Foods*
    B. Riboflavin   **riboflavin**
        1. Recommendations
        2. Deficiency
        3. Food sources   *O109 Riboflavin in Foods*
    C. Niacin   **niacin**
        1. Recommendations   **niacin equivalents (NE)**
        2. Deficiency   **pellegra, pellis, agra**
        3. Toxicity   **niacin flush**
                                                       pharmacological effect, physio, pharma
        4. Food sources   *O110 Niacin in Foods*
    D. Biotin   **biotin**
        1. Recommendations
        2. Deficiency   **avidin, avid**
        3. Food sources
    E. Pantothenic Acid   **pantothenic acid, pantos**
        1. Recommendations
        2. Deficiency
        3. Food sources
    F. Vitamin B6   **vitamin B6**
                                           serotonin
                                         antagonist
        1. Recommendations
        2. Deficiency
        3. Toxicity   **carpal tunnel syndrome**
        4. Food sources   *O111 Vitamin B6 in Foods*
    G. Folate   **folate**
        1. Recommendations   **dietary folate equivalents (DFE)**
        2. Folate and neural tube defects   **neural tube defects**
        3. Folate and heart disease
        4. Folate and cancer
        5. Deficiency   **anemia, an, emia**
                                         O114 Normal & Anemic Blood Cells
                                         macrocytic or megaloblastic anemia
                                         macro, cyte, mega
        6. Food sources   *O112 Folate in Foods*

SUMMARY AND OUTLINE: CHAPTER 10

H. Vitamin B12   **vitamin B12**
intrinsic factor, intrinsic

    1. Recommendations
    2. Deficiency   **atrophic gastritis,**
                                       atrophy,
                                         gastro, itis
                                 pernicious anemia,
                                         pernicious

    3. Food sources
I. Non-B Vitamins
    1. Choline   **choline**
    2. Inositol and carnitine   **inositol**
                                   carnitine

    3. Vitamin impostors
III. The B Vitamins-In Concert   *O115 Metabolic Pathways*
                                   Involving B Vitamins

A. Roles
B. Deficiencies   **glossitis**
                                 cheilosis, glosis, cheilos

C. Toxicities
D. Food sources
IV. Vitamin C   **scurvy**
                                 purgative
                                 antiscorbutic factor, anti,
                                       corbutic
                                 ascorbic acid, a, scorbic

A. Roles
    1. Antioxidant   **antioxidant**
                                 oxidative stress
    2. Collagen formation   **cofactor**
    3. Co-factor in other reactions
    4. In stress
    5. Cure for common cold   **histamine**
    6. Disease prevention
B. Recommendations   *O116 Vitamin C Intake*
                                 (mg/day)

C. Deficiency
D. Toxicity   **false positive**
                                 false negative
                                 withdrawal reaction
E. Food sources   *O113 Vitamin C in Foods*

SUMMARY AND OUTLINE: CHAPTER 10

V. Highlight: Vitamin and Mineral
    Supplements

A. Arguments for Supplements
    1. Correct overt deficiencies
    2. Improve nutrition status
    3. Reduce disease risk
    4. Support increased nutrient needs
    5. Improve the body's defenses
    6. Who needs supplements?
B. Arguments Against Supplements
    1. Toxicity
    2. Life-threatening misinformation
    3. Unknown needs
    4. False sense of security
    5. Other invalid reasons
    6. Bioavailability and antagonistic
        actions
C. Selection of Supplements

    1. Form
    2. Contents
    3. Misleading claims
    4. Cost
D. Regulation of Supplements
    1. Nutritional labeling
    2. FDA approval

    3. Health claims

    4. Relationship to disease
    5. Nutrient information

supplements
H10-1 Vitamin/Mineral
Supplement Evaluation

H10-2 Factors that
Destroy Vitamins

high potency

**FDA (Food and Drug
Administration)
FTC (Federal Trade
Commission)
structure-function
claims**

The Fat-Soluble Vitamins:
A, D, E, and K
Chapter 11

Chapter Summary

The fat-soluble vitamins include Vitamin A, D, E and K. Vitamin A is important to vision, healthy epithelial tissues, immunity and bone growth. Deficiency leads to infections, blindness, and keratinization of epithelial tissues. Preformed Vitamin A is found primarily in animal products and beta-carotene is found in bright orange and dark green leafy vegetables. Vitamin D is synthesized in the body with the help of sunlight. Vitamin D supports bone formation and maintenance. Deficiency causes rickets in children and osteomalacia in adults. Fortified milk is an important source of Vitamin D. Vitamin E serves as an antioxidant and is found primarily in vegetables oils. Deficiencies are rare. Vitamin K helps with blood clotting. Half of Vitamin K is obtained from bacterial synthesis in the intestine and half is obtained from foods such as liver, leafy green vegetables, and the cabbage family vegetables.

Fat-soluble vitamins are important to the growth and maintenance of the body. Toxicity is possible especially when supplements are used. Interrelationships of fat-soluble vitamins with each other and with minerals are important.

Highlight 11 explores the research on antioxidants and phytochemicals explaining their functions and relationships to disease. Food claims are mentioned.

Chapter Outline   Terms/Overheads/Handouts

I.   Vitamin A and Beta-Carotene   **vitamin A**
                                                 beta-carotene
                                                 retinoids
                                                 carotenoids
                                                 vitamin A activity

54

A. Roles
   1. Vision

retinol-binding protein
  (RBP)
O117 Forms of Vitamin A.

cornea
retina
pigment
rhodopsin, rhod, opsin
rods
opsin
*O118 Vitamin A's Role in
  Vision*

   2. Protein synthesis and cell
      differentiation

differentiation
epithelial cells
epithelial tissue
mucous membranes
*O119 Mucous Membrane
  Integrity*

   3. Reproduction and growth

remodeling
osteoclasts
osteoblasts, osteo, clast,
  blast
lysosomes

   4. Beta-carotene as an antioxidant

B. Deficiency
   1. Infectious diseases
   2. Night blindness
   3. Blindness (xerophthalmia)

night blindness
xerophthalmia, xero,
  ophthalm
xerosis
keratomalacia

   4. Keratinization

keratin
keratinization

C. Toxicity
   1. Birth defects
   2. Not for acne

teratogenic, terato, genic
acne

D. Recommendations
E. Food Sources

retinol equivalents (RE)
*O120 Vitamin A and
  Betacarotene in Foods*

   1. Food colors

chlorophyll
xanthophylls

   2. Vitamin A-poor fast foods
   3. Vitamin A-rich liver

II. Vitamin D

O121 Vitamin D Synthesis and Activation
O123 Vitamin D Synthesis and Latitude

  A. Roles
    1. Bone growth
    2. Other roles
  B. Deficiency
    1. Rickets

rickets
O122 Vitamin D Deficiency Syndrome-The Bowed Legs of Rickets

    2. Osteomalacia

osteomalacia, osteo, malacia

    3. Osteoporosis
    4. Elderly
  C. Toxicity

hypercalcemia

  D. Recommendations and Sources

cholecalciferol (Vitamin D3)
ergocalciferol (vitamin D2)

    1. Foods
    2. Sunlight

III. Vitamin E

tocopherol
alpha-tocopherol

  A. Antioxidant
  B. Deficiency

erthrocyte hemolysis, erthro, cyte, hemo, lysis
hemolytic anemia
muscular dystrophy
fibrocystic breast disease, fibro, cyst
intermittent claudication, intermittent, claudicare

  C. Toxicity
  D. Recommendations

tocopherol equivalents (TE)

  E. Food Sources

IV. Vitamin K

phylloquinone
menadione

  A. Roles

hemorrhagic disease
hemophillia
O126 Blood-Clotting Process

SUMMARY AND OUTLINE: CHAPTER 11

56

SUMMARY AND OUTLINE: CHAPTER 11

Water and the Major Minerals
Chapter 12

Chapter Summary

Water is an important nutrient responsible for carrying other nutrients and waste throughout the body. It participates in chemical reactions and helps to form macromolecules. It acts as a lubricant, shock absorber, and solvent, and aids in temperature regulation.

Imbalances of fluids cause dehydration or water intoxication. The body has specific mechanisms for regulating water balance and excretion. It uses minerals to help regulate the distribution of body fluids and electrolytes.

Sodium, chloride, potassium, calcium, phosphorus, magnesium, and sulfur are reviewed along with their specific functions, deficiency and toxicity symptoms, recommendations, significant food sources and unique characteristics. Interrelationships with other nutrients are explained.

Highlight 12 explores the role of calcium and health with emphasis on osteoporosis.

Chapter Outline	Terms/Overheads/Handouts
I. Water and the Body Fluids	**intracellular fluid, intra interstitial fluid, extracellular fluid, inter, extra water balance**
A. Water Balance and Recommended Intakes	
1. Water intake	**thirst dehydration water intoxication obligatory water excretion**

58

    2.   Water sources
    3.   Water losses
    4.   Water recommendations
B. Blood Volume and Blood Pressure

                                                                   O127 A Nephron, One of the Kidney's Many Functioning Units
O128 How the Body Regulates Blood Volume

    1.   ADH and water retention   **antidiuretic hormone (ADH), anti, di, ure, vasopressin, vaso, press**

    2.   Renin and sodium retention   **renin**
    3.   Angiotensin and blood vessel constriction   **angiotensin, angiotensinogen vasoconstrictor**

    4.   Aldosterone and sodium retention   **aldosterone adrenal glands**

C. Fluid and Electrolyte Balance
    1.   Dissociation of salt in water   *O129 Water Dissolves Salts and Follows Electrolytes*
salt
dissociates
ions
cations
anions
electrolytes
electrolyte solutions
millequivalents (mEq)

    2.   Electrolytes attract water
    3.   Water follows electrolytes   *O130 Examples of Osmosis*
solutes
solute concentration
osmosis

    4.   Proteins regulate flow of fluids and ions
    5.   Regulation of fluid and electrolyte balance
D. Fluid and Electrolyte Imbalance
    1.   Sodium and chloride most easily lost
    2.   Different solutes lost by different routes

SUMMARY AND OUTLINE: CHAPTER 12

    3. Replacing lost fluids and
       electrolytes **oral rehydration therapy (ORT)**

  E. Acid-Base Balance **pH**
O131 The pH Scale
carbonic acid

    1. Regulation by buffers
    2. Regulation by the lungs
    3. Regulation by the kidneys

II. The Minerals-An Overview **major minerals, macrominerals**

  A. Inorganic Elements
  B. The Body's Handling of Minerals
  C. Variable Bioavailability **binders, phytates, oxalates**

  D. Nutrient Interactions
  E. Varied Roles

III. Sodium **sodium**
  A. Sodium Roles in the Body
  B. Sodium Recommendations
  C. Sodium and Hypertension **salt sensitivity**
  D. Sodium and Osteoporosis
  E. Sodium in Foods *H12-1 Spices to Enhance Salt-Free Dishes*

  F. Sodium Deficiency
  G. Sodium Toxicity and Excessive Intakes

IV. Chloride **chloride**
  A. Chloride Roles in the Body
  B. Chloride Recommendations and Intakes
  C. Chloride Deficiency and Toxicity

V. Potassium **potassium**
  A. Potassium Roles in the Body
  B. Potassium Recommendations and Intakes *O137 Potassium in Selected Foods*

  C. Potassium and Hypertension
  D. Potassium Deficiency
  E. Potassium Toxicity

VI. Calcium **calcium**
  A. Calcium Roles in the Body
    1. Calcium in bones **hydroxapatite mineralization**
    2. Calcium in body fluids **calmodulin**
    3. Calcium and disease prevention

SUMMARY AND OUTLINE: CHAPTER 12

60

4. Calcium balance	**parathormone**
	parathyroid hormone
	calcitonin
	calcium rigor
	calcium tetany
	O132 Calcium Balance in Bone
5. Calcium absorption	**calcium-binding protein**
B. Calcium Recommendations and Sources	
1. Calcium recommedations	
2. Calcium sources	*O133 Calcium in Selected Foods*
3. Nonmilk sources	
C. Calcium Deficiency	**peak bone mass**
	osteoporosis, adult bone loss, osteo, porosis
	O134 Healthy and Osteoporotic Trabecular Bones

VII. Phosphorus — **phosphorus**
- A. Phosphorus Roles in the Body
- B. Phosphorus Recommendations
- C. Phosphorus Sources

VIII. Magnesium — **magnesium**
- A. Magnesium Roles in the Body
- B. Magnesium Intakes
- C. Magnesium Deficiency
- D. Magnesium and Hypertension
- E. Magnesium Toxicity

IX. Sulfur — **sulfur**

X. Highlight: Osteoporosis and Calcium
   A. Bone Development and Disintegration

cortical bone
trabecular bone
type I osteoporosis
type II osteoporosis
bone density

   B. Age and Bone Calcium

O135 Loss of Height in a
*   Woman Caused by*
*   Osteoporosis*
O136 Bone Losses Over
*   Time Compared*

      1. Maximizing bone mass
      2. Minimizing bone loss
   C. Gender and Hormones
   D. Genetics
   E. Physical Activity and Body Weight
   F. Smoking and Alcohol
   G. Calcium - Key to Prevention
   H. Supplements
   I. Summary

SUMMARY AND OUTLINE: CHAPTER 12

SUMMARY AND OUTLINE: CHAPTER 12

The Trace Minerals
Chapter 13

Chapter Summary

Each of the trace minerals fulfills a vital role in the body. A deficiency or an excess could be fatal. Well-balanced diets normally supply the right amount of each trace mineral to maintain health.

Each of the following trace minerals are reviewed: iron, zinc, iodine, selenium, copper, manganese, fluoride, chromium, molybdenum, and others. Chief functions in the body, deficiency and toxicity symptoms, and significant food sources are included. Recommendations are listed for RDAs or Estimated Safe and Adequate Intakes. Factors affecting absorption and utilization are presented. Additionally, environmental contamination, supplementation, and fortification is examined. Information is provided about interactions.

Highlight 13 explores the fast growing trend of functional foods.

Chapter Outline	Terms/Overheads/Handouts
I. Trace Minerals Overview	**trace minerals** **microminerals**

A. Food Sources
    B. Deficiencies
    C. Toxicities
    D. Interactions	

II. Iron	
A. Roles in the Body	**ferrous iron** **ferric iron** **myoglobin, myo**
B. Absorption and Metabolism	*O138 Iron Routes in the Body*
1. Iron absorption	**mucosa** **mucosal**

2. Heme and nonheme iron   **heme**
                                                             non-heme

3. Absorption-enhancing factors   **MFP factor**
4. Absorption-inhibiting factors
5. Dietary factors combined
6. Individuals variations
7. Iron transport and storage   **ferritin**
                                                             hemosiderin

8. Iron recycling

C. Deficiency   **iron deficiency**
                                            iron-deficiency anemia

1. Vulnerable stages in life
2. Blood losses
3. Assessment of iron deficiency   **erthrocyte**
                                                               protoporphyrin
                                             hematocrit

4. Iron deficiency and anemia   **iron-deficiency anemia**
                                                       microcytic hypochromic
                                                           anemia, micro, cytic,
                                                               hypo, chrom

5. Iron deficiency and behavior
6. Iron deficiency and pica   **pica**
                                               geophagia
                                               pagophagia
                                                     picus, geo, phagein,
                                               pago

D. Toxicity
   1. Iron overload   **iron overload**
                                               hemochromatosis
                                               hemosiderosis

   2. Iron and heart disease
   3. Iron and cancer
   4. Iron poisoning

E. Recommendations and Sources
   1. Recommended iron intakes
   2. Iron in foods   *O139 Heme & Nonheme*
                                                       Iron in Foods
                                         O140 Iron in Selected
                                                         Foods

   3. Iron-enriched foods
   4. Maximizing iron absorption
F. Contamination and Supplemental Iron
   1. Contamination iron   **contamination iron**
   2. Iron supplements   **chelate, chele**

SUMMARY AND OUTLINE: CHAPTER 13

III. Zinc   **metalloenzymes**
   A. Roles in the Body
   B. Absorption and Metabolism   *O141 Zinc Routes in the Body*

     1. Zinc absorption   **metallothionein, metallo, thio, ein**

     2. Enteropancreatic circulation   **enteropancreatic circulation**

     3. Zinc transport by albumin
     4. Zinc interactions with iron and copper
     5. Zinc losses
   C. Deficiency
     1. Zinc-deficiency symptoms   *O142 Zinc Deficiency Syndrome-The Stunted Growth of Dwarfism*

     2. Vulnerable stages in life
   D. Toxicity
   E. Recommendations and Sources   *O143 Zinc in Selected Foods*

   F. Contamination and Supplemental Zinc   **galvanized**
IV. Iodine
   A. Iodine Roles in the Body   **thyroxin**
   B. Iodine Deficiency   **goiter**
     goitrogen
     cretinism

   C. Iodine Toxicity
   D. Iodine Sources
   E. Iodine Intakes
   F. Iodine Recommendations
V. Selenium   **selenium**
   A. Selenium Deficiency   **Keshan disease**
   B. Selenium and Cancer
   C. Selenium Intakes
   D. Selenium Toxicity
VI. Copper
   A. Copper Roles in the Body
   B. Copper Deficiency and Toxicity
   C. Copper Recommendations and Intakes
VII. Manganese
   A. Manganese Deficiency
   B. Manganese Toxicity

SUMMARY AND OUTLINE: CHAPTER 13

VIII. Fluoride   **fluorapatite**
- A. Fluoride Roles in the Body
- B. Fluoridation and Dental Caries
- C. Fluoride Toxicity
- D. Fluorosis   **fluorosis**
- E. Fluoride Intakes

IX. Chromium
- A. Chromium Roles in the Body   **glucose tolerance factors**
- B. Chromium Recommendations and Intakes
- C. Chromium Picilinate Supplements

X. Molybdenum   **molybdenum**

XI. Other Trace Minerals

XII. Contaminate Minerals   **heavy metals**

XIII. Closing Thoughts on the Nutrients

XIV. Highlight: Functional Foods - Are They Really Different?   **functional foods**
- A. Traditional Foods
- B. Functional Foods   **yogurt**
                                            probiotics
  1. Unanswered questions
  2. Regulations
     - a) Health claims
     - b) Structure-function claims
     - c) Advertising
  3. Foods as pharmacy
- C. Future Foods

SUMMARY AND OUTLINE: CHAPTER 13

Fitness: Physical Activity, Nutrients, and Body Adaptations
Chapter 14

Chapter Summary

Regular physical activity benefits a person physically, psychologically and socially and provides many health benefits. Flexibility, strength, muscle endurance and cardiorespiratory endurance are components of fitness.

Training conditions the human body to be more fit. Muscle cells adapt in size and work capacity in response to demands. Cardiovascular conditioning improves heart and lung functioning to bring more oxygen to the cells. Both strength and endurance activities need to be included in a balanced fitness program.

A mixture of fuels is required for physical activity. During intense activity, muscles use glucose primarily. Low to moderate activity uses more fat. Protein is needed to build and maintain lean body tissue. Vitamins and minerals must be provided to support energy metabolism and tissue building. Water helps to distribute the fuels and eliminate waste. Water is especially important during training and competition.

The most common problems of female athletes include eating disorders, iron deficiency, amenorrhea and osteoporosis.

A suggested diet for physically active people must provide ample fluids, and a variety of nutrient-dense foods in quantities that meet energy needs.

A healthful diet surpasses the need for pills and powders to enhance athletic performance. Highlight 14 addresses the issues of supplements as ergogenic aids.

Chapter Outline	**Terms/Overheads/Handouts**

I. Fitness

O144 Guidelines for Physical Fitness

   A. Definition of Fitness

fitness
sedentary
O145 Physical Activity Pyramid

   B. Benefits of Fitness
      1. Restful sleep
      2. Nutritional health
      3. Optimal body composition
      4. Optimal bone density
      5. Resistance to colds and other infectious diseases
      6. Low risk of some cancers
      7. Strong circulation and lung function
      8. Low risk of cardiovascular disease
      9. Low risk of type 2 diabetes
     10. Reduced risk of gallbladder disease in women
     11. Low incidence of severity of anxiety and depression
     12. Strong self-image
     13. Long life and high quality of life in later years

   C. Components of Fitness

flexibility
muscle strength
muscle endurance
cardiorespiratory endurance

   D. Conditioning by Training

conditioning
training

      1. The overload principle

progressive overload principle
frequency
intensity
duration

      2. Applying overload

warm-up
cool-down

      3. Cautions on starting
      4. The body's response to physical activity

moderate exercise

hypertrophy
atrophy

      5. Weight training

weight training
resistance training

   E. Cardiorespiratory Endurance

VO2 max
O146 Delivery of Oxygen

SUMMARY AND OUTLINE: CHAPTER 14

    1. Cardiorespiratory conditioning   **cardiorespiratory conditioning**
                                                     cardiac output

    2. Muscle conditioning
    3. Balanced fitness program

II. Energy Systems, Fuels, and Nutrients
      to Support Activity   *O147 The Effect of Diets*
                                              on Physical Endurance

    A. The Energy Systems of Physical
          Activity-ATP and CP
       1. ATP
       2. CP   **CP, creatine phosphate**
                                               phosphocreatine

       3. Energy-yielding nutrients
    B. Glucose Use During Physical Activity   *O148 Recycling of*
                                               Glucose

       1. Diet affects glycogen storage and use
       2. Intensity of activity affects glycogen use
       3. Lactic acid
       4. Duration of activity affects glycogen use
       5. Glucose depletion
       6. Glucose during activity
       7. Glucose after activity
       8. Training affects glycogen use
    C. Fat Use During Physical Activity
       1. Duration of activity affects fat use
       2. Intensity of activity affects fat use
       3. Training affects fat use
       4. Recommended intensities and durations
       5. Choosing an activity
    D. Protein Use During Physical Activity and Between Times
       1. Protein used in muscle building
       2. Protein used as fuel
       3. Diet affects protein use during activity
       4. Intensity and duration of activity affect protein use during activity
       5. Training affects protein use
       6. Protein recommendations for active people
    E. Vitamins and Minerals to Support Activity
       1. Supplements
       2. Iron
       3. Iron deficiency
       4. Iron-deficiency anemia
       5. Sports anemia   **sports anemia**
       6. Iron recommendations for athletes
    F. Fluids and Electrolytes to Support Activity
       1. Fluid losses via sweat

SUMMARY AND OUTLINE: CHAPTER 14

2. Hyperthermia	**hyperthermia** **heat stroke**
3. Hypothermia	**hypothermia**
4. Fluid replacement via hydration	
5. Electrolyte losses and replacement	

G. Poor Beverage Choices: Caffeine and Alcohol
    1. Caffeine
    2. Alcohol

III. Diets for Physically Active People

A. Choosing a Diet to Support Fitness	*O149 An Athlete's Meal Selection*

    1. Water
    2. Nutrient density
    3. Carbohydrate
    4. Protein
    5. Example of a performance diet

B. Meals Before and After Competition
    1. Pregame meals
    2. Postgame meals

IV. Highlight: Supplements As Ergogenic Aids

A. Ergogenic Aids	**ergogenic acids, ergo, genic**
B. Dietary Supplements	
1. Protein powders	**whey protein**
2. Amino acid supplements	**branched-chain amino acids**
3. Carnitine	**carnitine**
4. Vitamin E	
5. Chromium picolinate	**chromium picolinate**
6. Complete nutrition supplements	
7. Creatine	**creatine**
8. Caffeine	**caffeine**
C. Hormonal Supplements	
1. Anabolic steroids	**anabolic steroids, anabolic, sterols**
2. DHEA and androstenedione	**DHEA (dehydroepiandros-terone)**
3. Human growth hormone	**hGH (human growth hormone)**

Life Cycle Nutrition:
Pregnancy and Lactation
Chapter 15

Chapter Summary

Adequate nutrient and energy intake is important for the normal growth and development of the fetus and the health of the mother. Energy needs increase during pregnancy, especially during the second and third trimester. There is also increased need for protein, thiamin, riboflavin, niacin, vitamin B6, folate, vitamin B12, vitamin D, iron and zinc. These needs can be met by consuming a balanced diet with additional servings of nutrient dense foods from the five food groups. Iron supplementation may be required.

Many nutrition-related problems can occur during pregnancy. These include nausea, constipation, hemorrhoids, heartburn, food cravings and aversions and nonfood cravings.

High risk pregnancies result from various conditions. Maternal weight (either low or high), nutritional deficiencies or toxicities, improper weight gain, poor socioeconomic status, preexisting or gestational diabetes, preexisting or transient hypertension, adolescent pregnancy and alcohol/drug abuse all increase risk to pregnancy. The mother's age may influence the course of a pregnancy. The most common outcome of high risk pregnancy is a low birth weight infant. Practices incompatible with pregnancy include alcohol and drug use, herbal supplements and tobacco use.

Lactation is a physiological process. Breastfeeding is a learned behavior that needs a supportive environment. Nutrient needs of the mother during breastfeeding include increased need for energy, vitamins and minerals, and water. Iron supplements may be necessary. Exercise is important.

Breastfeeding mothers need to be concerned about the use of alcohol, caffeine, smoking, colds, HIV infections, chronic diseases and environmental contaminants.

Highlight 15 describes the result of excess alcohol consumption during pregnancy. Fetal Alcohol Syndrome is characterized by growth retardation, brain and nerve impairment, facial and skull abnormalities and increased frequency of

72

major birth defects. It is preventable and the damages are irreversible. Women should be advised not to drink alcohol during pregnancy.

Chapter Outline	Terms/Overheads/Handouts
I. Growth and Development During Pregnancy	
A. Placenta Development	**conception**
	O150 The Placenta and Associated Structures
	placenta
	uterus
	amniotic sac
	umbilical cord, umbilicus
B. Fetal Growth and Development	*O151 Stages of Embryonic and Fetal Development*
	ovum
	sperm
1. Zygote	**zygote**
	implantation
2. Embryo	**embryo**
3. Fetus	**fetus**
C. Critical Periods	*O152 The Concept of Critical Periods*
	O153 Critical Periods of Development
	critical periods
	gestation, trimesters
1. Neural tube defects	**spina bifida, spina, bifida**
	O157 Spina-Bifidia - A Neural Tube Defect
	anencephaly, an, anencephaly
2. Folate supplementation	
3. Chronic diseases	
II. Maternal Weight	
A. Weight Prior to Conception	
1. Underweight	**preterm, term**
	premature infant
2. Overweight	**macrosomia**
	post term
	cesarean section
B. Weight Gain During Pregnancy	

SUMMARY AND OUTLINE: CHAPTER 15

      1.   Recommended weight gain   *O154 Recommended Prenatal Weight Gain based on Prepregnancy Weight*

      2.   Weight-gain patterns
      3.   Components of weight gain
      4.   Weight loss after pregnancy
   C. Exercise During Pregnancy

III. Nutrition During Pregnancy   *O155 Comparison of Nutrient Recommendations for Nonpregnant, Pregnant, and Lactating Women*

   A. Energy and Nutrient Needs During Pregnancy
      1.   Energy
      2.   Protein
      3.   Essential fatty acids
      4.   Nutrients for blood production and cell growth
      5.   Nutrients for bone development
      6.   Other nutrients
      7.   Nutrient supplements
   B. Common Nutrition-Related Concerns of Pregnancy
      1.   Nausea
      2.   Constipation and hemorrhoids
      3.   Heartburn
      4.   Food cravings and aversions   **food cravings**
                                                   food aversions
      5.   Nonfood cravings

IV. High-Risk Pregnancies   **high-risk pregnancy**
                                                 low-risk pregnancy
   A. Malnutrition and Pregnancy   *H15-1 Effects of Nutrient Deficiencies During Pregnancy*
      1.   Malnutrition and fertility   **fertility**
      2.   Malnutrition and early pregnancy
      3.   Malnutrition and fetal development
   B. Infant's Birthweight   **low birthweight (LBW)**
                                                     appropriate for gestational age (AGA)
                                                  small for gestational age (SGA)
   C. Maternal Health
      1.   Preexisting diabetes
      2.   Gestational diabetes   **gestational diabetes**

SUMMARY AND OUTLINE: CHAPTER 15

3. Preexisting hypertension
4. Transient hypertension of pregnancy **transient hypertension of pregnancy**

5. Preeclampsia and eclampsia **preeclampsia eclampsia**

D. Mother's Age
   1. Pregnancy in adolescents
   2. Pregnancy in older women **Down syndrome**
E. Practices Incompatible with Pregnancy
   1. Alcohol
   2. Medicinal drugs
   3. Illicit drugs
   4. Smoking and chewing tobacco **sudden infant death syndrome (SIDS)**

   5. Environmental contaminants
   6. Vitamin-mineral megadoses
   7. Caffeine
   8. Weight-loss dieting
   9. Sugar substitutes

V. Nutrition During Lactation **lactation**
  A. Lactation: A Physiological Process **mammary glands**
prolactin, pro, lacto
oxytocin
let-down reflex

B. Breastfeeding: A Learned Behavior
C. Mother's Nutrient Needs
   1. Energy intake and exercise
   2. Vitamins and minerals
   3. Water
   4. Nutrient supplements
   5. Particular foods
D. Practices Incompatible with Lactation
   1. Alcohol
   2. Medicinal drugs
   3. Illicit drugs
   4. Smoking
   5. Environmental contaminants
   6. Caffeine
E. Maternal Health
   1. HIV infection and AIDS
   2. Diabetes
   3. Postpartum amenorrhea **postpartum amenorrhea**
   4. Breast health

SUMMARY AND OUTLINE: CHAPTER 15

VI. Highlight: Fetal Alcohol Syndrome

fetal alcohol syndrome (FAS)
alcohol-related birth defects (ARBD)
fetal alcohol effects (FAE)
O156 Typical Facial Characteristics of FAS

A. Drinking During Pregnancy
B. Quantity of Alcohol
C. Damage from Alcohol

SUMMARY AND OUTLINE: CHAPTER 15

Life Cycle Nutrition:
Infancy, Childhood, and Adolescence
Chapter 16

Chapter Summary

An infant's rapid weight gain during the first year of life requires an ample supply of all nutrients. Breast milk provides nutrients needed for the first four to six months plus immunological protection. Iron-fortified infant formulas closely resemble breast milk and are appropriate for feeding to infants.

Solid foods can be introduced when the infant gives indications for readiness - approximately four to six months. New foods should be introduced slowly. At one year of age, an infant should be drinking from a cup and eating many of the same foods as the rest of the family. High Vitamin C and high iron foods are important. Mealtime should be a pleasant experience.

Healthful food choices and regular physical activity promote growth, develop healthy habits and help prevent diseases in later life. Nutrient needs of children vary, depending on their growth and physical activity. Malnutrition is common in children. Food intolerances and food allergies need to be specifically identified so nutrient deficiencies do not occur.

Children's eating behaviors are shaped both at home and at school. Balanced meals are important to provide adequate nutrients. Honoring children's preferences is also important. Mealtime should be a pleasant experience, devoid of conflict. Healthful snacks need to be provided. The timing of meals can affect children's behavior and academic performance. School meals and nutrition education at school are teaching tools to help children make healthy choices regarding food. Parents serve as important role models.

Several studies have found no correlation between the intake of sugar and hyperactivity. Caffeine and inconsistent care is often the source of "hyper" behavior. The prevalence of childhood obesity is correlated with the hours of television viewing which encourages inactivity and overconsumption of snack foods.

Nutrient needs rise rapidly during adolescence. There are gender differences in growth and development. Energy intakes vary depending on activity levels. Iron and calcium are crucial at this age. Busy lifestyles, peer influence and irregular eating habits add to the challenge of making wise food choices. Drug, tobacco and alcohol abuse can affect nutritional status.

Highlight 16 describes the early development for atherosclerosis, high blood cholesterol, and high blood pressure in children. Dietary recommendations for children are given.

Chapter Outline	Terms/Overheads/Handouts
I. Nutrition During Infancy	O158 *Weight Gain of Infants and Children in their First Five Years of Life*
A. Energy and Nutrient Needs	O159 *Weight-For-Age Percentiles: Girls Birth to 36 Months*
1. Energy intake and activity	O160 *Recommended Intakes of an Infant and an Adult Compared on the Basis of Body Weight*
2. Protein	
3. Vitamins and minerals	
4. Water	
B. Breast Milk	**alpha-lactalbumin, casein**
1. Energy nutrients	
2. Vitamins	
3. Minerals	
4. Nutrient supplements	
5. Immunological protection	**colostrum** **bifidus factors** **lactoferrin** **lactaherin**
6. Allergy protection	
C. Infant Formula	**wean**
1. Infant formula composition	
2. Risks of formula feeding	
3. Infant formula standards	
4. Special formulas	
5. Inappropriate formulas	
6. Nursing bottle tooth decay	**nursing bottle tooth decay**
D. Special Needs of Preterm Infants	**osteopenia** **rickets of prematurity**
E. Introducing Cow's Milk	

SUMMARY AND OUTLINE: CHAPTER 16

F. Introducing Solid Foods   **beikost**
 1. When to begin
 2. Food allergies
 3. Choice of infant foods
 4. Foods to provide iron
 5. Foods to provide vitamin C
 6. Foods to omit   **botulism**
 7. Food at one year   **milk anemia**
G. Mealtimes with Toddlers

II. Nutrition During Childhood   *O161 Body Shapes of One-Year-Old and Two-Year-Old Compared*

 A. Energy and Nutrient Needs
 1. Energy intake and activity
 2. Protein
 3. Vitamins and minerals
 4. Planning children's meals
 B. Hunger and Malnutrition in Children
 1. Hunger and behavior
 2. Iron deficiency and behavior
 3. Other nutrient deficiencies and behavior
 C. Malnutrition-Lead Connection
 D. Hyperactivity and "Hyper"-Behavior   **hyperactivity**
           attention-deficit /hyperactivity disorder (ADHD)

 1. Hyperactivity
 2. Misbehaving
 E. Adverse Reaction to Foods   **adverse reactions**
 1. Food intolerances   **food intolerances**
 2. Food allergies   **asymptomatic allergy**
           symptomatic allergy
           food allergies
           histamine
 F. Childhood Obesity   *O162 Body Mass Index for Age Percentiles: Boys and Girls Age 2-20*

 1. Growth
 2. Physical health
 3. Psychological development
 4. Diet
 5. Physical activity
 6. Psychological support
 7. Behavioral changes
 G. Mealtimes at Home   **gatekeepers**
 1. Honoring children's preferences

SUMMARY AND OUTLINE: CHAPTER 16

80

    2.   Learning through participation
    3.   Avoiding power struggles
    4.   Choking prevention
    5.   Play first
    6.   Snacks
    7.   Preventing dental caries
    8.   Serving as role models
  H. Nutrition at School
    1.   School meals
    2.   Competing influences at school
    3.   Nutrition education at school

H16-1 Supervised Food Activities for Preschoolers

III. Nutrition During Adolescence
  A. Growth and Development

adolescence
puberty

  B. Energy and Nutrient Needs
    1.   Energy intake and activity
    2.   Vitamins
    3.   Iron
    4.   Calcium
  C. Food Choices and Health Habits
    1.   Snacks
    2.   Beverages
    3.   Eating away from home
    4.   Peer influence
  D. Problems Adolescents Face
    1.   Marijuana
    2.   Cocaine
    3.   Ecstasy
    4.   General drug abuse
    5.   Alcohol abuse
    6.   Smoking
    7.   Smokeless tobacco

IV. Highlight: The Early Development of Chronic Diseases
    A. Early Development of Heart Disease
        1. Atheroschlerosis

cardiovascular disease (CVD), cardio, vascular
atheroschlerosis, athero, scleros, osis
fatty streaks
fibrous plaques

        2. Blood cholesterol
        3. Blood pressure
    B. Physical Activity
    C. Dietary Recommendations for Children
        1. Not before two
        2. Moderation, not deprivation
        3. Diet first, drugs later
    D. Smoking

SUMMARY AND OUTLINE: CHAPTER 16

Chapter 17
Illness and Nutrition Status

CHAPTER SUMMARY

The nutrition care process is used to identify and meet the nutrient and nutrition education needs of a client. By interrupting data collected from historical information, physical examinations, anthropometric data, and laboratory tests, health care professionals can search for nutrition imbalances.

Historical information, such as past health problems, prescription medications, and eating habits, helps health care professionals by providing the basis for developing realistic nutrition care plans. By gathering food intake data, a health care professional creates a record of foods a client eats and then uses the information to identify possible nutrient abnormalities. Several techniques used to collect food intake data include 24-hour recall, usual intake, food frequency questionnaire, and food records.

Physical and laboratory measurements are used in nutrition assessment to identify nutrient imbalances and to determine nutrient needs. Anthropometric measures such as length, height, weight, and head circumference are used in diagnosing abnormalities in growth and development. Additionally, physical signs observed by the health care team can justify the need for further tests. Assessment of laboratory data provides information as to what is happening internally in the body. For example, laboratory tests of serum albumin, serum transferrin, lymphocytes, transthyretin, and retinol-binding protein are routinely used to determine protein status.

Highlight 17 discusses the relationship between nutrition and mental health.

LEARNING OBJECTIVES

1. List the five steps of the nutrition care process.
2. Discuss how historical information is used in nutrition assessment.
3. Compare and contrast methods for gathering food intake data.
4. Give examples of anthropometric measurements commonly used to monitor growth and development in both children and adults.
5. Discuss several biochemical tests and indicators used in nutrition assessment and tell how the outcomes can be influenced.
6. Give examples of physical signs that can reflect nutrition status.
7. Describe the relationship between nutrition and mental health.

CHAPTER OUTLINE

I. Nutrition in Health Care

   A. Health Problems
      1. Immobility and Pressure Sores
      2. Indirect Effects
   B. The Nutrition Care Process
      1. Steps of the Nutrition Care Process
      2. Applications
   C. Roles of Health Care Professionals
      1. Physicians
      2. Clinical Dietitians
      3. Nurses
      4. Dietetic Technicians
      5. Other Health Care Professionals

II. Nutrition Assessment

   A. Complete Nutrition Assessments
   B. Nutrition Screening

III. Historical Information

   A. Health History
   B. Medication History
   C. Personal History
   D. Diet History

IV. Food Intake Data

   A. Identifying Potential Food Intake Problems
      1. Information from Clients
      2. Observation of Food Intake in Health Care Facilities
   B. Other Tools for Gathering Food Intake Data
      1. The 24-Hour Recall and Usual Intake Method
      2. Food Frequency Questionnaire
      3. Food Records
      4. Applying Food Intake Information

V. Body Measurements

   A. Anthropometric Measurements
      1. Length, Height, and Weight
      2. Head Circumference

Chapter 18
Nutrition, Medications, and
Complementary Therapies

CHAPTER SUMMARY

People spend billions of dollars every year for medications, dietary supplements, and herbs. New medications are made available each year after extensive research and approval by the FDA; however, dietary supplements and herbs can be marketed without such evaluation. Health care professionals play an active role in evaluating clients' risk for adverse nutrition-related side effects from both complementary and conventional therapies. Diet-drug interactions can reduce or heighten food intake, affect absorption, metabolism, and excretion.

Highlight 18 discusses nutrition and the immune system.

LEARNING OBJECTIVES

1. Compare and contrast conventional and complementary therapies.
2. Identify conditions that put clients at high risk for diet-drug interactions.
3. Discuss the ways medications can affect food intake.
4. Explain how diet-drug interactions can affect absorption.
5. Describe how metabolism is affected by diet-drug interactions.
6. Give examples of how diet-drug interactions can affect excretion.

CHAPTER OUTLINE

I.   Overview of Conventional and Complementary Therapies

    A. Medications
       1. Prescription Medications
       2. Over-the-Counter Medications
    B. Dietary Supplements
       1. Marketing of Dietary Supplements
       2. Other Problems Associated with Dietary Supplements

II. Weighing Risks and Benefits

    A. Learning about Benefits and Risks

      B. Evaluating Risks
      C. Limiting Risks

III.   Diet-Drug Interrelationships

      A. Medications and Food Intake
         1. Altering the Appetite
         2. Causing or Alleviating Complications
      B. Diet-Drug Interactions and Absorption
         1. Diet Effects on Medication Absorption
         2. Medication Effects on Nutrient Absorption
         3. Other Absorption-Related Interactions
      C. Diet-Drug Interactions and Metabolism
         1. Interactions Affecting Medications
         2. Interactions Affecting Nutrients
         3. Other Interactions
      D. Diet-Drug Interactions and Excretion
         1. Nutrient Effects on Medication Excretion
         2. Medication Effects on Nutrient Excretion
      E. Other Ingredients in Medications

IV.   Highlight: Nutrition and Immunity

Chapter 19
Nutrition Intervention

CHAPTER SUMMARY

A nutrition care plan is individualized to a client's needs and clearly defines both immediate and long-term nutrient recommendations, including strategies for meeting those needs. Effective communication is essential between health care professionals to relay diet instructions and ensure accurate health care. Several communication techniques used in medical nutrition therapy include diet orders, diet manuals, and medical records for professional communication.

When regular diet fails to meet the nutritional needs of a client, a modification of the diet is required. This may involve simply changing the consistency of the diet; adjusting the amounts energy, individual nutrients, or fluid; altering the number of meals; or eliminating certain foods. In all cases, the goal for diet modification is to support adequate nutrition status. A physician may order a client to be placed on a progressive diet, beginning with liquid foods and ultimately progressing to solid foods. This allows the diet to change as the client's tolerance improves. If a client is unable to achieve adequate nutrition from oral diet alone, tube and intravenous feedings can be used.

Highlight 19 discusses food and foodservice in Health Care Facilities.

LEARNING OBJECTIVES

1. Identify the goals of the nutrition care plan and identify the means for obtaining them.
2. Describe the use of medical nutrition therapy, including standard and modified diets, tube feedings, parenteral nutrition, diet orders, and diet manuals.
3. Discuss routine progressive diets and give examples of when they are used by health care facilities.
4. Discuss how medical records are used by health care professionals to communicate the needs of their clients.

CHAPTER OUTLINE

I.   Nutrition Care Plans

A. Goals and Interventions
B. Addressing Nutrition-Related Problems
C. Addressing Nutrition Education Needs

Chapter 20
Nutrition and Disorders of
the Upper GI Tract

CHAPTER SUMMARY

Disruption of the GI tract can affect the body's ability to ingest, digest, and absorb nutrients. Disorders associated with the mouth and esophagus include mouth ulcers, dry mouth, and dysphagia. In order to provide adequate nutrients, a health care team of speech therapists, dietitians, physicians, and nurses collaborate to develop an individualized diet based on the patient's swallowing ability. Disorders of the stomach range from indigestion to gastritis and ulcers. Gastric surgery including gastrectomy, pyloroplasty, and vagotomy are procedures commonly used for treatment that directly affect the functions of the stomach. When the pyloric sphincter is removed, bypassed, or disrupted, dumping syndrome may develop, which can lead to malabsorption and ultimately malnutrition.

Highlight 20 discusses ways to help people with feeding disabilities.

LEARNING OBJECTIVES

1. List several conditions that may lead to dysphagia and describe dietary therapy that is used for treatment.
2. Discuss the causes and consequences of reflux esophagitis.
3. Describe dietary and pharmacological intervention prescribed for treating nausea, vomiting, gastritis, and ulcers.
4. Give specific examples of how disorders of the upper GI tract can affect nutrition status.
5. Describe dietary recommendations for a patient who undergoes gastric partitioning for severe obesity.
6. Outline common nutritional problems and related therapies associated with gastric surgery.

CHAPTER OUTLINE

I.   Disorders of the Mouth and Esophagus

     A.   Difficulties Chewing
         1.   Diet Options
         2.   Cautious Use of Pureed Foods
         3.   Mouth and Throat Pain

           4.   Reduced Flow of Saliva
    B.   Difficulties Swallowing
            1.   Subtle and Dangerous
            2.   Signs of Dysphagia
            3.   Dietary Interventions for Dysphagia
            4.   Tube Feedings

II.   Disorders of the Stomach

    A.   Indigestion and Reflux Esophagitis
            1.   Causes of Esophageal Reflux
            2.   Consequences of Esophageal Reflux
            3.   Prevention and Treatment
            4.   Drug Therapy
    B.   Nausea and Vomiting
            1.   Treatment of Nausea and Vomiting
            2.   Dietary Interventions for Vomiting
    C.   Gastritis
            1.   Acute Gastritis
            2.   Chronic Gastritis
    D.   Ulcers
            1.   Causes of Ulcers
            2.   Treatment for Ulcers
    E.   Gastric Surgery
            1.   Dumping Syndrome
            2.   Postsurgical Care
            3.   The Postgastrectomy Diet
            4.   Weight Loss and Nutrient Deficiencies
            5.   Anemia
            6.   Bone Disease
            7.   Gastric Partitioning
            8.   Diet following Gastric Partitioning
            9.   Food Selections

III.   Highlight: Helping People with Feeding Disabilites

Chapter 21
Nutrition and Lower GI Tract Disorders

CHAPTER SUMMARY

A common characteristic associated with lower GI disorders is diarrhea, resulting from malabsorption of food or liquids. However, the causes of the malabsorption vary and some are unknown. The lower GI disorders that disrupt fat absorption possesses severe repercussions including weight loss, malnutrition, increased risk of bone disease, and increased risk of oxalate stone formation. Development of a proper diet is essential for patients with fat malabsorption syndromes to ensure adequate food energy, absorption of fat-soluble vitamins, calcium, and magnesium. Other causes of malabsorption include conditions of pancreatitis, cystic fibrosis, inflammatory bowel diseases, bacterial overgrowth, and disorders of the large intestine.

Highlight 21 points out strategies that promote intestinal adaptation.

LEARNING OBJECTIVES

1. Describe the nutritional management of motility disorders such as constipation, diarrhea, and irritable bowel syndrome.
2. Identify the causes and treatment of lactose intolerance.
3. Discuss the affects of fat malabsorption and describe effective methods used for treatment.
4. Discuss various condition that can lead to malabsorption.
5. Explain how nutrition can play a role in the treatment of malabsorption syndromes.
6. Describe the complications associated with inflammatory bowel diseases.
7. Identify specific conditions that affect the colon and its functions.

CHAPTER OUTLINE

I.   Common Problems of the Lower Intestine

    A.   Constipation
        1.   Causes of Constipation
        2.   Treatment of Constipation
        3.   High-Fiber Diet
        4.   Intestinal Gas
    B.   Diarrhea and Dehydration
        1.   Causes of Diarrhea

Chapter 22
Enteral Formulas

CHAPTER SUMMARY

Health care professionals use enteral formulas as a means of supplying adequate nutrients to clients who are unable to ingest a sufficient amount of food. Formulas have many characteristics that distinguish one from another. For example, standard formulas contain complete proteins, whereas hydrolyzed formulas contain protein fragments. In contrast to complete formulas that satisfy all the nutrient needs of a client, modular formulas provide a single nutrient. In choosing a formula, physicians and dietitians select the formula that meets the client's nutrient needs with the least complications. Based on the client's ability to eat, enteral formulas can be provided either orally or by tube feeding. To avoid possible complications, special attention should be given to the appropriate formula preparation, selection of the tube, delivery schedule, and administration of medications.

Highlight 22 addresses enteral formulas and inborn errors of metabolism.

LEARNING OBJECTIVES

1. Describe factors that should be considered when selecting oral or tube feeding formulas.
2. Differentiate between standard formulas, complete formulas, hydrolyzed formulas, and modular formulas.
3. Identify examples of conditions that make clients candidates for tube feeding.
4. Discuss various feeding tube placements and their advantages and disadvantages.
5. Describe alternative ways to administer tube feeding.
6. Identify complications that may develop with tube feeding.

CHAPTER OUTLINE

I.   Enteral Formulas: What Are They?

    A.   Types of Formulas
        1.   Standard Formulas
        2.   Hydrolyzed Formulas
        3.   Modular Formulas
    B.   Distinguishing Characteristics
        1.   Nutrient Density
        2.   Residue and Fiber

3.　　Osmolality
4.　　Costs

II.　　Enteral Formulas: Who Needs What?

A.　　Enteral Formulas Provided Orally
B.　　Tube Feedings
　　1.　　Feeding Tube Placement
　　2.　　Gastric Feedings
　　3.　　Feeding Tubes
C.　　Formula Selection

III.　　Tube Feedings: How Are They Given?

A.　　Safe Handling
　　1.　　At the Nursing Station
　　2.　　At Bedside
B.　　Initiating and Progressing a Tube Feeding
　　1.　　Formula Delivery Techniques
　　2.　　Intermittent Feedings
　　3.　　Continuous Feedings
　　4.　　Formula Volume and Strength
　　5.　　Supplemental Water
　　6.　　Gastric Residuals
C.　　Delivering Medications through Feeding Tubes
　　1.　　Medication Forms
　　2.　　GI Side Effects
　　3.　　Additional Considerations
D.　　Addressing Tube Feeding Complications
　　1.　　Types of Complications
　　2.　　What to Chart

III.　　From Tube Feedings to Table Foods

IV.　　Highlight: Enteral Formulas and Inborn Errors of Metabolism

Chapter 23
Parenteral Nutrition

CHAPTER SUMMARY

Nutrition solutions delivered by the vein are known as intravenous (IV) solutions. These solutions can contain any or all of the essential nutrients: water, amino acids, carbohydrate, fat, vitamins, and minerals. Dependent on the client's nutrient needs, IV solutions are provided in several ways. For example, simple IV solutions are used in well-nourished individuals to maintain body's fluid and electrolyte and acid-base balances. Clients who are malnourished, lack strong veins necessary for PPN, and who have high nutrient needs require TPN support to meet all their nutrient needs. Clients on PPN and TPN are monitored carefully to ensure their bodies are adapting probably. In certain circumstances, patients may require continued nutrition support to maintain adequate nutrition status. For example, individuals with AIDS, cancer, Crohn's disease, or other intestinal disorders may benefit from long-term home enteral and parenteral nutrition programs.

Highlight 23 examines trends in nutrition services and controlling costs.

LEARNING OBJECTIVES

1. Identify the components of a parenteral nutrition solution.
2. Describe conditions that warrant the use of simple IV solutions versus TPN.
3. Compare and contrast the characteristics of PPN versus central TPN.
4. Calculate the energy nutrient content of IV solutions.
5. Explain the possible complications that can accompany TPN and related intervention.
6. Explain the transition process from parenteral to enteral nutrition.
7. Discuss the benefits of home enteral and parenteral nutrition programs.

CHAPTER OUTLINE

I.   Intravenous Solutions: What Are They?

      A.   Intravenous Nutrients
            1.   Amino Acids
            2.   Carbohydrate
            3.   Lipid
            4.   Micronutrients
            5.   Other Additives

      B.   Types of Intravenous Solutions
          1.   Simple Intravenous Solutions
          2.   Complete Nutrient Solutions

II.   Intravenous Nutrition: Who Needs What?

      A.   Simple Intravenous Infusions
      B.   Peripheral Parenteral Nutrition (PPN)
      C.   Central Total Parenteral Nutrition (Central TPN)

III.   Intravenous Solutions: How Are They Given?

      A.   Insertion and Care of Intravenous Catheters
      B.   Administration of Complete Nutrient Solutions
          1.   Intravenous Lipid Infusion
          2.   Cyclic Infusion
      C.   Discontinuing Intravenous Nutrition
          1.   Transitional Feedings
          2.   Psychological Effects

IV.   Specialized Nutrition Support at Home

      A.   The Basics of Home Programs
          1.   Candidates for Home Nutrition Support
          2.   Roles of Health Care Professionals
          3.   Cost Considerations
          4.   Adjustments for Clients
      B.   How Home Enteral and Parenteral Nutrition Programs Work
          1.   Home Enteral Nutrition
          2.   Home TPN

V.   Highlight: Nutrition and Cost-Conscious Health Care

Chapter 24
Nutrition in Severe Stress

CHAPTER SUMMARY

When a person undergoes a period of stress from something, such as an infection, heart attack, stroke, surgery, burn, or fracture, the body attempts to sustain life with a protective stress response. This response enables the body to borrow energy from one system to help keep another system functioning, at least temporarily. However, it does not take long for vital organs to deteriorate from the vicious cycle of borrowing and lending. Even if the heart and lungs continue to function at some level, the immune system is severely compromised and an infection can develop.

The nurse and dietitian work together to provide nutritional support to persons under severe stress. The challenge is to nourish adequately, without underfeeding, which hinders the body's ability to respond to the stress, or overfeeding, which puts the body at risk of further damage. Therefore, careful assessment of nutritional needs and gradual progression from intravenous feeding to provision of regular food are essential.

Highlight 24 discusses the importance of nutrition and multiple organ failure.

LEARNING OBJECTIVES

1. Describe the body's responses to stress.
2. Compare and contrast the metabolic responses of fasting versus severe stress.
3. Discuss the effects of nutrition status on stress.
4. Outline the nutritional needs during stress.
5. Analyze the barriers associated with nutrient delivery following stress.
6. Estimate energy and protein needs following severe stress.
7. Design and plan to meet the nutrient needs of clients experiencing the following stressors: infection/fever, trauma, organ transplant, and burn.

CHAPTER OUTLINE

I.   The Body's Responses to Stress

    A.   Immune System Responses
    B.   Hormonal Responses

Chapter 25
Nutrition and Diabetes Mellitus

CHAPTER SUMMARY

Diabetes mellitus occurs when either the pancreas loses the ability to synthesize insulin (type 1 diabetes) or when insulin cell receptors become less sensitive or resistant to insulin (type 2 diabetes). Acute complications of diabetes include hyperglycemia, dehydration, and ketosis. Chronic complications include cardiovascular disease, microangiopathies, and neuropathy.

Consistent control of glucose levels through diet modification, physical activity, and drug therapy helps to prevent and/or retard these complications. Meal-planning strategies utilize the exchange lists and carbohydrate counting to carefully control protein, fat, and carbohydrate intake at specific times to coincide with insulin onset and peak. Blood glucose control has been shown to improve with a regular program of physical activity for clients with type 2 diabetes. Although this has not been proven to be true for clients with type 1 diabetes, the benefits of weight loss, improved blood lipid levels, and lower blood pressure is favorable to both types of diabetes. For type 1 diabetes, the use of insulin and insulin analogs are used to simulate a normally functioning pancreas. If clients with type 2 diabetes are unable to control their disease through diet modification and physical activity, then oral antidiabetic agents are used to stimulate insulin production and lessen peripheral insulin resistance.

Highlight 25 discusses how clients with diabetes can manage the disease.

LEARNING OBJECTIVES

1. Differentiate between the pathophysiology of type 1 and type 2 diabetes.
2. Discuss acute and chronic complications associated with diabetes mellitus.
3. Explain how protein, carbohydrate, and fat intakes should be modified for a diabetic client and why these modifications aid in glucose control.
4. List the physiological tests that measure glucose control.
5. Develop a plan for detecting and treating hyperglycemia and hypoglycemia in a diabetic client.
6. Plan a diet for a client with diabetes and illustrate how exchange lists and carbohydrate counting can be used.
7. Describe the desired balance between activity, drug therapy, and food intake in diabetes mellitus.
8. Describe the prenatal care for women with existing diabetes and gestational diabetes.

CHAPTER OUTLINE

I.   What is Diabetes Mellitus

    A.   Types of Diabetes
        1.   Type 1 Diabetes
        2.   Type 2 Diabetes
    B.   Acute Complications of Diabetes
        1.   Hyperglycemia and Glycosuria
        2.   Ketosis and Acidosis
        3.   Dehydration and Fluid and Electrolyte Imbalances
        4.   Coma in Diabetes
        5.   Hyperglycemia in Untreated Diabetes
        6.   Causes of Hyperglycemia in Treated Diabetes
        7.   Hypoglycemia
    C.   Chronic Complications of Diabetes
        1.   Cardiovascular Diseases
        2.   Small Blood Vessel Disorders
        3.   Neuropathy

II.   Treatment of Diabetes Mellitus

    A.   Treatment Goals
        1.   Benefits of Intensive Therapy
        2.   Evaluating Diabetes Control
        3.   Treatment Plans
    B.   Medical Nutrition Therapy for Diabetes
        1.   Energy
        2.   Protein
        3.   Carbohydrate
        4.   Complex versus Simple Sugars
        5.   Glycemic Index
        6.   Fat
        7.   Sodium
        8.   Alcohol
        9.   Micronutrients
        10.   Missed Meals and Illness
        11.   Treating Hypoglycemia
        12.   Enteral and Parenteral Formulas
    C.   Meal-Planning Strategies
        1.   Exchange Lists
        2.   Carbohydrate Counting
    D.   Drug Therapy for Diabetes
        1.   Oral Antidiabetic Agents
        2.   Insulin and Insulin Analogs
        3.   Insulin Therapy

Chapter 26
Nutrition and Disorders of the Heart,
Blood Vessels, and Lungs

CHAPTER SUMMARY

Atherosclerosis and hypertension are two conditions that are involved in the development of coronary heart disease (CHD). Left untreated, this condition can lead to severe consequences—heart attacks, chronic heart failure, and strokes. Major risk factors associated with the development of CHD are interrelated and include male gender, increasing age, elevated blood cholesterol, hypertension, tobacco smoke, diabetes mellitus, heredity, obesity, and physical inactivity. Preventive measures such as diet, physical activity, avoidance of tobacco smoke, and medications can act directly to reduce the risk of CHD.

Other disorders that have direct affect on organ function include disorders of the lungs. Without proper delivery of oxygen to the cells and removal of metabolic waste, gas exchange becomes inadequate to maintain an optimal level of health. As a result, it is important for health care professionals to closely monitor nutrition status in clients suffering with acute respiratory failure and chronic obstructive pulmonary disease.

Highlight 26 discusses the mechanisms of the metabolic syndrome.

LEARNING OBJECTIVES

1. Describe the interrelationship between atherosclerosis and hypertension and explain how they contribute to the development of CHD.
2. Identify modifiable and non-modifiable risk factors associated with CHD.
3. Discuss diet strategies for preventing and treating.
4. Describe both immediate care and long-term therapy used with clients following a heart attack.
5. Discuss the consequences and treatment of CHF.
6. Explain how nutrition status can be affected by stroke and describe medical therapies used to assist stroke patients.
7. Compare and contrast acute respiratory failure and chronic obstructive pulmonary disease.

CHAPTER OUTLINE

I.   Cardiovascular Diseases
     A.   Atherosclerosis

        1.   Causes of Atherosclerosis
        2.   Blood Lipids and Atherosclerosis
        3.   Consequences of Atherosclerosis
  B.   Hypertension
        1.   Consequences of Hypertension
        2.   Interrelationships between Hypertension and Atherosclerosis

II.   Risk Factors for Coronary Heart Disease

  A.   Prevalence of Risk Factors
  B.   Age, Gender, and Heredity
  C.   Tobacco Smoke
  D.   Physical Inactivity
  E.   Diet-Related Risk Factors

III.   Prevention and Treatment of Coronary Heart Disease

  A.   Diet Strategies
        1.   A Healthy Eating Pattern
        2.   A Healthy Body Weight
        3.   A Desirable Blood Cholesterol and Lipoprotein Profile
        4.   Achieve and Maintain a Normal Blood Pressure
        5.   A Word about Alcohol
        6.   Plant Sterols
        7.   Soy Protein and Isoflavones
  B.   Drug Therapy
        1.   Medications
        2.   Dietary Supplements

IV.   Heart Failure and Strokes

  A.   Heart Attacks
        1.   Immediate Care
        2.   Long-Term Diet Therapy
        3.   Encourage Lifestyle Changes
  B.   Chronic Heart Failure
        1.   Consequences of CHF
        2.   CHF and Nutrition Status
        3.   Treatment of CHF
        4.   Medical Nutrition Therapy
  C.   Strokes
        1.   Complications Affecting Food Intake
        2.   Medical Nutrition Therapy

V.   Disorders of the Lungs

Chapter 27
Nutrition and Renal Diseases

CHAPTER SUMMARY

The kidneys are primarily responsible for eliminating waste products and maintaining fluid and electrolyte balance; however, under circumstances when kidney function is altered, severe side affects develop. Disorders that affect the kidneys include kidney stones, the nephrotic syndrome, and acute and chronic renal failure.

Acute renal failure has a sudden onset and is usually precipitated by physiological stress that decreases glomerular filtration rate. Symptoms that hallmark the onset of acute renal failure are a sudden drop in urine output, hyperglycemia, and uremic syndrome. Associated signs of nausea, vomiting, and anorexia, make nutritional support a primary concern. In contrast, chronic renal failure has a gradual onset with extensive damage to nephrons before symptoms appear. Edema, metabolic acidosis, hypertension, and hyperglycemia are hallmarks of this condition. Clients have an altered nutritional status due to loss of nutrients, nausea, vomiting, diarrhea, and altered absorption ability. A renal diet is high in energy with individualized restrictions on protein, phosphorus, sodium, potassium, fluids, and often supplements of vitamins and minerals are recommended.

Clients in severe renal failure require dialysis to take over the function of the kidneys. An alternative to dialysis is a kidney transplant, which brings about a new set of dietary challenges. Because kidney recipients receive immunosuppressive drug therapy, they experience fluid retention, carbohydrate intolerance, and muscle wasting. Diet interventions are centered on restricting sodium and providing enough protein to prevent protein catabolism.

Highlight 27 examines how dialysis affects nutrient requirements.

LEARNING OBJECTIVES

1. Describe how kidney stones develop and explain what diet therapy can be used for treatment and prevention.
2. Explain the diet interventions for clients with nephrotic syndrome.
3. Differentiate between the symptoms and treatment of acute and chronic renal failure.
4. Explain the therapeutic options in acute renal failure and their impact on nutritional support.
5. Describe the long-term nutritional problems associated with chronic renal

failure and appropriate interventions for treatment.
6. Plan a diet for a client in chronic renal failure and discuss how protein, carbohydrates, and sodium intakes are modified.
7. Explain diet interventions following a kidney transplant.

CHAPTER OUTLINE

I.   Kidney Stones

    A.   Causes of Kidney Stones
        1.   Calcium Stones
        2.   Uric Acid Stones
        3.   Cystine Stones
    B.   Consequences of Kidney Stones
        1.   Renal Colic
        2.   Urinary Tract Complications
    C.   Prevention and Treatment of Kidney Stones
        1.   Drug Therapy
        2.   Medical Nutrition Therapy for Calcium and Oxalate Stones
        3.   Uric Acid Stones
        4.   Cystine Stones

II.   The Nephrotic Syndrome

    A.   Consequences of the Nephrotic Syndrome
        1.   Loss of Blood Proteins
        2.   Edema
        3.   Altered Blood Lipids
    B.   Treatment of the Nephrotic Syndrome
        1.   Energy
        2.   Protein
        3.   Fat
        4.   Sodium

III. Acute Renal Failure

    A.   Consequences of Acute Renal Failure
        1.   Electrolyte Levels Rise
        2.   Blood Volume Changes
    B.   Treatment of Acute Renal Failure
        1.   Energy
        2.   Protein
        3.   Fluids
        4.   Electrolytes
        5.   Enteral and Parenteral Nutrition
        6.   Drug Therapy

IV.   Chronic Renal Failure

     A.   Consequences of Chronic Renal Failure
          1.   Uremic Syndrome
          2.   Blood Chemistry Alterations
          3.   Other Complications
          4.   Growth Failure and Wasting
     B.   Treatment of Chronic Renal Failure
          1.   Energy
          2.   Protein
          3.   Lipid and Carbohydrate
          4.   Sodium and Fluids
          5.   Potassium
          6.   Phosphorus, Calcium, and Vitamin D
          7.   Other Vitamins
          8.   Trace Minerals
          9.   Enteral and Parenteral Nutrition
         10.   Diet Planning
         11.   Diet Compliance
     C.   Kidney Transplants and Diet
          1.   Immunosuppressant Drug Therapy
          2.   Dietary Interventions

V.   Highlight: Dialysis and Nutrition

Chapter 28
Nutrition and Liver Disorders

CHAPTER SUMMARY

Clients suffering from liver disorders, including fatty liver and hepatitis, experience metabolic derangement, physiological consequences, and alterations in nutritional requirements. Medical nutrition therapy plays an important role and is dependent on the cause of the liver dysfunction as well as the present nutritional status of the client. If liver disorders continue to the point in which liver cells are unable to regenerate, cirrhosis develops and can ultimately lead to liver failure. Alterations in protein metabolism are of paramount importance in liver disease. As liver disease progresses, the ability to metabolize and tolerate protein diminish and the provision of dietary protein declines; however, the need for protein remains. Energy requirements remain high to protect its functioning cells and to prevent protein catabolism. Many clients with liver disease develop malnutrition secondary to dietary restrictions as well as anorexia. Esophageal varices, ascites, and elevated blood ammonia levels add additional dietary modification and complexity to the regimen. At the final stages of liver failure, liver transplantation is inevitable and special attention is made to the nutritional status before and after the transplant.

Highlight 28 looks at the consequences and treatments for gallstones.

LEARNING OBJECTIVES

1. Describe the metabolic alterations associated with fatty liver and hepatitis and the appropriate nutritional therapy for each.
2. Discuss the conditions associated with the development of cirrhosis and the physiological and metabolic consequences of the disease.
3. State the kcalorie and protein requirements of clients with liver disease and explain why modifications of these requirements might be made.
4. Organize a diet for clients with liver failure including carbohydrate, fat, sodium, and fluid needs.
5. Describe diet therapy for clients before and after liver transplant.

CHAPTER OUTLINE

I.   Fatty Liver and Hepatitis

    A.   Fatty Liver
        1.   Consequences of Fatty Liver

Chapter 29
Nutrition, Cancer, and HIV Infection

CHAPTER SUMMARY

Cancer and HIV infection are conditions that affect multiple systems, which can interfere with nutrition status. Anorexia and inadequate nutrient intake in people with cancer have various causes. For example, cancer patients often suffer from fatigue, pain, or stress. Additionally, cancer therapies, such as surgery, chemotherapy, bone marrow transplants, and radiation therapy can further decrease nutrient intake by causing nausea, vomiting, stomatitis, mouth blindness, and food aversions. When a cancer patient does eat, nutrients are often lost due to malabsorption, vomiting, diarrhea, and inadequate digestion. Proper nutrition therapy can be used to help cancer patients maintain their strength and prevent wasting.

In regards to clients with HIV infection, treatments aim to slow the course of the infection, control associated symptoms, and alleviate pain. Anorexia and inadequate nutrient intake are common in clients with HIV infection. Severe psychological stress, thrush, respiratory infection, medication side effects, fatigue, and dementia all contribute to the problem. As the disease progresses, a person with AIDS may experience severe wasting. Nutrition therapy focuses on providing adequate amounts of energy and protein. If the client is unable to meet the nutrient needs through oral diet, tube feeding and TPN can be used to prevent nutrition complications and weight loss.

Highlight 29 focuses on ethical issue in nutrition care.

LEARNING OBJECTIVES

1. Explain how cancer develops and discuss factors that can influence its occurrence.
2. Differentiate between dietary factors that initiate, promote, and fight against cancer. Give examples of each.
3. Describe the consequences of cancer and its direct and indirect affects on nutrition status.
4. List recommendations for reducing the risk of cancer.
5. Discuss treatments typically used in fighting cancer and the nutrition support required.
6. Explain what HIV infection is and its progression to AIDS.
7. Describe factors that lead to alterations in nutrient status in people with HIV infection.
8. Discuss the importance of adequate nutrition support and how it might alter the

course of HIV infection.

CHAPTER OUTLINE

I. Cancer

    A.   How Cancers Develops
        1.   Genetic Factors
        2.   Immune Factors
        3.   Environmental Factors
        4.   Dietary Factors—Cancer Initiators
        5.   Dietary Factors—Cancer Promoters
        6.   Dietary Factors—Antipromoters
    B.   Consequences of Cancer
        1.   Wasting Associated with Cancer
        2.   Anorexia and Reduced Food Intake
        3.   Metabolic Alterations
        4.   Nutrient Losses
    C.   Treatments for Cancer
        1.   Medications to Combat Anorexia and Wasting
        2.   Other Medications
        3.   Alternative Therapies
    D.   Medical Nutrition Therapy
        1.   Early Nutrition Intervention
        2.   Oral Diets
        3.   Tube Feedings and TPN
        4.   Nutrition Support and Bone Marrow Transplants
        5.   Ethical Issues

II. HIV Infection

    A.   How HIV Develops
        1.   HIV Stages
        2.   Monitoring HIV Progression
    B.   Consequences of HIV Infection
        1.   Lipodystrophy
        2.   Weight Loss and Wasting
        3.   Anorexia and Reduced Nutrient Intake
        4.   Metabolic Alterations and Nutrient Losses
    C.   Treatments for HIV Infection
        1.   Medications to Combat Anorexia and Wasting
        2.   Other Medications
    D.   Medical Nutrition Therapy
        1.   Oral Diets
        2.   Vitamins and Minerals
        3.   Food Safety

4.   Tube Feedings and TPN

III.   Highlight: Ethical Issues in Nutrition Care

Transparency Acetate List

1. Fig. 17-2   Examples of Conditions Associated with Illness That Can Affect Nutrition Status
2. Fig. 17-3   The Nutrition Care Process
3. Fig. 17-4   Interrelationships among Health, Medications, Nutrition Status and Personal Factors
4. Table 17-4   Body Measurements Useful in Assessing Nutrition Status
5. Enrichment   How to Measure Triceps Fatfold
6. Enrichment   How to Measure Midarm Circumference
7. Fig. 18-1   Folate and Methotrexate
8. Fig. H18-1   Immune Cells of the Intestinal Villi
9. Fig. H18-2   Immune System Cells
10. Table 19-2   Foods Indicated on Liquid Diets
11. Table 19-3   Foods Included on Soft Diets
12. Fig. 20-1   The Upper GI Tract
13. Fig. 20-2   The Upper GI Tract, Acid Reflux, and Hiatal Hernia
14. Fig. 20-3   Typical Gastric Surgery Resections
15. Fig. 20-4   The Dumping Syndrome
16. Fig. H20-1   Examples of Adaptive Feeding Devices
17. Fig. 21-1   The Lower GI Tract and Related Organs
18. Fig. 21-2   The Consequences of Fat Malabsorption
19. Fig. 21-3   Nutrient Absorption and Consequences of Intestinal Surgeries
20. Fig. 21-4   Colostomy and Illeostomy
21. Fig. 21-5   Diverticula
22. Fig. 22-1   Feeding Tube Placement Sites
23. Fig. 22-2   Selecting a Formula
24. Fig H22-1   Biochemical Pathway: Normal
25. Fig H22-1   Biochemical Alterations in PKU
26. Photo p 688   Feeding Tubes
27. Fig. 23-1   Selecting a Feeding Route
28. Fig. 23-2   Central TPN
29. Table 23-1   Possible Indications for Central TPN
30. Fig. H23-1   The Nutrition Support Team
31. Fig. 24-1   Inflammatory Responses
32. Fig. 24-2   Inflammation and Tissue Damage
33. Fig. 24-3   Metabolic Responses to Fasting and Stress
34. Fig. H24-1   Effects and Potential Consequences of Severe Stress on the GI Tract
35. Page 746   The Obesity Cycle
36. Fig. 25-1   Acute Metabolic Consequences and Clinical Manifestations of Untreated or Uncontrolled Diabetes
37. Table 25-1   Features of Type 1 and Type 2 Diabetes
38. Fig. 25-2   Actions of Insulin Types
39. Fig. 26-1   The Heart, Blood Vessels, and Lungs
40. Fig. 26-2   Blood Pressure and Fluid Exchange
41. Fig. H26-1   Insulin Resistance and the Metabolic Syndrome
42. Fig. 27-1   The Kidneys and Urinary Tract
43. Fig. 27-2   Consequences of Urinary Protein Losses in the Nephrotic Syndrome
44. Fig. 28-1   The Liver, Biliary Tract, and Associated Blood Vessels
45. Fig. 28-2   The Consequences of Cirrhosis
46. Fig. 28-3   Ammonia Production in the Body
47. Table 28-3   Diet Guidelines for Liver Failure
48. Fig. H28-1   The Gallbladder and Bile Duct
49. Fig. 29-1   Tumor Formation
50. Fig. 29-2   The Cancer Cachexia Syndrome: Contributing Factors

Handouts

Prepared by Lori Turner, Ph.D., R.D.

University of Arkansas--Fayetteville

HANDOUTS
Prepared by Lori W. Turner, PhD, RD

Literature Critique: Critical Evaluation of Published Nutrition Information--"Should I Believe What I Just Read?"

Assignment for discussion: Carefully read a journal article and answer the following questions:

1. Summarize the basic idea of the article in a short paragraph.
2a. What are the credentials of the author(s)? What do the abbreviations after the name(s) mean? Do they enhance the authors' credibility? Explain.
 b. Is the author affiliated with an organization or institution? Does the affiliation with the organization or institution enhance the authors' credibility? Briefly explain.
 c. Does the periodical have an editorial board? Do the editors' credentials enhance the article's credibility? Where does one look in a periodical for the editorial board?
3a. Is scientific research being presented or discussed? Is the research current?
 b. If so, what specific kinds of research or data are presented or cited to support the ideas?
 c. Were references listed to allow readers to investigate the information's original source? Were full citations provided?
4a. What is the underlying hypothesis (if/then, cause/effect, etc.)?
 b. What are the article's conclusions/recommendations?
 c. Are the conclusions or recommendations supported by the research discussion? Explain briefly why or why not.
5a. Design and describe in depth additional research that could more decisively test the hypothesis identified. Pay particular attention to details and controls.
 b. Indicate what will be measured.
 c. State the type of experimental design and type of experiment.
6. Identify the statements in the article that you believe and those that you do not believe, and discuss why or why not for each.
7. What sources other than those listed in the periodical would you refer to if you were to research the article's topic further?

Source: Adapted with permission of: Deborah Fleurant, MOE Thesis, University of New Hampshire, 1989 (Thesis Advisor Sam Smith)

Evaluation of Published Nutrition Information

Research Project Using the Internet

This research project will employ the use of the Internet as a research tool. The student will be expected to become familiar with the diversity of Internet resources. Students will also be expected to participate in on-line discussions about nutrition and related topics in class-based listserve groups. The purpose of this project is to develop Internet and on-line participation skills.

1. Obtain your name and password. Change your password to one that cannot be hacked. Log onto e-mail. Send your instructor an e-mail message. Print it off and attach it to the assignment.
2. Borrow a book about Unix. Read as much as you can understand. Write down the 10 most important commands for users. Explain why these commands have been useful for you (1 page).
3. Use the Unix newsreader (TIN) to find a usenet newsgroup that is of interest to you and relevant to nutrition. Describe or print off some relevant comments (1-2 pages).
4. Use GOPHER to find something interesting. Browse both the Ryerson gopher and other gophers. Discuss what you found (1 page).
5. Telnet to a remote site on the Internet. Attach the telnet address. Describe or print off what you found (1 page).
6. Find a listserve to join. Demonstrate that you have made at least 3 comments over the semester. Print these off and attach to your assignment.
7. Access the world wide web. Document how you accessed the web and the address of the website accessed. Print off and discuss what you found. Attach this to the assignment.
8. Go to a library and obtain a recent edition of an Internet journal (such as NetGuide). Browse through it and report on what you found.
9. Borrow a book about the Internet. List 10 items that are most important for education and research and explain why (1-2 pages).
10. Enter the library computer system. Use a system to conduct a literature search regarding a topic (for example, vitamin A). Discuss your findings (1-2 pages).

Research Project Using the Internet

Tufts University Nutrition Navigator

The purpose of this assignment is to help familiarize the student with the *Tufts University Nutrition Navigator*, an online rating and review guide. The *Tufts University Nutrition Navigator* is designed to help with identifying reliable and accurate sources of nutrition information. Web sites are reviewed by Tufts nutritionists, who apply rating and evaluation criteria developed by the Tufts University Navigation Advisory Board, a prestigious panel of leading U.S. and Canadian nutrition experts. Site reviews are updated quarterly to ensure that ratings take into account the ever changing Internet and nutrition environments.

Assignment

1. Go to any library, or use your home computer and get online.
2. Enter this location address: http://navigator.tufts.edu/
   Be sure to carefully enter the address; pay close attention to spelling, punctuation and do not capitalize any of the letters.
3. If you have correctly entered the above address and you go online, then you will find the Tufts University Nutrition Navigator home page displayed on your monitor.
4. Select one of the generalized topic areas displayed on your screen: Educators, General Nutrition, Journalists, Kids, Health Professionals, Special Dietary Needs, Parents, Women. Begin your search with one of these selections. Alternatively, you may search for information on another specific topic that interests you such as: antioxidants, vitamin B_{12}, osteoporosis, HIV, cancer, etc.
5. Describe your findings on the topic that was researched.

Contributed by: Marvin Parent, Oakland Community College

Compare Your Food Intake to the Daily Food Guide (Pyramid)

List Food Item and Amount

Indicate Number of Servings From Each Food Group

Food Item	Bread/ Cereal	Fruit	Vege- table	Meat	Milk	Other
Breakfast ———— ———— ————						
Snack ———— ————						
Lunch ———— ———— ———— ————						
Snack ———— ————						
Dinner ———— ———— ———— ————						
Snack ———— ————						
TOTAL:						

HANDOUT 2-1

Compare Your Food Intake to the Daily Food Guide

Most Frequently Eaten Raw Fruits, Vegetables, and Seafood

The FDA's voluntary nutrition labeling program applies to the 20 most frequently consumed members of each category: raw fruits, vegetables, and seafood. They are listed here in descending order of consumption.

Fruits	Vegetables	Seafood
Bananas	Potatoes	Shrimp
Apples	Iceberg lettuce	Cod
Watermelons	Tomatoes	Pollock
Oranges	Onions	Catfish
Cantaloupes	Carrots	Scallops
Grapes	Celery	Salmon
Grapefruits	Corn	Flounder
Strawberries	Broccoli	Sole
Peaches	Cabbage	Oysters
Pears	Cucumbers	Orange roughly
Nectarines	Bell peppers	Mackerel
Honeydew melons	Cauliflower	Ocean perch
Plums	Leaf lettuce	Rockfish
Avocados	Sweet potatoes	Whiting
Lemons	Mushrooms	Clams
Pineapples	Green onions	Haddock
Tangerines	Green beans	Blue crabs
Cherries	Radishes	Rainbow trout
Kiwi fruit	Summer squash	Halibut
Limes	Asparagus	Lobster

HANDOUT 2-2

Most Frequently Eaten Raw Fruits, Vegetables, and Seafood

Transport of Nutrients Into Blood

Nutrient	Transport Into Blood
☞ **Water-soluble nutrients**	
Carbohydrates	
Monosaccharides	Directly into blood
Lipids	
Glycerol	Directly into blood
Short-chain fatty acids	Directly into blood
Medium-chain fatty acids	Directly into blood
Proteins	
Amino Acids	Directly into blood
Vitamins	
Vitamins B and C	Directly into blood
Minerals	Directly into blood
☞ **Fat-soluble nutrients**	
Lipids	
Long-chain fatty acids	Made into triglycerides
Monoglycerides	Made into triglycerides
Triglycerides	To lymph, then blood
Cholesterol	To lymph, then blood
Phospholipids	To lymph, then blood
Vitamins	
Vitamins A, D, E, K	To lymph, then blood

Transport of Nutrients Into Blood

Characteristics of Fiber

Dietary fibers are classified according to a number of characteristics, including their solubility in water and whether they are a polysaccharide. These differences influence their physiological effect on the body.

	Water Soluble	Water Insoluble
Polysaccharides	Gums Hemicellulose[a] Mucilages Pectins	Cellulose Hemicellulose[a]
Nonpolysaccharides		Lignins
Food Sources	Fruits Oats Barley Legumes	Vegetables Wheat Grains
Health Effects	Lower blood cholesterol Lower rate of glucose absorption	Softened stools Acceleration of intestinal transit time

[a]Some hemicelluloses are water soluble and others are water insoluble.

How to Modify a Recipe (Lasagna)

Original	Modified
1/3 c olive oil (to sauté vegetables)	[omit oil]
1-1/2 c diced onions	1-1/2 c onion, 1 green pepper, 1/2 lb mushrooms
2 cloves garlic	2 cloves garlic
1-1/2 lb ground chuck	3/4 lb ground round
2 t salt	[omit salt]
2 lb tomato sauce	use no-added-salt type tomato sauce
28 oz canned tomatoes	use no-added-salt type canned tomatoes
6 oz canned tomato paste	use no-added-salt type tomato paste
1 tbsp oregano	2 t oregano, 2 t basil, 1/4 c fresh parsley
2 tsp onion salt	[omit salt]
1 lb lasagna noodles	1 lb whole wheat lasagna noodles
2 tbsp olive oil (to cook noodles)	[omit oil]
16 oz ricotta	16 oz low-fat cottage cheese, pureed
8 oz mozzarella	8 oz part skim mozzarella
10 oz parmesan	4 oz parmesan
oil to grease pan	spray to grease pan

Yield 16 servings (2 9" x 12" pans)

Analysis	Original	Modified
Energy (kcal)	513	281
Protein (gm)	35	21
Fat (gm)	29 (6 t)	7 (1.4 t)
Sodium (mg)	1121	380
Cholesterol (mg)	73	32
% of calories from fat	51	24

Source: Culinary Hearts Kitchen Course, Tallahassee, Florida, as taught by Sandra Woodruff, M.S., R.D., with permission.

HANDOUT 5-1

How to Modify a Recipe

Plant Proteins in Human Nutrition: Myths and Realities

Myth	Reality
Plant proteins are not complete; they lack certain amino acids.	Most dietary combinations of proteins are complete; certain food proteins may be low in specific amino acids.
Plant proteins are lower in quality to animal proteins.	Protein quality depends not only on the source but also on the dietary mixture of plant proteins; plant proteins can be as high quality as animal proteins.
Proteins from different plant foods must be carefully mixed and eaten together in the same meal.	Proteins do not have to been eaten at the same meal; the mixture over a day is important for nutritional value.
Animal procedures can provide good indexes of the human nutritional value of food proteins.	Animal procedures may underestimate plant protein quality for humans.
Plant proteins are difficult to digest.	Depending on the source and method of food preparation, plant proteins can be easy to digest.
People cannot meet protein needs with plant proteins alone.	Plant protein or animal protein can provide adequate protein for human needs.
Plant proteins are lacking in nutritional value because they are not balanced.	Plant proteins do not create a practical problem in terms of balance; possible imbalances are observed in amino acid supplementation.

Alcohol's Effects on Nutrients in the Body

Nutrient	Effect	Possible Consequence
Vitamin A	Increased mobilization	liver alteration, enhanced carcinogenesis
Vitamin D	Less vitamin D converted to active form in liver, malabsorption	altered calcium metabolism, increased bone fractures
Thiamin	Decreased absorption, increased destruction and excretion	nerve damage, psychosis related to Wernicke-Korsakoff syndrome
Pyridoxine	Increased breakdown, decreased formation of active cofactor	possible abnormal amino acid measures and nitrogen balance
Folate	Decreased absorption, utilization	megaloblastic anemia
Vitamin C	Decreased absorption	decreased protection from ethanol toxicity
Iron	Possible overload, possible increased absorption	buildup damage to liver
Magnesium	Increased excretion	electrocardiogram changes, delirium tremens (DTs)
Zinc	Increased excretion	slow wound healing
Potassium	Increased excretion	muscle weakness

Source: Adapted from M. S. Meskin, Alcohol-Nutrient Interactions, Nutrition and the MD, December 1992, p. 4.

Alcohol's Effects on Nutrients in the Body

Medical Problems Associated With Obesity

- ☞Hypertension

- ☞Renal Disease

- ☞Gallbladder Disease

- ☞Pulmonary Disease

- ☞Problems With Anesthesia During Surgery

- ☞Osteoarthritis and Gout

- ☞Breast and Endometrial Cancer

- ☞Abnormal Plasma Lipid and Lipoprotein Concentrations

- ☞Impairment of Cardiac Function

- ☞Menstrual Irregularities and Toxemia of Pregnancy

- ☞Psychological Trauma

- ☞Flat Feet and Infection in Fatfolds

- ☞Organ Compression by Adipose Tissue

- ☞Impaired Heat Tolerance

Source: Art Gilbert, Director, Wellness Fitness Institute, University of California, Santa Barbara, with permission.

Medical Problems Associated With Obesity

Evaluation of a Commercial Weight-Loss Program

1.   Describe the food program promoted by the organization. Is the program flexible enough to allow people with different foodways and lifestyles to use it successfully? Is it adaptable and easy to follow? Does it provide variety? Does the program provide for weight maintenance after goal weight is achieved?

_____

_____

2.   Describe how the plan works. Does it require substantial registration fees, mandatory purchase of various items or foods, attendance at a minimum number of meetings?

_____

_____

3.   Evaluate whether the plan offers a nutritionally sound way to lose weight. What characteristics make it sound or unsound?

_____

_____

4.   Describe any "case histories" you might overhear or learn about and your impressions of them. Do the stories sound authentic? Do they sound as though the person's weight loss was achieved sensibly? Do they present facts? Do they contain any "magic bullets?"

_____

_____

5.   Describe your overall impressions of the meeting, telling whether they were positive or negative and why. If you had a weight problem, would you consider membership in this organization?

_____

_____

HANDOUT 9-1

Evaluation of a Weight-Loss Program

Eating Attitudes Test

Answer these questions using the following responses:
A=Always   U=Usually   O=Often   S=Sometimes   R=Rarely   N=Never

1. I am terrified about being overweight.
2. I avoid eating when I am hungry.
3. I find myself preoccupied with food.
4. I have gone on eating binges where I feel that I may not be able to stop.
5. I cut my food into very small pieces.
6. I am aware of the calorie content of the foods I eat.
7. I particularly avoid foods with a high carbohydrate content.
8. I feel that others would prefer if I ate more.
9. I vomit after I have eaten.
10. I feel extremely guilty after eating.
11. I am preoccupied with a desire to be thinner.
12. I think about burning up calories when I exercise.
13. Other people think I am too thin.
14. I am preoccupied with the thought of having fat on my body.
15. I take longer than other people to eat my meals.
16. I avoid foods with sugar in them.
17. I eat diet foods.
18. I feel that food controls my life.
19. I display self-control around food.
20. I feel that others pressure me to eat.
21. I give too much time and thought to food.
22. I feel uncomfortable after eating sweets.
23. I engage in dieting behavior.
24. I like my stomach to be empty.
25. I enjoy trying new rich foods.
26. I have the impulse to vomit after meals.

<u>Scoring</u>: 3 for never, 2 for rarely, 1 for sometimes, 1 for always, usually and often. Total scores under 20 points indicate abnormal eating behavior.

Source: J. A. McSherry, Progress in the diagnosis of anorexia nervosa, *Journal of the Royal Society of Health* 106 (1986): 8-9. (Eating Attitudes Test developed by Dr. Paul Garfinkel.)

Eating Attitudes Test

Exploring Eating Habits

To explore your eating habits, check all the answers that describe your food intake patterns. Then, consider possible areas for improvement.

When do I usually eat?

_____ At meatime.

_____ While studying.

_____ While preparing meals or clearing the table.

_____ When spending time with friends.

_____ While watching TV or participating in other activities.

_____ Anytime.

Where do I usually eat?

_____ At home at the kitchen or dining room table.

_____ In the school cafeteria.

_____ In fast-food places.

_____ In front of the TV or while studying.

_____ Wherever I happen to be when I'm hungry.

Why do I usually eat?

_____ It's time to eat.

_____ I'm hungry.

_____ Foods look tempting.

_____ Everyone else is eating.

_____ Food will get thrown away if I don't eat it.

_____ I'm bored or frustrated.

Changes I want to make:

_____

_____

Source: U.S. Department of Agriculture, Dietary Guidelines and Your Health: Health Educator's Guide to Nutrition and Fitness (Washington, DC, US Government Printing Office, 1992).

HANDOUT 9-3

Exploring Eating Habits

Vitamin/Mineral Supplement Evaluation

Complete the supplement evaluation form about a selected supplement.

Vitamin/Mineral Supplement Evaluation Form

1. What is the name of the supplement?_____

2. What is the cost per pill?_____

3. Is the supplement complete (does it contain all vitamins and minerals with established RDIs)? If no, what is missing?

   _____

   _____

4. Are most vitamins and minerals present at or near 100% of the RDIs? Exceptions include biotin, calcium, magnesium, and phosphorus, which are rarely found in amounts near 100% of the RDIs. List any vitamins or minerals that are present in low amounts or dangerously high amounts.

   _____

   _____

5. Does the supplement contain unnecessary nutrients or nonnutrients? If yes, list them.

   _____

   _____

6. Is there "hype" on the label? Does the label use the terms "natural," "organic," "chelated," "no sugar," "stress-reliever," etc.? List any terms used.

   _____

   _____

HANDOUT 10-1

Vitamin/Mineral Supplement Evaluation

Factors That Destroy Vitamins

Nutrient	Acid	Alkaline	Oxygen	UV Light	Heat
B Vitamins:					
Thiamin		X	X		X
Riboflavin		X		X	
Niacin	X				
Biotin	X	X	X	X	
Pantothenic acid	X	X			X
Vitamin B$_6$		X		X	X
Folate	X		X	X	X
Vitamin B$_{12}$	X			X	
Vitamin C		X	X		X
Vitamin A			X	X	X
Vitamin D	X		X	X	
Vitamin E			X	X	
Vitamin K		X		X	

Source: Adapted from C.D. Berdanier, Advanced Nutrition: Micronutrients (Boca Raton, Fla.: CRC Press, 1998).

Spices to Enhance Salt-Free Dishes

For general seasoning purposes, use these mixed herbs (place in shaker):

Saltless Surprise	2 tsp garlic powder; 1 tsp each of basil, oregano, and powdered lemon rind(or dehydrated lemon juice). Blend, mix well, store in glass container with rice to prevent caking.
Pungent Salt Substitute	3 tsp basil; 2 tsp each of savory, celery seed, ground cumin seed, marjoram, sage, lemon thyme. Mix well, then powder with a mortar and pestle.
Spicy Salt Substitute	1 tsp each of cloves, pepper, and crushed coriander seed; 2 tsp paprika; 1 tbsp rosemary. Mix in a blender and store in an airtight container.

For specific seasoning purposes, use these herbs. Store together mixtures of those you especially like, and label them "soup blend," "beef blend," etc.

When you serve:	Use:
Beef	Bay, chives, cloves, cumin, garlic, hot pepper, marjoram, rosemary, savory
Bread	Caraway, marjoram, oregano, poppy seed, rosemary, thyme
Cheese	Basil, chervil, chives, curry, dill, fennel, garlic chives, marjoram, oregano, parsley, sage, thyme
Fish	Chervil, dill, fennel, garlic, parsley, tarragon, thyme
Fruit	Anise, cinnamon, cloves, coriander, ginger, lemon verbena, mint, rose geranium
Lamb	Garlic, marjoram, oregano, rosemary, thyme
Pork	Coriander, cumin, garlic, ginger, hot peppers, pepper sage, savory, thyme
Poultry	Garlic, oregano, rosemary, sage, savory
Salads	Basil, borage, burnet, chives, garlic chives, parsley
Soups	Bay, chervil, marjoram, parsley, rosemary, savory
Vegetables	Basil, burnet, chervil, chives, dill, marjoram, mint, parsley, pepper, thyme

Source: Adapted from H. H. Shimizu, Do yourself a favor, *FDA Consumer*, April 1984, pp. 16-19.

Spices to Enhance Salt-Free Dishes

Effects of Nutrient Deficiencies During Pregnancy

Nutrient	Deficiency Effect
Energy	Low infant birthweight
Protein	Reduced infant head circumference
Folate	Miscarriage and neural tube defect
Vitamin D	Low infant birthweight
Calcium	Decreased infant bone density
Iron	Low infant birthweight and premature birth
Iodide	Cretinism (varying degrees of mental and physical retardation in the infant)
Zinc	Congenital malformations

Source: Adapted from L. K. DeBruyne and S. R. Rolfes, Life Cycle Nutrition: Conception Through Adolescence, ed. E. N. Whitney (St. Paul, Minn.: West, 1989), p. 68.

HANDOUT 15-1
Effects of Nutrient Deficiencies During Pregnancy

Supervised Food Activities For Preschoolers

Children's muscle development determines their abilities to perform activities involving foods. The ages listed here are average ages; individual children develop on their own schedules.

A two-year-old can use large muscles of the arms to:	☞scrub vegetables ☞tear lettuce ☞snap beans
A three-year-old can use hand muscles to:	☞wrap foods in foil; wrap cheese slices around bread sticks ☞pour beverages from a small pitcher into a cup ☞mix cereal snacks in a large bowl with clean hands ☞shake juices together in a small, sealed container ☞spread peanut butter, cream cheese, or jelly on bread with a dull butter knife or small spatula
A four-year-old can use the small muscles in the fingers to:	☞peel the shells from hard-boiled eggs or the skins from oranges ☞roll out a ball of ground meat or dough with clean hands ☞juice citrus fruit by pushing down and turning the fruit on a hand juicer ☞crack raw eggs by tapping the center of the egg against the side of a bowl ☞mash a bowl of cooked beans for dip
A five-year-old can use eye-hand coordination to:	☞measure ingredients with measuring spoons and cups ☞cut semi-soft foods such as soft cheese with a dull butter knife and practice keeping fingers away from the blade ☞grind chunky peanut butter or cooked meats in a hand-turned food grinder, or turn a hand-cranked ice cream maker ☞grate carrots or cheese on an upright grater with fingers far from the grater to avoid cuts

Source: Adapted from A. A. Hertzler, Preschoolers' food handling skills--motor development, Journal of Nutrition Education 21 (1989): 100B-100C.

Supervised Food Activities For Preschoolers

Functions of Cells of the Immune System

Phagocytes	Lymphocytes	
	T-Cells (Cell-mediated immunity)	B-Cells (Humoral immunity)
Engulf foreign organisms. Activate lymphocytes. Suppress appetite. Induce fever and malaise. Display antigens.	Recognize antiges and send chemical signals. Stimulate T-cell development. Release killer chemicals. Suppress immune response when battle against infection has been won.	Produce antibodies. Kill invaders directly or make them easy targets for phagocytosis.

Functions of Cells of the Immune System

Effects of Malnutrition on the Body's Immune Response

Immune System Component	Effects of Malnutrition
Skin	Thinned, with less connective tissue
Mucous membranes	Microvilli flattened; antibody secretions reduced
GI tract	Atrophy of intestinal cells
Lymph tissues	Thymus gland, lymph nodes, and spleen reduced in size; T-cell areas depleted of lymphocytes
Phagocytosis	Kill time delayed
Cell-mediated immunity	Circulating T-cells reduced
Humoral immunity	Circulating immunoglobulin levels normal; antibody response possibly impaired

Effects of Malnutrition on the Body's Immune Response

Causes of Malnutrition in HIV Infection

Reduced Food Intake	Accelerated Nutrient Losses
Drug therapy causes anorexia, nausea, and vomiting; food aversions arise	Cancers of the GI tract and cancer therapy lead to malabsorption
Lethargy and exhaustion drain the energy to eat	Chronic or recurrent diarrhea interferes with nutrient absorption
Fever, pain, and infection cause anorexia	Malabsorption limits nutrient absorption
Psychological sresses such as fever and depression make eating seem unimportant	Low serum albumin levels provide too few nutrient carriers
Oral infections (thrush) alter taste sensations, cause pain, and reduce saliva flow	PEM leads to diarrhea and malabsorption
Oral infections (herpes virus) cause painful mouth ulcers and problems with chewing and swallowing	Drug therapy causes diarrhea and malabsorption
Esophageal infections and lesions make swallowing difficult	High gastric pH limits absorption and promotes bacterial growth, leading to infections
Kaposi's sarcoma (a cancer associated with AIDS) causes esophageal lesions and obstructions	Infections and fever accelerate metabolism (high BMR)

Causes of Malnutrition in HIV Infection

How to Detect and Avoid Spoiled Foods

These Foods	Are Risky When
Fresh Poultry	☞ stored raw in the refrigerator for longer than 1-2 days, (3-4 days for cooked poultry) ☞ left unrefrigerated for more than 2 hours either before or after cooking
Fresh Meat	☞ stored raw in the refrigerator for longer than 3-5 days (1-2 days for hamburger) ☞ discolored, smelling, slimy ☞ left unrefrigerated for more than 2 hours either before or after cooking
Fresh Fish	☞ stored for longer than 1-2 days in the refrigerator ☞ dried at edges, smelly ☞ left unrefrigerated for more than 2 hours either before or after cooking
Milk, cream, egg products	☞ left unrefrigerated for more than 2 hours ☞ stored in the refrigerator longer than 5-7 days
Frozen meats, poultry, fish, casseroles	☞ thawed at room temperature ☞ allowed to thaw and be refrozen ☞ eaten without thorough cooking
Canned foods*	☞ liquid spurts out when can is opened ☞ can is corroded, rusty, or leaky, swollen on top or bottom, dented on side seams ☞ contents have off-odors, a foamy or mushy texture ☞ stored at temperatures above 100°F or allowed to freeze and thaw
Fresh fruits and vegetables	☞ unwashed, moldy
Cereal products, flour	☞ moldy, infested with insects

*Home canned foods should never be used in family day care, congregate meal sites, or other food service operations.

CANADIAN NUTRITION INFORMATION

Prepared by
MARGARET HEDLEY, MSc, RD
University of Guelph

CANADIAN NUTRITION INFORMATION

CONTENTS

* All subsequent chapters refer to Teaching Canadian Information

CANADIAN INFORMATION

INTRODUCTION

New technologies and increased global trade are affecting nutrition education in Canada. The world wide web gives Canadians increased access to information about food and nutrients around the world. Nutrition educators also have easy access to information about Canadian policy changes that affect social and health programs, as well as food availability, nutritional quality of foods and nutrition education. With increasing free trade, many policies and standards of Canada and the United States are becoming harmonized. Canadian nutrition educators have used a common research base for planning, implementing and evaluating programs with their colleagues in the United States. However, the countries still have so some differences in food intake patterns, health statistics, and health policy. These differences continue to influence the types and content of nutrition education programs in Canada. This section highlights Canadian regulations, standards, programs, and resources, according to the topics discussed in each chapter or highlight in *Understanding Nutrition, Ninth Edition*. It identifies readings and resources to support Canadian nutrition educators. Examples of the choice system of the Canadian Diabetes Association Good Health Eating Guide are given to help Canadian nutrition educators.

CANADIAN GOVERNMENT DEPARTMENTS

This section is an overview of general responsibilities of Canadian government departments that relate to food, nutrition, and health. Specific applications of legislation, e.g. nutrition labelling, will be described according to the chapters in *Understanding Nutrition, Ninth Edition.* Several departments work together to develop and administer regulations on food and nutrition. The Canadian government is using the internet to communicate with the public. Many of the documents, proposed policies, and structural changes are posted on the web. Consultation with the public is also done through the internet, as was done during the development of the proposed nutrition labelling policy.

HEALTH CANADA

Canadian instructors should visit the Health Canada web site (www.hc-sc.gc.ca) regularly and sign up for the Nutritional Sciences listserv to receive information about new policy documents. You can also encourage students to use the government web sites for assignments to help them learn about food and nutrition policy. The Minister of Health announced a new structure for Health Canada in 2000. Health Canada, in partnership with the provincial and territorial governments, provides national leadership in developing policy, enforcing health regulations, promoting disease prevention and enhancing healthy living for all Canadians. To meet this mandate Health Canada also works with other departments, such as Human Resources Canada and Environment Canada, or agencies, such as the Canadian Food Inspection Agency. A detailed description of the new Health Canada structure can be found at the Health Canada web site.

Health Products and Food Branch

The two main goals of the Health Products and Food Branch are "to promote good nutrition and informed use of drugs" and "to maximize the safety and efficacy of drugs, food, natural health products, medical devices, biologics and related biotechnology products in the Canadian marketplace and health system". This branch is responsible for developing and enforcing the health and safety aspects of the *Food and Drugs Act and Regulations*[1]. This legislation deals with food safety and quality, and economic fraud, and affects nutrient enrichment/composition, food additives, chemical contaminants, microbiological contaminants, nutrition labelling and health claims. The Food Directorate is responsible for program policies and standards related to food safety and nutritional value for this legislation and recommends standards for nutrient intake. Much of this work is done by the Nutrition Research Division and the Nutrition Evaluation Division of the Bureau of Nutritional Sciences. This bureau has been developing new policies on nutrition labelling and health claims for foods.

Natural Health Products Directorate

The Office of Natural Health Products was established in 2000, based on the recommendations of the Standing Committee on Health's report "Natural Health Products: A New Vision". The recommendations address concerns of Canadian consumers, health providers and industry. This directorate is developing a regulatory framework to ensure quality control of natural health products, and define evidence requirements and wording for health claims for the products. At the time of writing, the framework is undergoing public consultation. Visit www.hc-sc.gc.ca/hpb/onhp for the current status on the regulatory framework.

First Nations and Inuit Health Branch

The First Nations and Inuit Branch (FNIHB) was formerly called the Medical Services Branch. This branch works with the First Nations and Inuit peoples to improve their health status. Health services are provided to these peoples through Regional Offices and community-based programs. Nutritionists in the Regional Offices provide public health and health promotion programs to meet the regional needs.

The Nutrition Specialist is with Health Support Services, Indian and Northern Health Services within the Medical Services Branch and is a member of the Network of the Federal/Provincial/Territorial Group on Nutrition. Nutrition treatment services are also provided in areas which do not have access to other sources of service, such as provincial or territorial health services.

Population and Public Health Branch

The Population and Public Health Branch focuses on policies, programs, and systems relating to prevention, health promotion, disease surveillance, community action, and disease control. Within this branch the Centre for Healthy Human Development addresses prenatal and perinatal health, healthy child development, healthy families, healthy aging, healthy communities, rural health, and healthy lifestyles. In collaboration with health professions and health agencies, this centre provides health information on the internet through the Health Canada web site on the Canadian Health Network. Nutrition instructors and students will find relevant course information through this network.

AGRICULTURE AND AGRI-FOOD CANADA

Canadian Food Inspection Agency

The Canadian Food Inspection Agency (CFIA) is responsible for all inspection and associated activities related to food safety, economic fraud, trade related requirements, and animal and plant health programs. This federal agency reports to Parliament through the Minister of Agriculture and Agri-Food Canada. Instructors should be aware of this agency and the services it provides because it is the single contact for consumers, with questions and concerns about food products and their safety, and for food industry clients, who produce the foods and must meet food inspection requirements.

The CFIA is responsible for administering labelling, packaging, and advertising aspects of the *Food and Drugs Act and Regulations* and *Consumer Packaging and Labelling Act.* In 1996 Agriculture and Agri-Food Canada published the interpretation of the legislation and regulations for labelling and advertising foods, *Guide to Food Labelling and Advertising*[2]. This publication presents the guidelines for nutrition labelling and claims which comply with the *Guidelines in Nutrition Labelling* in the *Food and Drugs Act and Regulations*[1]. Look for revisions to these guidelines at the Health Canada web site when the new nutrition labelling policy is adopted.

Information about CFIA is at www.cfia-acia.agr.ca or toll-free phone at 1-800-442-2342.

PROVINCIAL, TERRITORIAL AND MUNICIPAL GOVERNMENTS

Health services are the responsibility of the provincial and territorial governments and are implemented at the municipal level. Each of the ten provinces and three territories has specific legislation for the provision of health services and programs. Public health nutrition issues across Canada are identified and discussed by the Network of the Federal/Provincial/Territorial Group on Nutrition. This group is comprised of the chief nutritionists from the provinces and territories and representatives from three branches of Health Canada. The network has supported the development of national guidelines for stages in the life cycle, such as pregnancy and preschool years. Information on nutrition and health services provided by the provinces and territories can be accessed through their government's web sites.

Information on nutrition and health services provided by the provinces and territories can be accessed through each government's web site.

Public health departments provide health promotion programs, including nutrition education. Local offices provide educational materials, or information on how to get nutrition education resources, to support teaching nutrition in your locality. Many of the municipal health departments can be accessed through the internet.

TEACHING CANADIAN INFORMATION: CHAPTER 1
AN OVERVIEW OF NUTRITION

1.1 HOW TO CALCULATE THE ENERGY AVAILABLE FROM FOODS IN KILOJOULES

Food energy values in Canada are expressed as Calories (kilocalories) or kilojoules. To become more familiar with kilojoules, students could calculate the energy available in foods using the example in *How to Calculate the Energy Available from Foods* in Chapter 1 of the textbook and the conversion factors in the footnote of the previous page.

16 g carbohydrate x 17 kJ/g	= 272 kJ
7 g protein x 17 kJ/g	= 119 kJ
9 g fat x 37 kJ/g	= 333 kJ
Total	= 724 kJ

1.2 DIETARY REFERENCE INTAKES FOR CANADIANS

As Chapter 1 of the textbook indicates, Canada is participating in the development and implementation of the new Dietary Reference Intakes (DRI). Canadian nutrition scientists are represented on each of the review committees and panels. One advantage of Canada participating in the process is that there will be a single set of recommendations for both Canada and the United States, thus supporting harmonization of trade-related issues and freer trade of food. The bonus for Canadian nutrition educators is that consumers and students will find more consistency in learning about nutrition labelling and other nutrition issues, when they are exposed to nutrition information from both countries. Health Canada provides current information about the progress of the DRI on its web site (www.hc-sc.gc.ca). Nutrition instructors will find the *Question and Answers* paper particularly helpful for planning lectures on the DRI.

The Canadian participants on committees and panels for the DRI include:

Dr. Stephanie Atkinson, McMaster University, member of the Standing Committee on the Scientific Evaluation of DRI and chair of the Panel on Calcium and Related Nutrients

Dr. Ian Munro, CanTox Inc., chair of the Subcommittee on Upper Reference Levels of Intake (SURL)

Dr. Phillippe De Wals, University of Sherbrooke, member the Panel on Folate and Other B Vitamins

Dr. Alan Chan, University of Ottawa, member of the Panel on Dietary Antioxidants

Dr. Susan Barr, University of British Columbia, member of Subcommittee on Interpretation and Uses of DRI

Dr. Harriet Kuhnlein, McGill University, member of Subcommittee on Interpretation and Uses of DRI

Health Canada has not yet officially adopted the new DRIs. However, Peter Fischer, Chief, Nutrition Research Divisions, Food Directorate, Health Products and Food Branch, Health Canada, has indicated that as a co-sponsor of the DRI process, Health Canada recognizes the DRIs as the latest scientific information available o nutrient recommendations[3]. He noted that it is appropriate for dietitians to use the DRIs in their practice.

1.3 NUTRITION ASSESSMENT OF POPULATIONS

Canada does not have nutrient intake data available on a national basis, such as HANES and NFCS and NHANES. The most recent national survey of food intake was Nutrition Canada, completed from 1970 to 72. Under the Canadian Heart Health Initiatives, several provincial surveys were completed during the 1990's. Since methods of data collection vary with the different surveys, the results of these studies have not been compiled nationally or used for comparisons between regions. The Ontario Food Survey, which used similar methodology to most other provincial surveys, was completed in 1998 but the results have not yet been published. Check with your provincial or territorial health department to see if the results for your area are available, for example *Nutrition Report of the 1990 Ontario Health Survey*[4].

The most recent published Canadian food intake survey, "Food Habits of Canadian" collected data between August 1997 and July 1998 from five regions of Canada (Atlantic, Québec, Ontario, Prairies and British Columbia)[5]. The results of the survey showed that the percent of energy from fat was 29 to 31%, close to the recommended 30%. The mean intakes of milk products and vegetables and fruit were below the minimum recommended servings. Although intake of fat has decreased since Nutrition Canada, changes are needed to improve the eating habits of Canadians.

The National Population Health Survey (NPHS) is a 20-year longitudinal survey which collects data on the same individuals every two years[6]. The original sample was selected to be representative of the Canadian population. The 1994-95 NPHS contained a supplement to collect self-reported data on how Canadians, 12 years and over, have responded to the 1990 *Nutrition Recommendations and Canada's Guidelines to Healthy Eating.* The results indicate that people aged 45 to 64 were most concerned about the amount of fat they consume. Most of the population who were concerned about fat intake (86%) were taking action to lower it. The BMI was calculated for individuals using self-reported height and weight, and results were compared to the data collected in the 1990 NPHS. A lower percentage of people was in the underweight category (BMI <20) and acceptable weight category (BMI 20.0-25.0). A higher percentage was in the possibly overweight category (BMI 25.1-27.0) and overweight (BMI >27). Although many people reported taking action to reduce fat intake, overweight continues to be a growing problem. The summary report of this data, *Canadians and Healthy Eating: How Are We Doing?* can be downloaded from the web site: www.hc-sc.gc.ca/nutrition.

The 2001 Annual Report from Statistics Canada reported that in 1998/99, more women (80%) than men (63%) reported they were concerned about maintaining or improving their health when choosing food[7]. Women were more likely than men to be concerned about weight, heart disease, osteoporosis, high blood pressure, cancer, and diabetes when they selected foods.

Nutrition monitoring was addressed in *Nutrition for Health: An Agenda for Action* by identifying 16 nutrition indicators[8]. The rationale for using these indicators was described by Davis in *A Report on the Use of Indicators in Canada's National Nutrition Plan*[9]. Nutrition professionals use these documents to advocate for better data collection for assessing nutritional status of the Canadian population. Such data will also help in evaluating the success of nutrition education and health promotion programs.

Canadian Readings and Resources

National Institute of Nutrition. Tracking nutrition trends 1989-1994-1997. Ottawa, 1999. www.nin.ca/consumer/backtnt.

Edwards P. *Building a Healthy Future* Insert in *Can J Public Health*, 1999. www.hc-sc.gc.ca/hppb/phdd/resources/Building_e.pdf

1.4 MAKING IT CLICK WITH KILOJOULES

Canadian students can calculate the energy from rice in kilojoules (as follows):

Calculate the energy in food *in kilojoules* from its energy-nutrient contents. A cup of fried rice contains 5 g protein, 30 g carbohydrate and 11 g fat.

a.   How many kilojoules does the rice provide from these energy nutrients?

    _____ = _____kJ protein

    _____ = _____kJ carbohydrate

    _____ = _____kJ fat

                     Total = _____kJ

b.   What percentage of the energy in the fried rice comes from each of the energy-yielding nutrients? (Make sure that the percentages of energy add up to 100% Sometimes they add to 99% or 101% due to rounding errors. This is acceptable.)

    _____ = _____% kilojoules from protein

    _____ = _____% kilojoules from carbohydrate

    _____ = _____% kilojoules from fat

                Total = _____%

c.   Calculate how many of the 615 kJ provided by a 12-ounce can of beer come from alcohol, if the beer contains 1 gram protein and 13 grams carbohydrate. (Hint: The remaining kJ derive from alcohol.)

    1 g protein   = _____ kJ protein
    13 g carbohydrate   = _____ kJ carbohydrate
                           = _____ kJ from alcohol

    How many grams of alcohol does this represent?   _____ g alcohol

MAKING IT CLICK WITH KILOJOULES - Answers

a. 5 g protein X 17 kJ/g   = 85 kJ protein

30 g carbohydrate x 17 kJ/g   = 510 kJ carbohydrate

11 g fat x 37 kJ/g   = 407 kJ fat

Total   = 1002 kJ

b. 85 kJ/1002 kJ   = 8.5%

510 kJ/1002 kJ   = 50.9%

407 kJ/1002 kJ   = 40.6%

Total   = 100.0%

c. 1 g protein   = 17 kJ protein

13 g carbohydrate   = 221 kJ carbohydrate

= 377 kJ from alcohol

How many grams of alcohol does this represent?   13 g alcohol

HIGHLIGHT 1: NUTRITION INFORMATION - EXPERTS AND QUACKS, ON THE NET AND IN THE NEWS

DIETITIANS' CREDENTIALS IN CANADA

The qualifications for admission to Dietitians of Canada (formerly The Canadian Dietetic Association) are similar to those for the American Dietetic Association. Dietitians of Canada (DC) accredits university undergraduate programs and dietetic internship programs which qualify dietitians to practise. There is no single designation of title or initials for Canadian dietitians. Provincial government legislation determines the professional designation for health professionals who practise in the province. A number of the provinces have established colleges or regulatory bodies under their health professions legislation to ensure that the public receives quality care from dietitians. The public can take any complaints about dietetic practice to the college or regulatory body. Dietitians are registered to practise through the college. All provinces include the word "dietitian" or "diététiste" in the title and protect those titles from use by unqualified individuals. The following list provides the designation for dietitians in each of the provinces.

Alberta	- R.D. (Registered Dietitian)
British Columbia	- R.D.N. (Registered Dietitian Nutritionist)
Manitoba	- R.D. (Registered Dietitian)
New Brunswick	- P.Dt. (Professional Dietitian)
Newfoundland	- R.Dt. (Registered Dietitian)
Nova Scotia	- P.Dt. (Professional Dietitian)
Ontario	- RD (Registered Dietitian)/Dt.P. (diététiste professionnelle)
Prince Edward Island	- P.Dt. (Professional Dietitian)
Québec	- dt.p. (diététiste professionnelle)
Saskatchewan	- P.Dt. (Professional Dietitian)

The address for Dietitians of Canada is listed with the Resources at the end of this Section. Current addresses for the dietetic regulatory bodies can be found at the Dietitians of Canada web site, www.dietitians.ca.

Canadian Reading

National Institute of Nutrition. Promoting Balanced Perceptions. *NIN RAPPORT* Vol. 15 No. 3(2000):1-5.

TEACHING CANADIAN INFORMATION: CHAPTER 2
PLANNING A HEALTHY DIET

2.1 CANADA'S FOOD GUIDE TO HEALTHY EATING

Canada's Food Guide to Healthy Eating is based on Canada's Guidelines for Healthy Eating and includes many of the recommendations of the Health and Welfare Communications/Implementation Committee[10]. The Guidelines help individuals achieve the Scientific Review Committee's Nutrition Recommendations for Canadians[11]. The food guide uses a total diet approach with a broader range of servings to accommodate individuals with higher nutritional needs. This guide recognizes the use of foods that don't fit into the four food groups within the "Other foods" category. Canada's Food Guide to Healthy Eating is presented on a two-sided tear sheet. This is found in Appendix I of the textbook. You will find the rainbow design handy for emphasizing the grain products and vegetables and fruit food groups. This is particularly useful for athletes with higher energy needs who should include good sources of complex carbohydrate. If you have plastic food models available, use them to teach the concept of serving size. The number of servings recommended from the food groups often appear very high until students realize that their portion size may be equal to two or three "Canada's Food Guide Servings"

The consumer booklet, *Using the Food Guide,* describes the rationale for the Food Guide and how to use the range of servings to meet individual needs. This is an important handout for most nutrition courses since the food guide is such an important educational tool and many people need more than just the tear sheet to understand how to use it.

Food Guide Facts: Background for Educators and Communicators includes fact sheets to help you interpret the information in the guide to your students. The information will help you to teach the concepts of the guide and explain reasons for the recommendations. If you expect that your students may teach the Food Guide after they complete their program, you should consider ordering copies of this publication to give to the students.

Canada's Food Guide for Healthy Eating Focus on Preschoolers: Background for Educators and Communicators was published in 1995 to provide advice for feeding children under four years. It puts a priority on supplying energy and nutrients for growth, with less attention to decreasing fat intake.

Canada's Food Guide for Healthy Eating Focus on Children Six to Twelve Years: Background for Educators and Communicators was published in 1997 to provide ideas and information for people who work with children six to twelve years old, such as teachers and youth workers.

Some of the publications can be downloaded as pdf files from www.hc-sc.gc.ca/nutrition. Your local or provincial public health department may have copies of these publications for distributing to students.

Activity

Your students can compare Canada's Food Guide to Healthy Eating to the Food Guide Pyramid in the textbook. You will note that the Canadian guide has a single group for vegetables and fruit, while the Pyramid has separate groups. Students can also compare their food intake for one day to the recommendations of Canada's Food Guide to Healthy Eating.

2.2 NUTRIENT ENRICHMENT IN CANADA

Nutrient enrichment of foods is mentioned in the section about whole and enriched grain products, on page 47 of the textbook. You should alert students now to the differences between Canadian and United States policies on the addition of nutrients to foods, before they calculate their food intakes or read food labels. You may want to refer to this information when teaching individual vitamins and minerals in Chapters 10, 11, 12 and 13 or with Chapter 19, Consumer Concerns about Foods and Water.

The Canadian *Food and Drug Regulations*[1] specify the foods to which nutrients may or must be added and the amounts which may be added. The policy requires or permits the addition of a nutrient to a food when there is need to:[2]

- correct a demonstrated nutrient deficiency in the population using an appropriate food;

- replace nutrients which are lost when the food is processed; and

- ensure the nutritional quality of products sold as substitutes for traditional foods, e.g. egg substitutes, or as sole sources of nourishment. Nutrient composition of the substitute should be comparable to the food being replaced. Sole sources of nourishment, e.g. meal replacements, infant formulas, or formulated liquid diets, must contain essential nutrients, including energy, in amounts related to the purpose of the food.

The difference in the enrichment legislation means that the nutrient composition of some foods sold in Canada is significantly different from similar foods sold in the United States. Thus nutrient values from food composition tables and computerized nutrient analysis programs based on United States data, such as Diet Analysis Plus, do not accurately reflect Canadian foods and nutrient intakes. Breakfast cereals are common examples of this variation. This is especially true for vitamins A and D and iron which can be higher in the United States cereal products. Vitamins A and D are not permitted to be added to cereals in Canada. Detailed information about foods to which nutrients can be added is found in Annex 2, Section VI in Guide to Food Labelling and Advertising[2]. One example of the difference in content is that unenriched bread, which is shown in Figure 2-6 Nutrients in Bread on page 48 of the textbook, would not be available in Canada, since enrichment of white bread is mandatory. *Nutrient Value of Some Common Foods* was revised and published by Health Canada in 1999. It is a quick reference for Canadian foods using the 1997 Canadian Nutrient Data File.

With the harmonization to facilitate free trade with United States, the Canadian regulations about addition of nutrients are being reviewed. When mandatory enrichment of specific foods with folic acid was implemented in the United States, Canadian regulations were adapted so that Canadian foods could have the same level of the nutrient. Check the Health Canada web site for discussion papers and decisions about addition of nutrients to foods.

Canadian instructors might note here that in Canada, enrichment of all fluid milk with vitamin D is mandatory, as is the addition of vitamin A to a fat-reduced milk. In 1997, Health Canada permitted the voluntary addition of calcium and vitamin D to cereal beverages. Students should check labels for the addition of these nutrients.

2.3 GOOD HEALTH EATING GUIDE

The Canadian Diabetes Association Good Health Eating Guide involves a Food Group System using the exchange concept[12]. The food groups and their nutrient content differ from the United States exchange system. Table 2.1 summarizes the energy nutrient content of the food groups. The complete exchange or choice lists for the Good Health Eating Guide are in Appendix I.

If you refer to the exchange lists when teaching about carbohydrates, lipids and proteins, please remind students about the differences for the Good Health Eating Guide. This is especially important for the carbohydrate content for milk, which uses a 1/2 cup (125 mL) serving instead of 1 cup (250 mL) and fruits and vegetables, which are in a single group instead of separate groups.

The current Good Health Eating Guide was published in 1994. The addition of the Sugars Group was an important new concept for this guide. Sugar in moderation can be included in the eating plan of people with diabetes. Moderation means providing up to 10% of total energy intake. One sugar choice contains about 10 g carbohydrate, 167 kJ (40 Calories).

     1 Sugar choice = 1 Fruits and Vegetables choice
     3 Sugar choices = 2 Starch choices

Table 2.1 Energy Nutrient Content of Food Groups in the Good Health Eating Guide[12]

Food Group Choice	Protein (g)	Fat (g)	Carbohydrate (g)	Energy kJ (kcal)
Starchy Foods	2	-	15	290 (68)
Fruits and Vegetables	1	-	10	190 (44)
Milk: whole	4	4	6	319 (76)
2%	4	2	6	244 (58)
1%	4	1	6	206 (49)
skim	4	-	6	170 (40)
Protein Foods	7	3	-	230 (55)
Fats and Oils	-	5	-	190 (44)
Extras	-	-	< 2.5	< 60 (14)

There is also a section in the guide called "Combined Food Choices" that includes foods that represent more than one food choice group, such as donuts, lasagna and minestrone soup, as well as nuts and legumes. For example 250 mL (1 cup) of cooked lentils or chick peas is equivalent 2 Starch choices and 1 Protein choice. For peanuts, 50 mL (¼ c) is equivalent to 1 Protein choice and 2 Fat choices.

Materials have been developed to present the new Good Health Eating Guide approach: the Canadian Diabetes Association *Pocket Food Guide*, the *Good Health Eating Guide Poster Pin-Up,* and the *Good Health Eating Guide Resource.* Copies of the resources can be purchased from the Canadian Diabetes Association at the address listed under Resource in the Canadian Information Section. These will be important to use if you teach the exchange system which is used in Canada. Some food labels with Nutrition Information include the symbols and food choice servings (Appendix I). This type of labelling is voluntary.

Activity

If your Canadian students are using the Good Health Eating Guide choice system for this course, they could practise using the system for diet planning as described on page 46. They could use the servings of the Good Health Eating Guide and Canada's

Food Guide to Healthy Eating choices for:

- Table 2-4, Diet Planning with the Exchange System using the Daily Food Guide Pattern and

- Table 2.5 A Sample Diet Plan and Menu.

2.4 CANADIAN FOOD LABELLING

Food labelling in Canada is regulated under the *Food and Drugs Act and Regulations.* The Canadian Food Inspection Agency enforces the food labelling regulations. The *Consumer Packaging and Labelling Act and Regulations* also apply to food packaging and labels. All current regulations for labelling requirements and making nutrition claims are described in The *Guide to Food Labelling and Advertising*[2], which can usually be accessed through the web site of Food Program of the Health Canada, www.hc-sc.gc.ca/food-aliment/. All label information required by the regulations must appear in both English and French.

Food labelling policy is undergoing a major review, specifically about nutrition labelling (nutrition information panel), nutrient content claims and health claims for food. In October 2000, the Minister of Health introduced the proposal for nutrition labelling policy. The policy development process and proposals are available through the web site of the Food Program of the Health Canada, www.hc-sc.gc.ca/food-aliment/.

The Canadian labelling system has not used Daily Values on food labels, as described in the textbook. However, the proposed policy does include % Daily Value[13]. Canadian instructors and students should check the latest nutrient labelling proposal on the web site to be ready to handle the new food labels.

Food Ingredients

Food ingredients are listed, using their common name, in descending order of proportion or percentage of the packaged product. For some foods, such as vegetable oils or spices, the class rather than the common name is permitted. If an ingredient is optional or can be substituted for another one in a product, the label must list all the ingredients that are likely to be used in the product within a one-year period. The label must indicate that all of these specific ingredients may not be present in each package of the food. This is often seen on cracker labels when the source of oil or fat varies with the market availability of oil products. At this time there is no requirement to identify food products resulting from genetic engineering unless there is a significant change in nutrient or chemical content or there is potential health or safety risk for a population, such as allergic potential[14]. However, there is considerable pressure on the government for mandatory labelling for genetically modified foods.

Biological Role of Nutrients

The Food and Drugs Act and Regulations specify the nutrients for which claims of the biological activity are permitted[2]. These are being reviewed along with other proposed health claims. Canadian instructors should check the web site for the Food Program for the latest proposal abut biological and health claims for food before presenting information to students on this topic.

Food Labelling and Advertising

Canadian regulations for food advertising are similar to those for food labelling and more restrictive than those in the United States. Since many Canadians have access to United States radio and television stations, it is often difficult to know the source of the commercial. Students enjoy learning about the Canadian regulations by comparing commercials from each country.

Canadian Readings

National Institute of Nutrition. Food Labelling. *NIN RAPPORT* Vol.15 No. 4(2000):1-8. www.nin.ca

Organization of Nutrition Education. Nutrition labelling in Canada. *ONE Bulletin* Vol. 20 No. 1(2000):1-9.

2.5 MAKING IT CLICK WITH A CANADIAN LABEL

1. Read a Canadian cereal label with a Nutrition Information panel and answer the following questions.
   a) What is the size of a serving of cereal?
   b) How many Calories (kcalories) and kilojoules are in a serving?
   c) How much fat is in a serving?
   d) How many kcalories does the fat represent?
   e) What percentage of the kcalories does this represent?
   f) What does this tell you?
   g) Does this cereal meet the criteria of a low-fat product? (See Nutrition Labelling in Canada.)
   h) How much fibre is in a serving?
   i) Identify what, if any, claim can be made about dietary fibre content of the cereal?
   j) What is the predominant ingredient in the cereal?
   k) What, if any, nutrients have been added to the cereal?

2.6 CANADIAN STUDY QUESTIONS

Replace or change the following items from the Study Questions in Chapter 2 of the textbook.

2. What recommendations appear in *Canada's Guidelines for Healthy Eating*? How do they compare with the *Nutrition Recommendations for Canadians* in Chapter 1?

3. Name the four food groups of *Canada's Food Guide to Healthy Eating* and identify several foods typical of each group and the "other foods" category. (Answer the other parts of question 3.)

4. Name the choice lists of *Canada's Good Health Eating Guide* and identify a food typical of each list. (Answer the other parts of question 4.)

5. Review *Canada's Guidelines for Healthy Eating*. What types of grocery selections would you make to achieve those recommendations?

Omit questions 6., 7., and 8.

HIGHLIGHT 2: COLLEGE BOUND AND HUNGRY

FOLLOWING THE RAINBOW

Canadian students can think about following the rainbow of Canada's Food Guide to Healthy Eating, rather than a pyramid. Planning eating can start from the outer arcs of the rainbow with grain products, followed by vegetables and fruit. As with the pyramid, fewer servings or less food comes from the smaller, inner parts of the rainbow. Meat and alternatives is the smallest group. Although "other foods", such as sugars and oils, are mentioned in the food guide, they are not part of the rainbow picture. So students can use the same foods that are discussed in the pyramid in Highlight 2 but use the rainbow concept instead.

TEACHING CANADIAN INFORMATION: CHAPTER 4
THE CARBOHYDRATES: SUGARS, STARCHES AND FIBRES

4.1 CANADIAN RECOMMENDATIONS FOR CARBOHYDRATE AND DIETARY FIBRE

The *Nutrition Recommendations for Canadians* state that "the Canadian diet should provide 55% of energy as carbohydrate (138 g/1000 kcal or 165 g/5000 kJ) from a variety of sources"[11]. They recommend including sources of carbohydrate which provide complex carbohydrates and a variety of dietary fibre. There is no numerical recommendation for dietary fibre or sugar. However, the recommendations assume that the increase in carbohydrate intake will lead to the desired increase in dietary fibre intake. It is recommended that any increase in dietary fibre be a gradual one. Canada's Guidelines for Healthy Eating[10] encourage an increased dietary fibre intake by promoting the intake of cereals, breads, other grain products, vegetables and fruits. The guidelines for claims on dietary fibre content are based on the Report of the Expert Committee on Dietary Fibre[15]. The proposed nutrition labelling policy sets the Reference Daily Intake for carbohydrate as 300 mg and fibre as 25 mg[13].

4.2 HOW TO USE THE GOOD HEALTH EATING GUIDE TO ESTIMATE CARBOHYDRATE

The food groups for the Good Health Eating Guide[12] are different from the Exchange lists. (See Appendix I.) Table 4.1 shows the carbohydrate content for each of the food groups.

Table 4.1 Carbohydrate Content of One Food Choice

One Food Choice[a]	Carbohydrate (g)
Starchy Foods	15
Fruits & Vegetables	10
Milk	6
Protein Foods	-
Fats & Oils	-
Extras	<2.5
Sugars	5

Students who are required to learn the Good Health Eating Guide food choice system could estimate the carbohydrate content of the breakfast in the How To section on page 118 of the textbook, using the Canadian system. Table 4.2 shows the estimates using the Good Health Eating Guide.

Table 4.2 How to Use the Good Health Eating Guide to Estimate Carbohydrate in Breakfast

Breakfast	Food Group Choices[a]	Carbohydrate (g)	
		Estimate	Actual
1 cup shredded wheat	2 Starch	30	34
1 c milk	2 Milk	12	12
½ banana	1 Fruits & Vegetables	10	13
		52	59

[a] Based on Food Group Choices from Canadian Diabetes Association Good Health Eating Guide Resource[12].

4.3 MAKING IT CLICK

Canadian students will benefit from completing the *Making it Click* exercise in this chapter. The calculations are similar to the Canadian proposed labelling which will provide the % Daily Value for carbohydrate[13].

TEACHING CANADIAN INFORMATION: CHAPTER 5
THE LIPIDS: TRIGLYCERIDES, PHOSPHOLIPIDS, AND STEROLS

5.1 CANADIAN RECOMMENDATIONS ABOUT FATS

The *Nutrition Recommendations for Canadians* state that "The Canadian diet should include no more than 30% energy as fat" and "no more than 10% as saturated fat"[11] They also recommend that n-6 fatty acids be at least 3% of energy and n-3 fatty acids at least 0.5% of energy with a ratio of n-6 to n-3 fatty acids in the range of 4:1 to 10:1. Although no numeric recommendation was made for cholesterol in the Nutrition Recommendations for Canadians, the proposed Canadian labelling policy uses 300 mg as the Daily Reference Intake[13].

The Joint Working Group of the Canadian Paediatric Society and Health Canada published their report *Nutrition Recommendations Update... Dietary Fat and Children*[16] in 1993. Considering whether the fat intake of growing children should be restricted, the Working Group concluded the following[16] .

1. Providing adequate energy and nutrients to ensure adequate growth and development remains the most important consideration in the nutrition of children. Small frequent feedings play a significant role in providing energy in the diets of children.

2. During the preschool years nutritious food choices should not be eliminated or restricted because of fat content. During early adolescence an energy intake adequate to sustain growth should be emphasized with a gradual lowering of fat intake. Once linear growth has stopped, fat intake as

currently recommended is appropriate.

3. Food patterns which emphasize variety, complex carbohydrate and include lower fat choices are appropriate and desirable for children.

4. Physical activity and healthy eating are important lifestyle habits for children.

The following recommendations were made[16].

From the age of two until the end of linear growth, there should be a transition from the high fat diet of infancy to a diet which includes no more than 30% energy as fat and no more than 10% of energy as saturated fat.

During this transition, energy intake should be sufficient to achieve normal growth and development. Food patterns should emphasize variety and complex carbohydrate, and include lower fat foods. Physical activity should be stressed.

You may introduce this report during this chapter or with Chapter 16, Life Cycle Nutrition: Infancy, Childhood, and Adolescence.

5.2 CANADIAN LIPID PROFILE FOR ASSESSING CARDIOVASCULAR DISEASE RISK

The Canadian Medical Association published Recommendations for the Management and Treatment of Dyslipidemia[17]. These recommendations do not provide single profile values for the blood lipid components similar to those shown in the margin on page 148 of the textbook. Instead, the target values for the lipid components are listed according to the level of risk based on the patient's history. A person's risk for cardiovascular disease is assessed using more than the blood lipid profile.

Canadian Reading

McDonald BE. Dietary Fat and Cholesterol Lessons Learned from the Past Decade. *National Institute of Nutrition Review.* No. 30, 2000 (www.nin.ca)

5.3 HOW TO USE THE GOOD HEALTH EATING GUIDE TO ESTIMATE FAT

Students can estimate the fat content of the meal on page 154 of the textbook, using the Good Health Eating Guide. Some of the foods might be considered Starch choices but because of fat content are listed under "Combined Food Choices" (Appendix I). For example, a small bran muffin (45 g) is one Starch choice, one Sugar choice, and one Fat choice. Higher fat choices from Protein Food are listed at the end of the Protein foods section, e.g. cheese and peanut butter. For example, one piece of regular cheese (25 g) is one Protein choice and one Fat choice. The fat content of the Canadian Food Choice Groups is listed in Table 5.1. The estimate for fat intake for the foods *in How to Use the Exchange System to Estimate Fat* in the textbook has been calculated using the Good Health Eating Guide in Table 5.2.

Table 5.1 Fat Content of One Food Choice

One Food Choice[a]	Fat (g)
Starchy Foods	-
Fruits & Vegetables	-
Milk	
Whole	4
2%	2
1%	1
Skim	-
Protein Foods	3
Fats & Oils	5
Extras	-

Table 5.2 How to Use the Good Health Eating Guide to Estimate Fat in Dinner

Dinner	Food Group Choices[a]	Fat (g)	
		Estimate	Actual
Salad:			
1 c raw spinach leaves, shredded carrots, and sliced mushrooms	1 Fruits & Vegetables	0	0
½ c garbanzo beans	1 Starch + ½ Protein	1.5	2
1 tbsp sunflower seeds	½ Fat	2.5	4
2 tsp ranch salad dressing	1 Fat	5	3
Entree:			
Spaghetti with meat sauce			
1 c pasta (cooked)	2 Starch	0	1
1 c tomato sauce	3 Fruits & Vegetables	0	1
90 g lean ground beef	3 Protein	9	12
½ c green beans	1 Extras	0	0
1 medium corn on the cob	2 Starch	0	0
2 tsp butter	2 Fat	10	8
Dessert:			
1/12 angel food cake	½ Starch + 2½ Sugar	0	0
Beverage:			
1 c 1% low-fat milk	2 Milk (1%)	2	3
		30.0	34

[a] Based on Food Group Choices from Canadian Diabetes Association Good Health Eating Guide Resource[12].

5.4 HOW TO CALCULATE A PERSONAL DAILY VALUE FOR FAT

Canadian students would benefit from doing the exercise in this *How To* section, even though the Daily Value concept is different from the Canadian labelling system. Many people have difficulty translating the recommendation of no more than 30% energy from fat into amount of fat per day. The calculation in this section will help to clarify this.

HIGHLIGHT 5: ALTERNATIVES TO FATS

Simplesse has been approved for use in Canada. At the time of writing this section, Olestra has not been approved for use in Canada. Look on the labels of low-fat and fat-free products to see if a fat alternative has been used. Starch derivatives are often used to improve the texture of the lower fat products.

TEACHING CANADIAN INFORMATION: CHAPTER 6
PROTEIN: AMINO ACIDS

6.1 CANADIAN RECOMMENDED INTAKES OF PROTEIN

The *Nutrition Recommendations*[11] address the issue of protein recommendations beyond the level of preventing protein deficiency. The recommended safe and adequate level of protein intake for adults is 0.86 g/kg BW. Thich is lower than the RDA. It is more accurate to estimate protein RNI using the RNI based on g/kg BW than to use RNI for the average person in your age and sex group from the tables in Appendix I. This is the intake level which minimizes the risk of a deficiency.

The recommendations recognize that the current average protein intake in Canada is considerably higher. Because there is no evidence that this higher intake has damaging effects on healthy individuals, the committee emphasized maintaining current patterns of protein intake rather than making drastic changes to the lower safe intake. The recommended proportion of protein is 13-15% of energy throughout adulthood, with an increase for female seniors to 15-20% of energy.

6.2 HOW TO CALCULATE THE RECOMMENDED PROTEIN INTAKES

The protein RNI for adolescents and adults are:
  0.98 g/kg for males 12-19 yr.,
  0.95 g/kg for females 12-19 yr., and
  0.86 g/kg for adults over 19 yr.

For students to determine their protein RNI they should follow the first step in the

How to Calculate Recommended Protein Intakes in Chapter 6 of the textbook to find the appropriate weight in kilograms. Then students should multiply their weight in kilograms by 0.86 (or the appropriate number, if they are under 20 years).
For example:

Weight　　　　　　　= 68 kg

68 kg x 0.86 g/kg　　= 58 g protein (rounded off)

Printouts from *Diet Analysis Plus 4.0, Canadian Version* use the Canadian RNIs.

6.3 HOW TO USE THE GOOD HEALTH EATING GUIDE TO ESTIMATE PROTEIN

Since the protein content of the food groups in the Good Health Eating Guide is different from the United States Exchange Lists, you could have students complete the estimate using the Canadian food choices (Appendix I). Note the slight differences in protein content of the food groups between the U.S. and the Canadian Systems. Also remember that the size of a Milk choice is ½ cup of milk. Table 6.2 shows the lunch example from *How To Use the Exchange System to Estimate Protein* in Chapter 6 of the textbook, using the Good Health Eating Guide.

Table 6.1 Protein Content of One Food Choice

One Food Choice[a]	Protein (g)
Starchy Foods	2
Fruits & Vegetables	0
Milk	4
Protein Foods	7
Fats & Oils	-
Extras	-

Table 6. 2 How to Use the Good Health Eating Guide to Estimate Protein in Lunch

Lunch	Food Group Choices[a]	Protein (g)	
		Estimate	Actual
1 c pinto beans	1 Protein + 2 Starches	11	14
25 g cheese	1 Protein + 1 Fat	7	7
1 tortilla	1 Starch	2	2
1 c milk	2 Milk	8	8
1 apple	1 Fruits & Vegetables	-	1
		28	32

[a] Based on Food Group Choices from Canadian Diabetes Association Good Health Eating Guide Resource[12].

Please note the different serving sizes and choices for pinto beans and cheese compared to those with the US Exchange System.

6.5 MAKING IT CLICK

When completing the *Making it Click* section of this chapter of the textbook, Canadian students should use the Canadian RNI for protein as given above in *6.2 How To Calculate the Recommended Protein Intakes*.

A woman 5 ft. 8 in. tall is 68 in tall. From the table on the inside back cover, the midpoint in the blue area for this woman is 67 kg.

   0.86 g/kg x 67 kg   = 58 g protein per day

Calculations for 1. are:

a. A woman 5 feet 1 inch tall:

Weight: 54 kg

Recommended Intake   0.86 g/kg x 54 kg =   46 g protein per day

b. a. A man (18 years) 6 feet 4 inches tall:

Weight: 122 kg

Recommended Intake   0.98 g/kg x 122 kg = 120 g protein per day

HIGHLIGHT 7: ALCOHOL AND NUTRITION

The *Nutrition Recommendations for Canadians* state that "The Canadian diet should include no more than 5% of total energy as alcohol, or two drinks daily, whichever is less"[11]. This recommendation was not to encourage alcohol consumption. This indicates the need to limit alcohol intake. The rationale for the recommendation is described on pp. 181-2 of Nutrition Recommendations[11]. It is especially important to discuss limiting alcohol intake in relation to pregnancy and fetal alcohol syndrome. Please see Chapter 15 in this Canadian Information Section about Canada's recommendations on preventing fetal alcohol syndrome.

TEACHING CANADIAN INFORMATION: CHAPTER 8
ENERGY BALANCE AND BODY COMPOSITION

8.1 ENERGY IN - ENERGY OUT IN KILOJOULES

This chapter focuses on energy units involved with energy balance, using kcalories both as a unit and the term for energy. Since both kilocalories and kilojoules are used in Canada, you may choose the most appropriate terms for teaching energy concepts. If the students are likely to be involved in health care, e.g. dietetics, nursing, etc., it is appropriate to use kilojoules in calculations and the term "energy" to replace kcalories. Try calculating the energy value of the food described on page 242 of the textbook:

12 g carbohydrate @17 kJ/g	= 204 kJ
5 g fat @37 kJ/g	= 185 kJ
8 g protein@17 kJ/g	= 136 kJ

Total	= 525 kJ

Canadian students might practise thinking in kilojoules by estimating their BMR and exercise energy output in kilojoules.

8.2 BODY WEIGHT, BODY COMPOSITION AND HEALTH

The Body Mass Index (BMI) was adopted by Health Canada for assessing health risk from body composition to replace the concept of a single ideal weight[18]. The interpretation of the BMI in Canada is different from that described in Chapter 8 of the textbook.

Table 8.1 Canadian Interpretation of Body Mass Index (BMI) for Evaluation of Weight[a]

Under 20   A BMI under 20 may be associated with health problems for some
              individuals. It may be a good idea to consult a dietitian and physician,
              especially if there has been a sudden decline in BMI.

20 - 25   This zone is associated with lowest risk of illness for most people. This
              is a "generally acceptable range" of weight for health.

25 - 27   A BMI over 25 may be associated with health problems for some
              people. Caution is suggested if your BMI is in this zone. This is a
              "generally acceptable range" of weight for health.

Over 27   A BMI over 27 is associated with increased risk of health problems such
              as heart disease, high blood pressure and diabetes. It maybe a good
              idea to consult a dietitian and physician for advice.

[a] The Canadian Dietetic Association. *Healthy Eating Is... A Resource Manual for Health Professionals.*
Toronto: The Canadian Dietetic Association, 1988, p.20.

The Expert Committee on Weight Standards recommended that health professionals
also use Waist-Hip Ratio as an indicator of fat distribution when assessing health risk
with BMI[19]. Men with a waist-to-hip ratio greater than 1.0 and women with a waist-to-
hip ratio greater than 0.8 are at increased risk to health. The committee also noted
that the BMI is not appropriate to use for pregnant women, children and trained
athletes, and may have limitations for adolescents and adults over 65 years. Issues
related to body weight and prevention of weight problems are also addressed in
Promoting Healthy Weights: A Discussion Paper[19]. Some provincial health ministries
have published pamphlets which can be used as handouts for the topic of healthy
weights.

The Health Promotion and Programs Branch, Health Canada introduced the Vitality
program in 1991[20]. This program has three components: enjoyable, healthy eating;
enjoyable, physical activity; and positive self and body image. This program involves
providing information and promoting activities which support the three components.

TEACHING CANADIAN INFORMATION: CHAPTER 9
WEIGHT CONTROL: OVERWEIGHT AND UNDERWEIGHT

9.1 OVERWEIGHT IN CANADA

The 1994 National Population Health Survey found that 35.2% of men and 25.8% of women were obese (BMI>27)[6]. Overweight and obesity are also increasing among children (7 to 13 years)[21]. The direct cost of obesity in Canada for 1997 was reported to be $1.8 billion[22]. Thus, prevention and treatment of overweight and obesity are priorities in Canada. The suggested readings below present the recommendations of the Canadian Medical Association.

Canadian Readings

Douketis JD, Feightner JW, Attia J et al. Periodic health examination, 1999 update: 1. Detection, prevention and treatment of obesity. *Can Med Assoc J* 160(1999):513-525.

Leiter LA, Abbott D, Campbell NRC et al. 2. Recommendations on obesity and weight loss. *Can Med Assoc J* 160(9 Suppl)(1999) :S7-S12.

9.2 PHYSICAL ACTIVITY GUIDE TO HEALTHY ACTIVE LIVING

Health Canada and Canadian Society for Exercise Physiology published *Canada's Physical Activity Guide to Healthy Active Living* and *Canada's Physical Activity Guide to Healthy Active Living* for Older Adults. For each of these, there is a single tear sheet of the guide and a handbook to describe how to use the guide. The regular Physical Activity Guide is in Appendix I of this textbook. Copies of the guide and handbook can be printed from a pdf file or ordered on the internet from: www.paguide.com or by phone toll free from 1-888-334-9769. This guide provides a healthy approach for balancing physical activity with healthy eating. The graphics on the physical activity guide are consistent with those on Canada's Food Guide to Healthy Eating.

HIGHLIGHT 9: EATING DISORDERS

The National Eating Disorder Information Centre provides information about eating disorders and treatment in Canada. See the Resource Groups at the end of this section for its address and phone number.

<u>Canadian Resource</u>

Promoting Healthy Body Image from the Best Start Program (Ontario) - www.opc.on.ca/beststart/bodyimg

TEACHING CANADIAN INFORMATION: CHAPTER 10
THE WATER-SOLUBLE VITAMINS: B VITAMINS AND VITAMIN C

10.1 VITAMINS IN CANADIAN FOODS

The major differences in the vitamin content of foods sold in Canada are due to the differences in the regulations for nutrient enrichment. These were discussed in 2.2 Nutrient Enrichment in Canada of this section. A review of this topic may be appropriate with this chapter to help students connect the specific vitamins with foods. If the students are completing the self-study for the water-soluble vitamins, provide information or resources to assist them in finding the accurate Canadian values, e.g. Nutrient Value of Some Common Foods[24] or Nutrition Information on the food label. Watch the Health Canada web site (www.hc-sc.gc.ca) for changes to the nutrient enrichment regulations .

You should note that folic acid fortification in Canada is similar to that in the United States.

HIGHLIGHT 10: VITAMIN AND MINERAL SUPPLEMENTS

CANADIAN REGULATION OF SUPPLEMENTS

Vitamin and mineral supplements are regulated in Canada under Part D of *The Food and Drugs Act and Regulations*[1]. The regulations set minimum and maximum levels for vitamins in supplements. Some, such as vitamin K, can be sold only on prescription. Advertising of supplements is also controlled, preventing advertising which recommends high doses. The regulations affecting health claims for supplements are currently being reviewed because of the desires of manufacturers and consumers for identifying foods and nutrients which prevent or treat disease, often called nutriceuticals or functional foods. Check the Health Canada web site (www.hc-sc.gc.ca) before teaching this topic for information about the latest policies on health claims and natural health products.

If you are teaching Canadian students who live near the United States border, an interesting activity would be to compare the cost and the content of vitamin and mineral supplements from each country.

TEACHING CANADIAN INFORMATION: CHAPTER 11
THE FAT-SOLUBLE VITAMINS: A, D, E, AND K

11.1 FAT-SOLUBLE VITAMINS IN CANADIAN FOODS

The Canadian policy on enrichment differs from that of the United States for vitamins A and D. In Canada, neither vitamin A nor vitamin D can be added to cereals. One product sold in Canada on the same shelf as cereals does contain added vitamin A. However that product is called a "meal replacement" rather than a "cereal". It is mandatory for vitamin D to be added to all cow's milk which is sold as fluid milk, and vitamin A to be added to cow's milk which has had fat removed. Vitamins A and D must also be added to margarine.

Canadian regulations now allow fortification of soy beverages with calcium, vitamin D and vitamin B_{12}. Remind students who are using soy, rice or other cereal-based beverage as an alternative to milk to check to see if the product is fortified.

HIGHLIGHT 11: ANTIOXIDANT NUTRIENTS AND PHYTOCHEMICALS IN DISEASE PREVENTION

The Canadian Food and Drugs Act and Regulations[1] do not permit health claims for antioxidants in foods. Special regulations allowing disease prevention claims for functional foods or nutriceuticals have not yet been introduced. This topic is generating discussion among regulators and food manufacturers in Canada.

The 2001 Canadian campaign to promote consumption of fruits and vegetables is called "5 to 10 a Day".

TEACHING CANADIAN INFORMATION: CHAPTER 12
WATER AND THE MAJOR MINERALS

12.1 SODIUM CONTENT OF CANADIAN PACKAGED FOOD

The proposed Canada nutrition labelling policy includes sodium on the core list, which means that sodium content must be declared on the label[13]. The Reference Daily Intake proposed for the label is 2400 mg.

12.2 CALCIUM

Canadian students should note that the regulations allowing addition of calcium to foods and beverages (fortification) differ from those in the United States. In 1997, regulations were changed to allow voluntary fortification of cereal beverages, such as soy and rice, with calcium and vitamin D.

Some milk products contain added milk solids, increasing the amount of calcium in milk by up to 33%. Some fruit products have added milk solids or added calcium. Read the labels of these products carefully to compare calcium content and cost.

TEACHING CANADIAN INFORMATION: CHAPTER 13
THE TRACE MINERALS

13.1 IRON ENRICHMENT

If Canadian students are completing a nutrient analysis of their food intake, they should check the iron content of breakfast cereals. The iron content on the package label, as % RDI, may be lower than the value in the food composition tables in Appendix H of the textbook or the computer printout using *Diet Analysis Plus 4.0, Canadian Version.*

HIGHLIGHT 13: FUNCTIONAL FOODS ARE THEY REALLY DIFFERENT?

The regulations for functional foods in Canada are still in the developmental stages. Depending on the product and the health claim, these products may fall under the category of foods or natural health products. Watch the Health Canada web site (www.hc-sc.gc.ca) for announcements about these policies. Industry and scientists are forming liaisons to take advantage of development and marketing functional foods. The multi-disciplinary Canadian Functional Foods Network has the mission to improve human health through the development of a science-based, profitable functional foods and nutraceutical sector in Canada. The network can be contacted by email at cffn@ualberta.ca.

Canadian Resources and Readings

National Institute of Nutrition. *Consumer Awareness of and Attitudes Toward Functional Foods.* Ottawa: NIN, 2000.

National Institute of Nutrition. Functional Foods. *NIN RAPPORT* 15 No. 2(2000): 1-6.

TEACHING CANADIAN INFORMATION: CHAPTER 14
FITNESS: PHYSICAL ACTIVITY, NUTRIENTS, AND
BODY ADAPTATIONS

14.1 PHYSICAL ACTIVITY GUIDE TO HEALTHY ACTIVE LIVING

Health Canada recently launched the *Physical Activity Guide to Healthy Active Living* to encourage Canadians to be more active. A copy of this publication is in Appendix I of the textbook and would support the teaching of this section of the nutrition course, providing current Canadian Guidelines. The *Handbook for Physical Activity Guide to Healthy Active Living* provides more informationto support this publication and is available from the Physical Activity Guide web site at www.paguide.com.

14.2 CANADIAN STUDIES

The Canadian Fitness and Lifestyle Research Institute (CFLRI), Fitness/Active Living Unit of Health Canada, and the Interprovincial Sport and Research Council manages the Physical Activity Benchmarks program to monitor the physical activity of Canadians and assess the impact of programs aimed at reducing population levels of physical inactivity. The 1999 Physical Activity Monitor is being published by sections and are available on the CFLRI web site at www.cflri.ca/cflri/resources/pub.phb. The survey is completed through computer-assisted telephone interviews. The 1997 Physical Activity Monitor identified that the percentage of Canadians who reported being active increased from 21% in 1981 to 37% in 1995, with most of the increase occurring between 1981 and 1988. One in ten Canadians are considered truly sedentary[24]. Older Canadians are becoming less active. For details on the physical activity of Canadians, barriers to physical activity and benefits of physical activity, visit the CFLRI web site (www.cflri.ca/cflri/resources/pub.phb).

TEACHING CANADIAN INFORMATION: CHAPTER 15
LIFE CYCLE NUTRITION: PREGNANCY AND LACTATION

15.1 CANADIAN PRENATAL GUIDELINES

The Canadian recommendations for preconceptional and prenatal nutrition care are found in *Nutrition for a Healthy Pregnancy: National Guidelines for the Childbearing Years*, published by Health Canada[25]. The guidelines have been endorsed by Dietitians of Canada, The Society of Obstetricians and Gynaecologists of Canada, and members of the Federal/Provincial/Territorial Group on Nutrition. The guidelines recommend the following gestational weight gain, based on pre-pregnancy body mass index:

Table 15.1 Canadian Recommendations for Gestational Weight Gain[a]

BMI Category (Pre-Pregnancy)	Recommended Total Gestational Gain	
	kg	lb.
<20	12.5 - 18.0	28 - 40
20 - 25	11.5 - 16.0	25 - 35
>27	7.0 - 11.5	15 - 25

[a] Health Canada. *Nutrition for a Healthy Pregnancy: National Guidelines for the Childbearing Years.* Ottawa: Minister of Public Works and Government Services, 1999. www.hc-sc.gc.ca/nutrition.

The national guidelines discuss problem nutrients, suggested food patterns, and recommendations for problems such as gestational diabetes mellitus, pre-eclampsia, morning sickness, and constipation. The guidelines were summarized and discussed in the NIN Rapport Vol. 13, No. 1, Winter 1999. The Executive Summary or the full guidelines document should be standard reading for Canadian students so they can appreciate the food and nutrition issues and the Canadian recommendations for pregnancy.

15.2 CANADIAN PRENATAL PROGRAMS

Although Canada does not have a single nutrition program for pregnant women, supportive nutrition programs are available to them. One noted early program was established at the Montreal Diet Dispensary by Agnes Higgins[26]. Mendelson et al. described the results of the evaluation of the Healthiest Babies Possible program that was established in Toronto[27].

The Canadian Prenatal Nutrition Program (CPNP), announced by Health Canada in 1994, provides food supplementation, nutrition counselling, support, education, referral, and counselling on lifestyle issues for women who are most likely to have unhealthy babies[28]. The program supports community-based services by funding local community groups to establish and deliver services according to the local population needs and build on existing prenatal programs. The women targeted by this program include: pregnant adolescents, youth at risk of becoming pregnant, pregnant women who abuse alcohol or other substances, pregnant women living in violent situation, off-reserve aboriginals and Inuits, refugees, and pregnant women living in isolation or not having access to services. The CPNP is jointly managed by the Federal government, and Provincial/Territorial governments. In September 2000, there were 277 CPNP projects in more than 680 communities across Canada[29]. Students can get more information about the CPNP and its participants by going to the CPNP web site: www.hc-sc.gc.ca/hppb/childhood-youth/cbp/cpnp/

Many public health departments offer prenatal and postnatal education programs to interested members of the community. To find out about programs for pregnant women at nutritional risk in your locality, contact your local or provincial public health department.

15.3 CANADIAN RECOMMENDATIONS FOR LACTATION

Breastfeeding is discussed on pages 45 to 50 in the *Nutrition for a Healthy Pregnancy: National Guidelines for the Childbearing Years*[26]. Canada's Food Guide to Healthy Eating has sufficient range of recommended servings to cover lactating women. However, there is some concern about the nutritional adequacy of the food intake of women who are breastfeeding. One of the few studies about food intake by lactating women in low-income communities is provided by Doran and Evers[30].

Health Canada supports and promotes breastfeeding. However, many public health professionals are concerned about the promotion of infant formulas in Canada and its effect on breatfeeding rate and duration. Health Canada completed a study of the attitudes of mothers and their partners towards breastfeeding to help in planning programs to promote exclusive breastfeeding for infants for their first 4 to 6 months[31].

The Breastfeeding Committee of Canada, made up of representatives of Dietitians of Canada and other groups interested in breastfeeding, published a breast feeding statement to identify issues and make recommendations[32]. This breast feeding statement is an appropriate additional reading for Canadian students. Many health professionals support the concept of Baby-Friendly Hospital initiative to encourage breastfeeding. However few Canadian hospitals have achieved that designation.

Canadian Readings and Resources

Martens PJ, Phillips SJ, Cheang MS, Rosolowich V. How baby-friendly are Manitoba hospitals? The provincial infant feeding study. *Can. J. Public Health 91(2000):51-57.*

Maclean H. Breastfeeding in Canada: A demographic and experiential perspective. *J Can Diet Assoc* 59(1998):15-23.

Bourgoin GL, Lahaie NR, Rheume BA et al. Factors influencing the duration of breastfeeding in the Sudbury Region. *Can J Public Health* 88(1997):238-241.

Visit INFACT Canada on the internet at www.io.org/~infacto/internet.htm.

HIGHLIGHT 15: FETAL ALCOHOL SYNDROME

In 1996, Health Canada and the Canadian Paediatric Society released a joint statement on Fetal Alcohol Syndrome and Fetal Alcohol Effects[34]. The basis of the recommendations is that "the prudent choice for women who are or may become pregnant is to abstain from alcohol". It also recommends that health professionals inform pregnant women who have consumed small amounts of alcohol occasionally that the risk is minimal. They should also tell them that both mother and fetus will benefit if the mother stops drinking alcohol at any time during the pregnancy. This statement is available through the Health Canada Nutrition web site (www/hc-sc.gc.ca/nutrition) and is consistent with the 1999 *Nutrition for a Healthy Pregnancy: National Guidelines for the Childbearing Years*[26].

TEACHING CANADIAN INFORMATION: CHAPTER 16
LIFE CYCLE NUTRITION: INFANCY, CHILDHOOD, AND ADOLESCENCE

16.1 NUTRITION FOR HEALTHY TERM INFANTS

The current guidelines for infant feeding were prepared and approved by the Canadian Paediatric Society, Dietitians of Canada and Health Canada and are called *Nutrition for Healthy Term Infants*[34]. The Executive Summary and complete report can be downloaded from the Health Canada web site (www.hc-sc.gc.ca). The Executive Summary provides an excellent overview of issues involved with infant feeding and is useful as a framework for teaching this topic.

16.2 INFANT FORMULAS IN CANADA

The nutrient composition of infant formulas in Canada is regulated by the Food and Drugs Act and Regulations[1] and varies slightly from those in the United States. Both Canadian and United States consumers who live close to the border may buy infant formula in the nearby country. Health professionals should advise parents who are buying infant formulas in the other country to look at the labels carefully, especially for iron content, which may be labelled differently. If you have questions about this, contact local sales representative from infant formula companies.

16.3 IRON STATUS OF CANADIAN INFANTS

Iron status of infants continues to be a concern for infants, especially in low income communities and aboriginal and Inuit populations[35].

Canadian Readings and Resources for Infant Feeding

Canadian Egg Marketing Association. Child nutrition: A question of Balance *Nutrition in Your Practice* 11(2001):1-2. www.canadaegg.ca/english/nutrit/nutrit_prof_index.html

Yeung GS, Zlotkin SH. Efficacy of meat and iron-fortified commercial cereal to prevent iron depletion in cow milk-fed infants 6 to 12 months of age: A randomized controlled trial. *Can J Public Health 91(2000):263-267.*

Potter B, Sheeshka J, Valaitis R. Canadian analysis of infant feeding messages in a Canadian Women's Magazine, 1945 to 1995. *J Nutr Ed 32(2000):196-203.*

Williams PL, Innis SM, Vogel AMP, Stephen LJ. Factors influencing infant feeding practices of mothers in Vancouver. *Can J Public Health* 90(1999):114-119.

Hyewon LH, Wilkie J, Wade K, et al. Infant feeding practices in North York: Compliance with CPS guidelines. *J Can Diet Assoc.* 59(1998):24-29.

McKim E, Laryea M, Banoub-Baddour S. Infant feeding practices in coastal Labrador. *J Can Diet Assoc.* 59(1998):35-42.

Schwartz C, Evers S. Infant feeding practices in low-income communities in Ontario. *J Can Diet Assoc.* 59(1998):30-34.

Innis S, Nelson CM, Wadsworth LD, McLaren IA, Lwanga D. Incidence of iron-deficiency anaemia and depleted iron stores among nine-month-old Infants in Vancouver, Canada. *Can J Public Health* 88(1997):80-88.

Local public health offices often provide pamphlets and brochures on infant feeding which might be appropriate for class handouts.

The following preschooler food guide has been put on a single page so that you can copy it for a student handout, if you don't order copies for your class.

16.4 CANADA'S FOOD GUIDE FOR PRESCHOOLERS

In 1995, Health Canada published *Canada's Food Guide for Healthy Eating Focus on Preschoolers Background for Educators and Communicators*. This publication is available from your provincial or local health department. This resource promotes how to use Canada's Food Guide for Healthy Eating to help preschoolers learn to enjoy healthy eating. It offers suggestions to parents and caregivers about how to handle the feeding environment and how much to expect young children to eat. Table 16.1 summarizes the preschool recommendations for the size and number of servings from the food groups of Canada's Food Guide to Healthy Eating. You should note the recommendation for at least 2 cups of milk per day to ensure sufficient vitamin D.

Table 16.1 Canadian Preschool Food Guide to Healthy Eating[a]

Food Group	Number of Child-size Servings	Examples of One Child-size Serving
Grain Products	5-12	1/2-1 slice of bread 15-30 g cold cereal 75-175 mL (⅓-¾ cup) hot cereal ¼-½ bagel, pita or bun 50-125 mL (¼-½ cup) pasta or rice
Vegetables and Fruit	5-10	½-1 medium-size vegetable or fruit 50-125 mL (¼-½ cup) fresh, frozen or canned vegetables or fruit 125-250 mL (½-1 cup) salad 50-125 mL (¼-½ cup) juice
Milk Products	Preschoolers should consume 500 mL (2 cups) of milk every day (for vitamin D). They may also choose a child-size serving of other Milk Products, such as cheese or yogurt.	25-50 g cheese 75-175 mL (⅓-¾ cup) yogurt
Meat and Alternatives	2-3	25-50 g meat, fish or poultry 50-125 mL (¼-½ cup) beans 50-100 g (¼-⅓ cup) tofu 15-30 mL (1-2 Tbsp) peanut butter

[a] Health Canada. *Canada's Food Guide for Healthy Eating Focus on Preschoolers*. Ottawa: Minister of Supply and Services, 1995.

16.5 FOCUS ON CHILDREN SIX TO TWELVE YEARS

Canada's Food Guide for Healthy Eating Focus on Children Six to Twelve Years Background for Educators and Communicators gives background on issues for school-age children, recommendations for healthy eating for children and activities and resources for promoting healthy eating among children. This is an excellent handout for students who expect to be involved with feeding or educating children, such as teachers.

16.6 OBESITY AND CANADIAN CHILDREN

A review of the secular changes in body mass index of children has identified that Canadian children, aged 7 to 13 years, are becoming pregressively overweight and obese[21]. From 1981 to 1996, BMI increased at a rate of nearly 0.1 kg/m^2 per year for both sexes at most ages. Prevalence of overweight (>85th age- and sex-specific percentile) increased in boys from 15% in 1981 to 28.8% in 1996; in girls from 15% to 23.6%. During the same period, prevalence of obesity (>95th age- and sex-specific percentile) increased from 5% to 13.5% for boys and 5% to 11.8% for girls. Overweight among children is an important health issue in Canada.

16.7 SCHOOL FOOD POLICY

Canada has no national policy or program for feeding school children. Some provinces or local boards of education are developing school food policies to address availability and quality of food in schools and the nutrition curricula. Teacher associations are showing great concern for the hungry children in classrooms and many schools have developed some type of feeding program. Two resources, listed below, examine the issue of effectiveness of school-feeding programs, a good discussion topic for classes, especially if students have read one of these resources prior to the discussion. Instructors could check with the local board of education to get details on local programs and policies.

The Canadian Living Foundation for Families provides resources for breakfast programs for children. This foundation is collaborating with the Ontario government to support school feeding programs in that province. Check the Canadian Living Foundation for Families web site for information about the school feeding programs.

16.8 HEALTH OF CANADIAN YOUTH

Canada is participating in an international study of the World Health Organization that has been monitoring trends in the health of youth since 1990. The 2000 report, Trends in the Health of Canadian Youth: Health Behaviour of School-Aged Children Study is available at www.hc-sc.gc.ca/hppb.childhood-youth/spsc.html. Chapter 7 of this report describes the healthy eating and dieting data from this study. This report describes trends in intake of fruits and vegetables, whole wheat and rye bread, low fat milk, soft drinks, and other products in 1990, 1994 and 1998. Unhealthy dieting practices are also monitored. Dieting is one approach to addressing the increasing prevalence of obesity during childhood[22].

Canadian Readings and Resources on Childhood Nutrition

Hay, DI. *School-based Feeding Program: A Good Choice for Children.*Victoria, BC: Information Partnership, July 2000. www.infopartners.ca/index.html?feature/

McIntyre L, Travers K, Dayle JB. Children's feeding programs in Atlantic Canada: Reducing or reproducing inequities. *Can J Public Health* 90(1999):196-200.

Leaman M, Evers S. Dietary intake by food groups of preschool children in low-income communities in Ontario. *J Am Diet Assoc.* 97(1997):184-191.

Evers S, Hooper M. Dietary intake and anthropometric status of 7 to 9 year old children in economically disadvantaged communities in Ontario. *J Am Coll Nutr.* 14:595-603, 1995.

HIGHLIGHT 16: THE EARLY DEVELOPMENT OF CHRONIC DISEASES

DIETARY FAT AND CHILDREN

The Canadian perspective on children's fat intake is presented in Nutrition Recommendations Update... Dietary Fat and Children[16] and was discussed with Chapter 5, The Lipids: Triglycerides, Phospholipids, and Sterols, in this Canadian Information section. The recommendations should be discussed here in the context of the importance of young children meeting their energy needs to support normal growth and development. This was seen as a priority for children's health. Physical activity is encouraged in the recommendations to help prevent obesity and the development of chronic diseases.

TEACHING CANADIAN INFORMATION: CHAPTER 17
LIFE CYCLE NUTRITION: ADULTHOOD AND THE LATER YEARS

17.1 CANADIAN PROGRAMS FOR THE ELDERLY

As with other age groups, there are no Canadian national programs focused on nutrition for the elderly. However many of the provinces or municipalities have meals-on-wheels programs or other nutrition programs aimed at the aging population. Check with social service agencies and the public health department in your community to find examples of local sneior nutrition programs.

17.2 NUTRITION SCREENING TOOL FOR SENIORS

Seniors in the Community: Risk Evaluation for Eating and Nutrition (SCREEN) has been developed and validated among seniors of varying health status, living in the community[36,37]. This screening tool is being used to identify seniors at risk for nutrition problems and plan programs and services to address these problems in Guelph, Ontario and five other locations across Canada. This screening tool is available on the Dietitians of Canada web site (www.dietitians.ca).

Canadian Readings

Keller HH, Østbye T, Bright-See E, Campbell MK. Activity limitation and food intake in community-living seniors. *Can J Aging* 18(1999):47-63.

Moving the Seniors' Agenda Forward Nutrition and the 55+ Canadian. National Institute of Nutrition. *RAPPORT* 13(1998):1-2, 4-5.

Keller H, Østbye T, Bright-See E. Predictors of dietary intake in Ontario seniors. *Can J Public Health* 88(1997):305-309.

National Institute of Nutrition. *Food and Nutrition Opportunities in the Seniors' Market: A Situation Analysis Executive Summary.* Ottawa, 1996.

TEACHING CANADIAN INFORMATION: CHAPTER 18
DIET AND HEALTH

18.1 NUTRITION RECOMMENDATIONS

The 1990 Nutrition Recommendations address the role of nutrition in chronic disease and disease prevention[11]. This is a single set of recommendations, with supporting guidelines to address most chronic diseases. An overview is provided in Nutrition and Disease, pp.13-18. The relationships of specific nutrients to diseases are discussed in the sections for the individual nutrients. Alcohol and caffeine are addressed in Part III. This information may be helpful to Canadian instructors planning lectures on the topic of nutrition and disease.

18.2 CANADIAN RECOMMENDATIONS FOR DYSLIPIDEMIA AND HYPERTENSION

The Canadian Medical Association recommendations for managing and treating dyslipidemia, use a comprehensive risk evaluation approach to determine target lipid profiles and risk of cardiovascular diseases[17]. This comprehensive method has been found to be more effective for identifying individuals who would benefit from treatment for hypercholesterolemia and other dyslipidemias than a single lipid profile indicator. Consult the full paper (Canadian Resources) to address target lipid profile and nutrition treatment before planning your lecture on this topic.

The Canadian Medical Association has published recommendations for lifestyle modifications to prevent and control hypertension and for managing hypertension. Consult these documents (Canadian Resources) for information about recommendations about salt, other nutrients and weight loss before teaching this topic.

Canadian Resources

Fodor JG, Frolich JJ, Genest JG, McPherson PR. Recommendations for the management and treatment of dyslipidemia. Report of the Working Group on Hypercholesterolemia and Other Dyslipidemias. *Can Med Assoc J* 162(2000):1441-1447.

Canadian Medical Association. Lifestyle modifications to prevent and control hypertension. Supplement to *Can Med Assoc J 160(1999) 9 Suppl.*

Canadian Medical Association. 1999 Canadian recommendations for the management of hypertension including Case-based applications of the recommendations. Supplement to *Can Med Assoc J* 161(1999) 10 Suppl.

These resources are available from the Canadian Medical Association web site.

18.3 GOOD HEALTH EATING GUIDE RESOURCE

The Canadian exchange system, the *Good Health Eating Guide*, is published by the Canadian Diabetes Association[12]. This system is described in chapter 2 of this Canadian Information Section. The complete lists for the Good Health Eating Guide are in Appendix I of the textbook. Canadian students should use this system when developing meal patterns and food plans in this chapter.

HIGHLIGHT 18: COMPLEMENTARY AND ALTERNATIVE MEDICINE

The practice of health professions is regulated by the provinces. Groups which practice alternative therapies, such as naturopaths, are regulated by legislation in some provinces. There is a growing trend to consider other alternative practitioners, such as homeopaths, under health profession regulation to make them more accountable to the public. If this is of interest to your class, check about the regulations for alternative therapists in your province or territory.

The Office of Natural Health Products is developing a regulatory framework to manage herbs and other products recommended by alternative practitioners. Check the web site for the Office of Natural Health Products to find the current status of this regulatory framework (www.hc-sc.gc.ca/hpb/onhp/). This framework should fit with the overall framework for regulating food and drugs.

TEACHING CANADIAN INFORMATION: CHAPTER 19
CONSUMER CONCERNS ABOUT FOODS AND WATER

19.1 FOOD-BORNE ILLNESSES

The safety of foods is regulated by the Food and Drugs Act and Regulations[1] and provincial public health regulations. It is monitored by the Canadian Food Inspection Agency and provincial or municipal public health departments. Mishandling of foods during handling, storage and preparation often permit the growth of pathogens leading to food-borne illness. The Regulations define storage requirements and microbial specifications for foods to be offered for sale. Inspectors monitor foods for contamination from extraneous matter such as insects, insect fragments, rodent hair, animal droppings, metal or wood fragments, glass, etc. Educational material to promote food safety is available from the Canadian Food Inspection Agency or local public health departments.

Safe handling of foods by foodservice is required to ensure the safety of foods served in restaurants and institutions. These are monitored by provincial or municipal health departments. Some community colleges or health departments offer education programs on sanitation in foodservice operations for food handlers.

19.2 FOOD ADDITIVES AND ALLERGENS

Food additives are regulated in Canada under the *Food and Drugs Act and Regulations*. The approach and regulations are similar to those of the United States. The policy on the use of food additives in Canada is consistent with the FAO/WHO Joint Expert Committee on Food Additives.

The safety of food additives is a concern for individuals with allergies or hypersensitivities. The requirement that all ingredients and food additives be included on labels of prepackaged foods helps these individuals to select foods which they can tolerate. Health Canada publishes *Allergy Allerts* with *product recalls* when foods or beverages are recalled when nuts, or other foods which are common allergens, are found to be in them, but are not listed as ingredients.

19.3 FOOD IRRADIATION

Food irradiation has not gained the consumer acceptance in Canada which it has in the United States. Generally irradiated food products have not reached the market. Health Canada is currently reviewing requests to approve the sale of irradiated hamburger patties in Canada. Irradiated fresh fruit is not available in Canada.

Canadian Resources

Canadian Food Inspection Agency - www.cfia-acia.agr.ca/english/

Canadian General Standards Board. *Organic Agriculture* - www.pwgsc.gc.ca/cgsb/catalogue/standards/

HIGHLIGHT 19: FOOD BIOTECHNOLOGY

Considerable research is being conducted in Canada with food biotechnology and genetic engineering. Health Canada and the Canadian Food Inspection Agency have responsibilities for regulating products derived through biotechnology. Health Canada is responsible for assessing the human health and safety of products derived from biotechnology including foods, drugs, cosmetics,medical devices, and pest control products. CFIA is responsible for regulating products derived through biotechnology including plants, animal feeds and animal feed ingredients, fertilizers, and veterinary biologics. For genetically modified crop plants, CFIA assesses the potential risk of adverse envrionmental effects and authorizes and oversees import permits, confined trials, unconfined release and variety registration.

The topic of labelling foods derived from genetic engineering is an important one in Canada. At this time, labelling is mandatory for food produced involving genetic engineering if there is a significant change in nutrient or chemical content or if there is potential health or safety risk for a population, such as allergic potential[14]. Some European countries require all foods that have been derived through genetic engineering to be identified through labelling. Many consumer groups are demanding the same policy in Canada. The Canadian General Standards Board established a committee to set standards for voluntary labelling of genetically modified foods. The committee comprises representatives of stakeholders. The committee has not yet presented their final report. Visit the Canadian General Standards Board web site (www.pwgsc.gc.ca/cgsb/) for the latest report from this committee.

Canadian Readings and Resources

National Institute of Nutrition. *Voluntary Labelling of Foods from Biotechnology: Report on a Qualitative Study Among Consumers*. Ottawa, 1999. Available from the Office of Biotechnology, Canadian Food Inspection Agency.

National Institute of Nutrition. Views on Biotechnology. *NIN RAPPORT* 14 No. 2(1999):1-7.

Health Canada. *Guidelines for the Assessment of Novel Foods*, Vol. 1 and 2. Food Directorate, Health Protection Branch, 1998.

Visit the Biotechnology pages of the Agriculture and Agri-food Canada web site for the latest information on genetic engineered food products. www.agr.ca/biotece.html

The Food Biotechnology Communications Network provides toll-free balanced, science-based information for Canadians at 1-877-366-3246. Resource sheets on current topics about food biotechnology can be found at their web site: www.foodbiotech.org.

TEACHING CANADIAN INFORMATION: CHAPTER 20
HUNGER AND GLOBAL ENVIRONMENTAL PROBLEMS

20.1 HUNGER IN CANADA

Hunger is a concern in Canada. The Progress of Canada's Children, 1996 notes that one in five children live in poverty and 40% of welfare recipients are children[38]. There has been a huge increase in the number of food banks and emergency feeding programs. Helping at a local food bank, shelter, or emergency feeding centre provides students with an opportunity to gain an understanding of the hunger issue. The following readings provide some perspectives on hunger issues in Canada and the role of nutrition professionals. The research articles focus on two large cities, Montreal and Toronto.

The article by Tarasuk and Davis is a key reading for Canadian students because it links food security with Canadian government policy in a way which is particularly meaningful for nutrition educators[39]. It will help students understand why Canada does not have programs which are comparable to the United States programs listed in this chapter of the textbook.

Canadian Readings

Tarasuk V, Davis B. Responses to food insecurity in the changing Canadian welfare state. *J Nutr Ed.* 28:71-75, 1996.

Jacobs Starkey L, Kuhnlein H. Montreal food bank users' intakes compared with recommendations of Canada's Food Guide to Healthy Eating. *Can J Diet Prac Res 61(2000):73-75.*

Tarasuk VS, Beaton GH. Household food insecurity and hunger among families using food banks. *Can J Public Health* 90(1999):109-113.

Tarasuk VS, Beaton GH. Women's dietary intakes in the context of household food insecurity. *J Nutr.* 129(1999):672-679.

Jacob Starkey L, Kuhnlein H, Gray-Donald. Food bank users: sociodemographic and nutritional characteristics. *Can Med Assoc J.* 158(1998):1143-1149.

Tarasuk V, Reynolds R. A qualitative study of community kitchens as a response to income-related food insecurity. *Can J Diet Prac Res* 60(1999):11-116.

HIGHLIGHT 20: PROGRESS TOWARD SUSTAINABLE AGRICULTURE

Concerns about sustainable agriculture, food safety, and global economic conditions are leading to some changes in agriculture production methods in Canada. The Environment Bureau of Agriculture and Agri-food Canada Policy Branch has the mandate to integrate environmental sustainability into all of Agriculture and Agri-food Canada's lines of business. Activies of the bureau include policy development and implementation related to sustainable development strategies, environmental protection, and environmental assessment. Agriculture commodity groups are also concerned about a sustainable environment and are implementing programs to increase sustainability. The structure of the agriculture industry in Canada differs from that in the United States. If this topic is important to your course, check with your provincial ministry of agriculture to identify programs to support sustainable agriculture in your province.

Canadian Resource

Agriculture and Agri-food Canada. *Environment & Sustainability*
www.agr.ca/environ_e.phtml

RESOURCE GROUPS

Please note that offices may move or phone numbers may change from the date of printing. Check with the Telephone Information if you are unable to contact these offices.

GOVERNMENT

HEALTH CANADA

Bureau of Nutritional Sciences, Food Directorate, Health Protection Branch, Health Canada, Banting Building, Tunney's Pasture, Ottawa, Ontario K1A 0L2

Regional Offices:

Halifax: Ralston Building, 1557 Hollis Street, Halifax, NS B3J 1V5

Quebec: Complexe Guy-Favreau, East Tower, 200 René Lévesque Blvd West, Montreal QC H2Z 1X4

Toronto: 25 St. Clair Ave. East, 4th Floor, Toronto, ON M4T 1M2

Winnipeg: 391 York Ave., Suite 425, Winnipeg, MB R3C 0P4

Edmonton: Suite 815, Canada Place, 9700 Jasper Ave., Edmonton AB T5J 4C3

Vancouver: Suite 405, Winch Building, 757 West Hastings St., Vancouver BC V6C 1A1

First Nations and Inuit Health Branch:

First Nations and Inuit Health Branch, 20th Floor, Jeanne Mance Building, Address Locator: 1920B, Tunney's Pasture, Ottawa, ON K1A 0L3

Regional Offices:

Northern Secretariat Region (Yukon Territory, Northwest Territory, Nunavut): Jeanne Mance Building, Postal Locator: 1921B, Ottawa ON K1A 0L3

Pacific Region: Regional Nutritionist, Suite 540, 757 West Hastings Street, Vancouver, BC V6C 3E6

Alberta Region: Regional Nutritionist, Suite 730, 9700 Jasper Avenue, Edmonton, AB T5J 4C3

Saskatchewan Region: Regional Nutritionist, 18TH fLOOR - 1920 Broad Street, Regina, SK S4P 2N5

Manitoba Region: Regional Nutritionist, Room 300, 303 York Avenue, Winnipeg, Manitoba R3C 4W1

Ontario Region: Regional Nutritionist, 3rd Floor, 1547 Merivale Road, Nepean, ON K1A 0C3

Region Du Québec: Nutritionniste Regionale, Suite 202, 2nd floor, East Tower, Place Guy Favreau, 200 Ouest, boul. René Lévesque, Montreal, QC H2Z 1X3

Atlantic Region: Regional Nutritionist, Suite 634, Ralston Bldg, 1557 Hollis Street, Halifax, NS B3J 1V6

AGRICULTURE AND AGRI-FOOD CANADA

Agriculture and Agri-Food Canada, 59 Camelot Drive, Nepean, Ontario K1A 0Y9.

DIETETIC ASSOCIATION

Dietitians of Canada, 480 University Avenue, Suite 604, Toronto, Ontario M5G 1V2 - (416) 596-0857 (The ten provincial dietetic associations and the Canadian Dietetic Associations have merged into one organization to serve all dietitians in Canada.)

Information about dietetics in Canada and its regional areas can be found at the website - www.dietitians.ca.

Some provinces, such as Ontario, have a college which regulates the practice of dietetics. College of Dietitians of Ontario, 438 University Ave., Suite 1810, Box 40, Toronto, Ontario M5G 2K8 (416) 598-1725.
Information on the governing bodies for dietetics in specific provinces can be found through the Dietitians of Canada web site.

OTHER ORGANIZATIONS

Canadian Diabetes Association, National Office, Toronto Street, Suite 1001, Toronto, Ontario M5C 2E3 - (416) 363-3373.

Canadian Living Foundation for Families, 50 Holly Street, Toronto, Ontario M4S 3B3.

Canadian Produce Marketing Association, 310-1101 Prince of Wales Dr., Ottawa, Ontario K2C 3W7 - (613) 226-4187

Canadian Public Health Association, Publications, Suite 400, 1565 Carling Ave. Ottawa, Ontario K1Z 8R1 (613) 725-3769.

Canadian Restaurant and Foodservices Association, 80 Bloor Street West, Suite 1201, Toronto, Ontario M5S 2V1 - (416) 923-8416 or 1-800-387-5649.

Consumer's Association of Canada, 307 Gilmour St., Ottawa, Ontario K2P 0P7

National Eating Disorder Information Centre, 200 Elizabeth St., College Wing 1-328, Toronto, Ontario M5G 2C4 - (416) 340-4156.

National Institute of Nutrition, 302 - 265 Carling Avenue, Ottawa, Ontario K1S 2E1 - (613) 235-3355

For Canadian Cancer Society and Canadian Heart and Stroke Foundation, information and publications are available from local or provincial offices.

Educational nutrition material is also available from many of the food manufacturers, food producer organizations, provincial ministries of agriculture or health, or local public health departments.

REFERENCES

1. Health and Welfare Canada. *Departmental Consolidation of the Food and Drugs Act and Regulations.* Ottawa: Ministry of Supply and Services, 2001. The current regulations can be found at www.hc-sc.gc.ca/food-aliment/english/publications/acts_and_regulations/food_and_drugs_acts/

2. Food Division, Food Inspection Directorate, Agriculture and Agri-Food Canada. *Guide to Food Labelling and Advertising.* Ottawa: Agriculture and Agri-Food Canada,1996.

3. Dietitians of Canada. Health Canada puts stamp of approval on DRIs. *Members in Action,* April 2001, p. 2.

4. Hedley M, Chambers L, Tomasik HH et al. *Ontario Health Survey 1990 Working Paper No. 10 Nutrition Report.* Toronto: Ontario Ministry of Health, 1995.

5. Gray-Donald K, Jacobs-Starkey L, Johnson-Down L. Food habits of Canadians: Reduction in fat intake over a generation. *Can J Public Health* 91(2000):381-385.

6. Health Canada. *Canadians and Healthy Eating: How Are We Doing? Nutrition Highlights, National Population Health Survey, 1994-95.* Ottawa: Health Canada, 1998.

7. Health Statistics Division. *How Healthy are Canadians? A Summary - 2001 Annual Report.* Ottawa. Statistics Canada, 2001. www.statcan.ca/english/ads/82-003XIB/sim2001.pdf.

8. Joint Steering Committee. *Nutrition for Health: An Agenda for Action.* Ottawa: Health Canada, 1996. (www.hc-sc.gc.ca/datahpb/npu/index.html)

9. Davis BA. *A Report on the Use of Indicators in Canada's National Nutrition Plan.* Ottawa: Joint Steering Committee of Nutrition for Action: An Agenda for Action, 1996.

10. Health and Welfare Canada. *Action Towards Healthy Eating...Canada's Guidelines for Healthy Eating and Strategies for Implementation.* The Report of the Communications/ Implementation Committee. Ottawa: Minister of Supply and Services Canada, 1990.

11. Health and Welfare Canada. *Nutrition Recommendations.* Ottawa: Minister of Supply and Services Canada, 1990.

12. Canadian Diabetes Association. *Good Health Eating Guide Resource.* Toronto, 1994.

13. Bureau of Nutritional Science, Food Directorate, Health Protection Branch. *Principles of Proposed Policy for Nutrition Labelling.* Ottawa:Health Canada, 2000. www.hc-sc.gc.ca/english/proposed_policy_nutrition_labelling.html.

14. Agriculture and Agri-Food Canada. *Labelling of Foods Derived Through Genetic Engineering. Communiqué, Dec. 1995.* www.cfia-acia.agr.ca/english/ppc/biotech/.

15. Health and Welfare Canada. *Report of the Expert Committee on Dietary Fibre to the Health Protection Branch Health and Welfare Canada.* Ottawa: Minister of National Health and Welfare, 1985.

16. The Joint Working Group of the Canadian Paediatric Society and Health Canada. *Nutrition Recommendations Update... Dietary Fat and Children.* Ottawa: Minister of Supply and Services Canada, 1993.

17. Fodor JG, Frolich JJ, Genest JG, McPherson PR. Recommendations for the management and treatment of dyslipidemia. Report of the Working Group on Hypercholesterolemia and Other Dyslipidemias. *Can Med Assoc J* 162(2000):1441-1447.

18. Health and Welfare Canada. *Canadian Guidelines for Healthy Weights.* Ottawa: Minister of Supply and Services, 1988.

19. The Canadian Dietetic Association. *Healthy Eating Is... A Resource Manual for Health Professionals.* Toronto: The Canadian Dietetic Association, 1988, p.20.

20. Health and Welfare Canada. *Promoting Healthy Weights in Canada.* Ottawa: Minister of Supply and Services, 1988.

21. Health Canada. *The Vitality Approach: A guide for leaders.* Ottawa: Minister of Supply and Services Canada, 1999.

22. Tremblay MS, Willms JD. Secular trends in the body mass index of Canadian Children. *Can Med Assoc J* 163(2000):1429-1433.

23. Birmingham CL, Muller JL, Palepu A, Spinelli JJ, Anis AH. The cost of obesity in Canada. *Can Med Assoc J* 160(1999):483-488.

24. Health Canada. *Nutrient Value of Some Common Foods.* Ottawa: Public Works and Government Services Canada, 1999.

25. Canadian Fitness and Lifestyle Research Institute. *Foundation for Joint Action: Reducing Physical Inactivity* (1999). www.cflri.ca/cflri/resources/pub.php

26. Health Canada. *Nutrition for a Healthy Pregnancy: National Guidelines for the Childbearing Years.* Ottawa: Minister of Public Works and Government Services, 1999. www.hc-sc.gc.ca/nutrition.

27. Higgins, A.C. Nutritional status and the outcome of pregnancy. *J Can Diet Assoc* 37(1976):17-35.

28. Mendelson, R., Dollard, D., Hall, P., Zarrabi, S.Y., Desjardin, E. The impact of the Healthiest Babies Possible Program on maternal diet and pregnancy outcome in underweight and overweight clients. *J Can Diet Assoc* 52(1991):229-234.

29. Health Canada. *Canadian Nutrition Prenatal Program.* Ottawa. www.hc-sc.gc.ca/hppb/childhood-youth/cbp/cnpp/ 1999.

30. Health Canada. *Canadian Prenatal Nutrition Program: A Portrait of Participants, September 2000.* Ottawa. www.hc-sc.gc.ca/hppb/childhood-youth/cbp/cpnp/newsletter2.

31. Doran L and Evers S. Energy and nutrient inadequacies in the diets of low-income women who breast-feed. *J Am. Diet Assoc.* 97(1997):1283-1287.

32. Health Canada. *Study of Attitudes on Breastfeeding.* Ottawa: Health Canada, 1995.

33. Breastfeeding Committee for Canada. Breastfeeding statement of the Breastfeeding Committee of Canada. *J Can Diet Assoc.* 59(1998):11-13.

34. Health Canada and The Canadian Paediatric Society. *Joint Statement on Fetal Alcohol Syndrome and Fetal Alcohol Effects.* Ottawa, 1995

35. The Canadian Paediatric Society, Dietitians of Canada, Health Canada. Nutrition for healthy term infants. *Can J Diet Practice and Res* (formerly J Can Diet Assoc).59(1997):93-96. www.hc-sc.gc/hpb/cny/infantnutrition/nutritionforhealthyterminfants/index.html

36. Wollows ND, Dewailly E, Gray-Donald K. Anemia and iron status in Inuit infants from Northern Quebec. *Can J Public Health* 91(2000):407-410.

37. Keller HH, Hedley M, Wong Brownlee S. The development of SCREEN - Seniors in the community:Risk evaluation for eating and nutrition. *Can J Diet Pract Res* 61(2000):67-72.

38. Keller HH, McKenzie JD, Goy R. The construct validation study and test-retest reliability of SCREEN (Seniors in the community: Risk Evaluation for Eating and Nutrition). *J Geront Med Sci* (Accepted for publication July 2001).

39. Canadian Council of Social Development. *The Progress of Canada's Children, 1996.* Ottawa: 1996.

40. Tarasuk V, Davis B. Responses to food insecurity in the changing Canadian welfare state. *J Nutr Ed.* 28:71-75, 1996.

CHAPTER 1
AN OVERVIEW OF NUTRITION

a   2(A)   01.   A person who eats a bowl of oatmeal for breakfast every day would be displaying a food choice most likely based on

   a.   habit.
   b.   availability.
   c.   body image.
   d.   environmental concerns.

d   2(K)   02.   Excluding non-fast-food establishments, approximately what percentage of restaurants in the United States show an ethnic emphasis?

   a.   15
   b.   30
   c.   45
   d.   60

b   2(K)   03.   What is the chief reason people choose the foods they eat?

   a.   Cost
   b.   Taste
   c.   Convenience
   d.   Nutritional value

1

b   2(K)   04.   Characteristics of an acute disease include all of the following EXCEPT

      a.   it develops quickly.
      b.   it progresses slowly.
      c.   it runs a short course.
      d.   it causes sharp symptoms.

d   3(A)   05.   Which of the following represents a food choice based on negative association?

      a.   A tourist from China who rejects a hamburger due to unfamiliarity
      b.   A child who spits out his mashed potatoes because they taste too salty
      c.   A teenager who grudgingly accepts an offer for an ice cream cone to avoid offending a close friend
      d.   An elderly gentleman who refuses a peanut butter and jelly sandwich because he deems it a child's food

c   4(a)   06.   A person viewing an exciting sports match of her favorite team and eating because of nervousness would be displaying a food choice behavior most likely based on

      a.   habit.
      b.   availability.
      c.   emotional comfort.
      d.   positive association.

c   4(K)   07.   What is the term that defines foods that contain nonnutrient substances whose known action in the body is to promote well-being to a greater extent than that contributed by the food's nutrients?

      a.   Fortified foods
      b.   Enriched foods
      c.   Functional foods
      d.   Health enhancing foods

b   4(K)   08.   In the body, the chemical energy in food can be converted to any of the following EXCEPT

      a.   heat energy.
      b.   light energy.
      c.   electrical energy.
      d.   mechanical energy.

a   5(A)   09.   Which of the following is an example of a macronutrient?

                          a.   Protein
                          b.   Calcium
                          c.   Vitamin C
                          d.   Vitamin D

c   5(A)   10.   Which of the following is an example of a micronutrient?

                          a.   Fat
                          b.   Protein
                          c.   Vitamin C
                          d.   Carbohydrate

b   4-5(K)   11.   By chemical analysis, what nutrient is present in highest
                          amounts in most foods?

                          a.   Fats
                          b.   Water
                          c.   Proteins
                          d.   Carbohydrates

a   5(K)   12.   Which of the following is NOT one of the six classes of
                          nutrients?

                          a.   Fiber
                          b.   Protein
                          c.   Minerals
                          d.   Vitamins

b   5(K)   13.   What nutrient is usually consumed in greatest quantity from
                          the diet?

                          a.   Fat
                          b.   Water
                          c.   Protein
                          d.   Carbohydrate

c   5(A)   14.   Which of the following statements most accurately describes the composition of most foods?

     a.   Contain only one of the three energy nutrients although a few contain all of them
     b.   Contain equal amounts of the three energy nutrients, except for high fat foods
     c.   Contain mixtures of the three energy nutrients, although only one or two may predominate
     d.   Contain only two of the three energy nutrients although there are numerous other foods that contain only one

d   5(K)   15.   Which of the following is an organic compound?

     a.   Salt
     b.   Water
     c.   Calcium
     d.   Vitamin C

c   5(A)   16.   Which of the following is characteristic of an essential nutrient?

     a.   Cannot be found in food
     b.   Cannot be degraded by the body
     c.   Cannot be made in sufficient quantities by the body
     d.   Cannot be used to synthesize other compounds in the body

d   5(A)   17.   Which of the following most accurately describes the term organic?

     a.   Products sold at health food stores
     ·b.   Products grown without use of pesticides
     c.   Foods possessing superior nutrient qualities
     d.   Substances possessing carbon-carbon or carbon-hydrogen bonds

c   5(K)   18.   Approximately how many nutrients are considered indispensable from the diet?

     a.   15
     b.   25
     c.   40
     d.   55

a   5(A)   19.   Which of the following is an organic nutrient?

a.   Fat
b.   Water
c.   Oxygen
d.   Calcium

d   5(A)   20.   Which of the following CANNOT be "fattening" to the body?

a.   Alcohol
b.   Proteins
c.   Carbohydrates
d.   Inorganic nutrients

c   5(K)   21.   Which of the following nutrients does NOT yield energy during its metabolism?

a.   Fat
b.   Proteins
c.   Vitamins
d.   Carbohydrates

c   6(K)   22.   International units of energy are expressed in

a.   newtons.
b.   calories.
c.   kilojoules.
d.   kilocalories.

c   6(K)   23.   Approximately how many milliliters are contained in a half-cup of milk?

a.   50
b.   85
c.   125
d.   200

b   6(A)   24.   How much energy is required to raise the temperature of one liter of water 1°C?

a.   10 calories
b.   1 kilocalorie
c.   10,000 calories
d.   1000 kilocalories

c   6(K)   25.   A normal half-cup vegetable serving weighs approximately
                          how many grams?

                          a.   5
                          b.   50
                          c.   100
                          d.   200

c   7(A)   26.   A weight reduction regimen calls for a daily intake of 1400 kcal
                          which includes 30g of fat. Approximately what percentage of
                          the total energy is contributed by fat?

                          a.   8.5
                          b.   15
                          c.   19
                          d.   25.5

a   7(K)   27.   Gram for gram, which of the following provides the most
                          energy?

                          a.   Fats
                          b.   Alcohol
                          c.   Proteins
                          d.   Carbohydrates

a   7(A)   28.   Which of the following nutrient sources yields more than 4
                          kcalories per gram?

                          a.   Plant fats
                          b.   Plant proteins
                          c.   Animal proteins
                          d.   Plant carbohydrates

a   7(A)   29.   A diet provides a total of 2200 kcalories of which 40% of the
                          energy is from fat and 20% from protein. How many grams of
                          carbohydrate are contained in the diet?

                          a.   220
                          b.   285
                          c.   440
                          d.   880

d   7(A)   30.   What is the kcalorie value of a meal supplying 110 g of carbohydrates, 25 g of protein, 20 g of fat, and 5 g of alcohol?

    a.   160
    b.   345
    c.   560
    d.   755

d   7(K)   31.   When consumed in excess, all of the following can be converted to body fat and stored <u>EXCEPT</u>

    a.   sugar.
    b.   corn oil.
    c.   alcohol.
    d.   vitamin C.

a   7(A)   32.   Which of the following results from the metabolism of energy nutrients?

    a.   Energy is released
    b.   Body fat increases
    c.   Energy is destroyed
    d.   Body water decreases

c   8(K)   33.   Which of the following is a feature of the minerals as nutrients?

    a.   They are organic in form
    b.   They yield 4 kcal per gram
    c.   Some become dissolved in body fluids
    d.   Some may be destroyed during cooking

c   8(A)   34.   Which of the following is <u>NOT</u> a characteristic shared by minerals?

    a.   Yield no energy
    b.   Stable in cooked foods
    c.   Metabolized in the body
    d.   Structurally smaller than vitamins

b   7-8(K)   35.   Which of the following is <u>NOT</u> a characteristic of the vitamins?

    a.   Essential
    b.   Inorganic
    c.   Destructible
    d.   kcalorie-free

d   7-8(K)   36.   Which of the following is/are <u>NOT</u> fat-soluble?

a.   Vitamin A
b.   Vitamin K
c.   Vitamin D
d.   B vitamins

d   7(K)   37.   How many vitamins are known for human beings?

a.   5
b.   8
c.   10
d.   13

b   8(A)   38.   Overcooking a food is <u>LEAST</u> likely to affect the value of what group of nutrients?

a.   Vitamins
b.   Minerals
c.   Proteins
d.   Carbohydrates

c   8(K)   39.   How many minerals are known to be required in the diet of human beings?

a.   6
b.   12
c.   16
d.   24

b   9(K)   40.   In nutrition research, observations of the quantities and types of foods eaten by groups of people and the health status of those groups are known as

a.   case-control studies.
b.   epidemiological studies.
c.   human intervention trials.
d.   correlation-control studies.

d   10-11(A)   41.   What is the benefit of using controls in an experiment?

a.   The size of the groups can be very large
b.   The subjects do not know anything about the experiment
c.   The subjects who are treated are balanced against the placebos
d.   The subjects are similar in all respects except for the treatment being tested

b   10(A)   42.   What is the benefit of using placebos in an experiment?

a.   All subjects are similar
b.   All subjects receive a treatment
c.   Neither subjects nor researchers know who is receiving treatment
d.   One group of subjects receives a treatment and the other group receives nothing

b   10-11(K)   43.   What is the meaning of a double-blind experiment?

a.   Both subject groups take turns getting each treatment
b.   Neither subjects nor researchers know which subjects are in the control or experiment group
c.   Neither group of subjects knows whether they are in the control or experiment group but the researchers do know
d.   Both subject groups know whether they are in the control or experiment group but the researchers do not know

a   10(A)   44.   What is the benefit of using a large sample size in an experiment?

a.   Chance variation is ruled out
b.   There will be no placebo effect
c.   The experiment will be double-blind
d.   The control group will be similar to the experimental group

b   13-14(A)   45.   Recommended Dietary Allowances may be used to

a.   measure nutrient balance.
b.   assess dietary nutrient adequacy.
c.   treat persons with diet related illness.
d.   calculate exact food requirements for most individuals.

c   13(K)   46.   The RDAs (Recommended Dietary Allowances) for nutrients are generally

a.   more than twice as high as anyone needs.
b.   the minimum amounts that average people need.
c.   designed to be adequate for almost all healthy people.
d.   designed to prevent deficiency disease in half the population.

b   12(K)   47.   The lowest amount of a nutrient that is consumed over a prolonged period and that maintains a specific function is called the nutrient

a.   allowance.
b.   requirement.
c.   tolerable limit.
d.   adequate intake.

c   12(K)   48.   The Dietary Reference Intakes may be used to

a.   treat people with diet-related disorders.
b.   assess adequacy of all required nutrients.
c.   plan and evaluate diets for healthy people.
d.   assess adequacy of only vitamins and minerals.

d   13-14(K)   49.   The starting point to formulate a Recommended Dietary Allowance uses the

a.   lower Tolerable Limit.
b.   upper Tolerable Limit.
c.   subclinical Deficiency Value.
d.   estimated Average Requirement.

c   13(A)   50.   If a group of people consumed an amount of protein equal to the average requirement for their population group, what percentage would receive insufficient amounts?

a.   2
b.   33
c.   50
d.   98

d   13-14(A)   51.   Which of the following represents a rationale for setting the RDA for energy?

a.   Since protein is an energy nutrient, the figures for energy intake are set in proportion to protein intake
b.   Since a large number of people are overweight, the figures are set to induce a gradual weight loss in most individuals
c.   Since the energy needs within each population group show little variation, the figures are set to meet the needs of almost all individuals
d.   Since a margin of safety would result in excess energy intake for a large number of people, the figures are set at the average energy intake

b   13-14(K)   52.   How are the RDA figures for almost all nutrient intakes set?

a.   Low, so as not to risk toxicity
b.   High, to cover virtually all healthy individuals
c.   Extremely high, to cover every single person
d.   At the mean, to cover most healthy individuals

d   13-15(K)   53.   In setting Dietary Recommended Intakes for nutrients, the DRI Committee makes all of the following assumptions EXCEPT

a.   people generally are healthy.
b.   people generally consume protein of good quality.
c.   people generally consume diets adequate in kcalories.
d.   people buy their foods exclusively at health food stores.

a   13-15(K)   54.   Which of the following is a feature of the RDA and Adequate Intake?

a.   Useful to set nutrient goals for individuals
b.   Useful to identify toxic intakes of nutrients
c.   Useful to restore health of malnourished individuals
d.   Useful to develop nutrition programs for schoolchildren

d   13(K)   55.   The amount of a nutrient that meets the needs of about 98% of a population is termed the

a.   Adequate Intake.
b.   Daily Recommended Value.
c.   Tolerable Upper Intake Level.
d.   Recommended Dietary Allowance.

c   14(K)   56.   Which of the following is a feature of a nutrient's Tolerable Upper Intake Level?

a.   It represents the maximum amount allowed for fortifying a food
b.   It is a number calculated by taking twice the RDA or three times the AI
c.   It represents the total intake from food, water, and supplements
d.   It represents the maximum allowable amount available in supplement form

a   15(K)   57.   Which of the following is used to detect nutrient deficiencies?

                           a.   Assessment techniques
                           b.   Nutrient stages identification
                           c.   Overt symptoms identification
                           d.   Outward manifestations assessment

b   16(K)   58.   Which of the following is used to determine the presence of
                           abnormal functions inside the body due to a nutrient
                           deficiency?

                           a.   Diet history
                           b.   Laboratory tests
                           c.   Body weight loss
                           d.   Physical examination

d   16-17(K)   59.   Inspection of hair, eyes, skin, and posture is part of the
                           nutrition assessment component known as

                           a.   diet history.
                           b.   anthropometrics.
                           c.   biochemical testing.
                           d.   physical examination.

a   17(A)   60.   Which of the following would most likely lead to a primary
                           nutrient deficiency?

                           a.   Inadequate nutrient intake
                           b.   Reduced nutrient absorption
                           c.   Increased nutrient excretion
                           d.   Increased nutrient destruction

a   17-18(K)   61.   Which of the following represents the usual sequence of
                           stages in the development of a nutrient deficiency resulting
                           from inadequate intake?

                           a.   Declining nutrient stores, abnormal functions within the
                                body, and overt signs
                           b.   Abnormal functions within the body, declining nutrient
                                stores, and overt signs
                           c.   Abnormal functions within the body, overt signs, and
                                declining nutrient stores
                           d.   Declining nutrient stores, overt signs, and abnormal
                                functions within the body

c   17(K)   62.   What type of deficiency is caused by inadequate absorption of
                              a nutrient?

                              a.   Primary
                              b.   Clinical
                              c.   Secondary
                              d.   Subclinical

b   17-18(K)   63.   Which of the following is an <u>overt</u> symptom of iron deficiency?

                              a.   Anemia
                              b.   Headaches
                              c.   Skin dryness
                              d.   Decreased red blood cell count

b   18(K)   64.   What is the acronym that describes an ongoing national survey
                              of the diet histories, anthropometrics and physical and
                              laboratory tests of about 50,000 people?

                              a.   USNHG
                              b.   NHANES
                              c.   NNDAPL
                              d.   NUT2001

c   19-20(K)   65.   Which of the following statements defines the association
                              between a risk factor and the development of a disease?

                              a.   All people with the risk factor will develop the disease
                              b.   The absence of a risk factor guarantees freedom from the
                                   disease
                              c.   The more risk factors for a disease, the greater the chance
                                   of developing that disease
                              d.   The presence of a factor such as heredity can be modified
                                   to lower the risk of degenerative diseases

b   20(K)   66.   What is the major cause of death in the United States?

                              a.   Poor diet
                              b.   Tobacco use
                              c.   Alcohol intake
                              d.   Sexual behavior

c   19(K)   67.   The diseases most common today in the United States include all of the following EXCEPT

a.   cancer.
b.   diabetes.
c.   tuberculosis.
d.   diseases of the heart and blood vessels.

b   19(K)   68.   Of the ten leading causes of illness and death, how many are associated directly with nutrition?

a.   1
b.   4
c.   7
d.   10

a   19(K)   69.   Factors known to be related to a disease but not proven to be causal are called

a.   risk factors.
b.   genetic factors.
c.   degenerative factors.
d.   environmental factors.

d   19(K)   70.   Which of the following leading causes of death in the U.S. does NOT bear a relationship to diet?

a.   Cancer
b.   Heart disease
c.   Diabetes mellitus
d.   Pneumonia and influenza

a   26(K)   71.   Which of the following best describes a college-educated nutrition and food specialist who is qualified to make evaluations of the nutritional health of people?

a.   Registered dietitian
b.   Licensed nutritionist
c.   Master of nutrient utilization
d.   Doctor of food and nutritional sciences

b   26(K)   72.   All of the following are minimum requirements for becoming a Registered Dietitian <u>EXCEPT</u>

a.   earn an undergraduate degree.
b.   complete a three-week clinical internship or the equivalent.
c.   complete approximately 60 semester hours in nutrition and food science.
d.   pass a national examination administered by the American Dietetic Association.

c   25-27(A)   73.   Who would be the most appropriate person to consult regarding nutrition information?

a.   Chiropractor
b.   Medical doctor
c.   Registered dietitian
d.   Health food store manager

a   27-28(K)   74.   What section of a research article contains a detailed description of the study's findings, including any tables and figures?

a.   Results
b.   Abstract
c.   Conclusions
d.   Methodology

c   27(K)   75.   Which of the following describes the limitations, if any, for a person who disseminates dietary advice to the public?

a.   The title "dietitian" can be used by anyone in all states
b.   The title "nutritionist" can be used by anyone in all states
c.   A license to practice as a nutritionist or dietitian is required by some states
d.   A license to practice as a nutritionist or dietitian is mandatory in all states

a   28-29(K)   76.   All of the following are recognized, credible sources of nutrition information <u>EXCEPT</u>

a.   Who's Who in Nutrition.
b.   Food and Drug Administration.
c.   American Dietetic Association.
d.   United States Department of Agriculture.

Matching (Answers can be used only once)

G	5	77.	Substance containing no carbon, hydrogen or oxygen
D	5	78.	Number of indispensable nutrients for human beings
K	5	79.	Most substances containing carbon-hydrogen bonds
J	5	80.	Substance containing nitrogen
E	5	81.	Energy (kcal) required to increase temperature of 1 liter of water from $0^{\circ}C$ to $100^{\circ}C$
H	5	82.	Nutrient with the highest body concentration
F	6	83.	Nutrient with the highest energy density
C	6	84.	Energy (kcal) yield of five grams of sugar
A	7	85.	Energy (kcal) yield of one gram of alcohol
N	7	86.	A water-soluble vitamin
B	8	87.	Number of indispensable minerals for human beings
L	10	88.	An inert medication
M	13	89.	The RDA for this fat-soluble nutrient exceeds the population mean
I	13	90.	The RDA for this nutrient is set at the population mean
P	15	91.	Excess nutrient intake leads to this
O	15	92.	Deficient nutrient intake leads to this
Q	16	93.	Measurement of physical characteristics
S	16	94.	Inspection of skin, tongue, eyes, hair, and fingernails
R	17	95.	A nutrient deficiency showing outward signs
T	17	96.	A nutrient deficiency in the early stages

A.	7	K.	Organic
B.	16	L.	Placebo
C.	20	M.	Vitamin A
D.	40	N.	Vitamin C
E.	100	O.	Malnutrition
F.	Fat	P.	Overnutrition
G.	Iron	Q.	Anthropometrics
H.	Water	R.	Overt deficiency
I.	Energy	S.	Physical examination
J.	Protein	T.	Subclinical deficiency

Essay Questions

2-4   97.   Describe six behavioral or social motives governing people's food choices.

2-4   98.   Explain how food choices are influenced by habits, emotions, physical appearance, and ethnic background.

3   99.   Discuss some of the consequences of eating in response to emotions.

4-5   100.   What is the meaning and significance of the popular phrase "You are what you eat?"

5;7-8   101.   Define the term organic. How do the properties of vitamins relate to their organic nature? Contrast these points with the properties of inorganic compounds such as minerals.

10-11   102.   Explain the importance of the placebo and the double-blind technique in carrying out research studies.

13-14   103. What approach is taken in setting recommended allowances for energy intakes? Why is this approach taken? How does this approach differ from that taken for other nutrients?

12-14   104. Describe the steps involved in establishing nutrient values that make up the Dietary Reference Intakes.

13-14   105. Compare and contrast the meaning of Adequate Intakes, Recommended Dietary Allowances, Estimated Average Requirements, and Tolerable Upper Intakes Levels for nutrients.

15-17   106. A. List and discuss four methods commonly used to assess nutritional status of individuals.

             B. What types of individuals are qualified to evaluate nutritional health of individuals?

16-19   107. Compare and contrast the rationales underlying dietary recommendations for individuals versus the population.

18   108. List 10 goals of the Healthy People 2010 program.

25   109. List ways in which to identify a reliable nutrition information website.

26-27   110. A. Explain the requirements for education and training associated with obtaining registration as a dietitian.

            B. List several career areas in which registered dietitians are often employed.

27-30   111. A. List techniques that help identify nutrition quackery.

            B. Where can you find reliable sources of nutrition information?

CHAPTER 2
PLANNING A HEALTHY DIET

Ans   Page

d   33(K)   01.   What are the "ABCDMV" principles of diet planning?

a.   Abundance, B vitamins, kcalories, diet control, minerals, and variety
b.   Abundance, balance, conservative, diversity, moderation, and vitamins
c.   Adequacy, bone development, correction, vitamin density, master, and variety
d.   Adequacy, balance, kcalorie control, nutrient density, moderation, and variety

b   33-34(A)   02.   Which of the following is the most nutrient dense food relative to calcium content?

a.   Whole milk
b.   Nonfat milk
c.   Low-fat milk
d.   Cheddar cheese

c   33-34(K)   03.   Nutrient density refers to foods that

a.   carry the USDA nutrition labeling.
b.   are higher in weight relative to volume.
c.   provide more nutrients relative to kcalories.
d.   contain a mixture of carbohydrate, fat, and protein.

1

d   33-34(K)   04.   The concept of nutrient density is most helpful in achieving what principle of diet planning?

    a.   Variety
    b.   Balance
    c.   Moderation
    d.   kCalorie control

a   33-34(A)   05.   Which of the following is an expression of the nutrient density of a food?

    a.   0.01 mg iron per kcal
    b.   110 kcal per cup
    c.   0.5 mg iron per serving
    d.   110 kcal per serving

a   34(A)   06.   Applying the principle of variety in food planning also ensures the benefits of

    a.   dilution.
    b.   moderation.
    c.   vegetarianism.
    d.   nutrient density.

c   35-36(K)   07.   Which of the following is NOT a feature of a food group plan?

    a.   Excludes some foods
    b.   Considered a tool for diet-planning
    c.   Sorts foods of similar water content
    d.   Specifies the number of servings from each group

d   36(A)   08.   Which of the following is NOT characteristic of the Daily Food Guide?

    a.   Most foods can be placed into one of the five groups in the Guide
    b.   The Guide can be used with great flexibility once its intent is understood
    c.   The Guide specifies that a certain quantity of food must be consumed from each group
    d.   Following all of the Guide's rules ensures that the day's needs for all nutrients are met

a   36;38(A)   09.   Which of the following is an alternative choice for meats in the Daily Food Guide?

a.   Nuts
b.   Bacon
c.   Baked potatoes
d.   Sweet potatoes

b   36-38(K)   10.   What are two major nutrients supplied by the fruit and vegetable group?

a.   Vitamins D and E
b.   Vitamins A and C
c.   Protein and calcium
d.   B vitamins and iron

b   36-38(A)   11.   Consider the following menu from the point of view of the Daily Food Guide.

Breakfast	Lunch	Supper
2 eggs	2 oz tuna fish	3 oz hamburger
1 tsp margarine	lettuce	meat
2 slices enriched	1 tbsp mayonnaise	1 oz cheese
white bread	1 c whole milk	2 slices enriched
coffee	1 apple	white bread
		1/2 c cooked rice
		1/2 c carrots
		coffee

Which of the following describes the nutritional value of the fruits and vegetables in this menu?

a.   A source of vitamin A source is missing
b.   A source of vitamin C source is missing
c.   The Five Food Group recommendations are met
d.   The Five Food Group recommendations are exceeded

d   36-37(A)   12.   Which of the following is a feature of the Food Guide Pyramid?

    a.   The vegetable group includes legumes
    b.   Alcoholic beverages are listed at the top
    c.   The recommended number of milk and milk products servings is 4 to 6
    d.   A standard serving size is generally smaller than what people typically eat

b   37-38(A)   13.   Which of the following foods could help meet the iron needs of vegetarians who consume dairy?

    a.   Coconut
    b.   Legumes
    c.   Skim milk
    d.   Potato salad

d   37(K)   14   Which of the following is descriptive of the USDA Food Guide Pyramid?

    a.   An education tool for teaching nutrition to children which consists of food blocks that require stacking in a specific order
    b.   A three-dimensional structure designed to assist the average consumer in the use of the Food Exchange System
    c.   A system of specialized containers of several different sizes which allows for better storage and preservation of perishable food items
    d.   A graphic representation of the Dietary Guidelines that displays complex carbohydrates at the base and fats and sweets at the very top

b   37(K)   15.   According to the principles of the Daily Food Guide, the foundation of a healthful diet should consist of

    a.   dairy.
    b.   grains.
    c.   vegetables.
    d.   meats and alternatives.

a   37(K)   16.   In the Food Guide Pyramid, the small dots and triangles scattered in the background represent

    a.   fats and sugars.
    b.   salt and pepper.
    c.   calcium and iron.
    d.   vitamins and minerals.

a   37(A)   17.   Which of the following foods would be placed in the "miscellaneous" category of food group plans?

    a.   Jam
    b.   Watermelon
    c.   Raw carrots
    d.   Brussels sprouts

c   37(K)   18.   All of the following are examples of legumes EXCEPT

    a.   lentils.
    b.   peanuts.
    c.   potatoes.
    d.   garbanzo beans.

d   36-37(K)   19.   In the Daily Food Guide, consuming the lowest number of servings from each food group would provide the energy needs for

    a.   teenage girls.
    b.   most children.
    c.   sedentary men.
    d.   sedentary women.

c   37(K)   20.   According to the Food Guide Pyramid, approximately what percentage of the day's food servings should be derived from plant foods?

    a.   20
    b.   50
    c.   75
    d.   95

a   41(K)   21.   Food exchange systems were originally developed for people with

    a.   diabetes.
    b.   terminal diseases.
    c.   cardiovascular disease.
    d.   life- threatening obesity.

c   41(K)   22.   In food exchange lists, to what group is milk assigned?

    a.   Fat
    b.   Meat
    c.   Carbohydrate
    d.   Meat substitute

d   41(K)   23.   A diet survey of thousands of people has shown that adequate intake(s) from among the food groups occurred only for

    a.   bread.
    b.   milk/dairy.
    c.   fruit and dairy.
    d.   meat and vegetable.

d   42-43(A)   24.   Which of the following is a feature of the Food Exchange System?

    a.   Foods are grouped according to their source
    b.   Adequate intakes of minerals and vitamins are virtually guaranteed
    c.   A fat portion provides about twice the energy level as a carbohydrate portion
    d.   All foods are grouped into other carbohydrates, meats/meats substitutes, or fats

a   47(K)   25.   Which of the following is a characteristic of enriched grain products?

    a.   They have all of the added nutrients listed on the label
    b.   They have the fiber restored from the refining procedure
    c.   They have virtually all the nutrients restored from refining procedure
    d.   They have only 4 vitamins and 4 minerals added by the food processor

c   47(K)   26.   What nutrient makes up most of the endosperm section of grains such as wheat and rice?

  a. Fat
  b. Fiber
  c. Starch
  d. Protein

d   47-48(A)   27.   Which of the following breads has the highest fiber content?

  a. White
  b. Refined
  c. Enriched
  d. Whole-grain

d   46-47(K)   28.   The part of the grain that remains after being subjected to refining is the

  a. bran.
  b. germ.
  c. husk.
  d. endosperm.

b   47-48(K)   29.   All of the following are features of the process of nutrient enrichment of flours EXCEPT

  a. it includes products such as pastas.
  b. fiber levels are similar to those in the whole grains.
  c. it is required of all refined grain products that cross state lines.
  d. thiamin and riboflavin are added in amounts exceeding their levels in the whole grain.

a   47-48(K)   30.   What mineral is added in the enrichment process of refined flours?

  a. Iron
  b. Iodine
  c. Calcium
  d. Magnesium

CHAPTER 3
DIGESTION, ABSORPTION, AND TRANSPORT

Ans   Page

b   66(K)   01.   What structure prevents food from entering the trachea when you swallow?

a.   Tongue
b.   Epiglottis
c.   Esophagus
d.   Cardiac sphincter

c   66(K)   02.   A bolus is conducted past the diaphragm through the

a.   epiglottis.
b.   stomach.
c.   esophagus.
d.   large intestine.

c   66(K)   03.   What is one function of the pyloric sphincter?

a.   Secretes acid into the stomach
b.   Secretes hormones into the stomach
c.   Prevents the contents of the intestines from backing up into the stomach
d.   Prevents the contents of the intestine from emptying too quickly into the colon

b   66-67(K)   04.   What structure separates the colon from the small intestine?

       a.   Pylorus
       b.   Ileocecal valve
       c.   Gastric retainer
       d.   Rectal sphincter

d   66(K)   05.   Into what region of the intestinal tract does the stomach empty?

       a.   Ileum
       b.   Cecum
       c.   Jejunum
       d.   Duodenum

b   66(K)   06.   What is a bolus?

       a.   Enzyme that hydrolyzes starch
       b.   Portion of food swallowed at one time
       c.   Device used to analyze the contents of the stomach
       d.   Sphincter muscle separating the stomach from the small intestine

b   66(K)   07.   Which of the following is a description of chyme?

       a.   The semisolid mass of undigested food which passes through the ileocecal valve
       b.   A semiliquid mass of partially digested food released by the stomach into the intestines
       c.   The mixture of pancreatic juices containing enzymes for digestion of the macronutrients
       d.   A thick, viscous material synthesized by mucosal cells for protection against digestive juices

c   66(A)   08.   After swallowing, in what order does food pass through the regions of the GI tract?

       a.   Jejunum, duodenum, colon, ileum, rectum
       b.   Jejunum, ileum, duodenum, rectum, colon
       c.   Stomach, duodenum, jejunum, ileum, colon
       d.   Stomach, jejunum, duodenum, colon, ileum

b   66(K)   09.   What structure functions to prevent entrance of food into the trachea?

    a.   Tongue
    b.   Epiglottis
    c.   Cardiac sphincter
    d.   Trachea sphincter

b   67(K)   10.   What structure controls the passage of material from the small intestines to the large intestines?

    a.   Pyloric valve
    b.   Ileocecal valve
    c.   Colonic sphincter
    d.   Jejunal sphincter

c   66-67(K)   11.   What is the primary function of the rectum?

    a.   Controls functioning of the colon
    b.   Absorbs minerals from waste materials
    c.   Stores waste materials prior to evacuation
    d.   Absorbs excess water from waste materials

a   66(K)   12.   What is the name given to partially digested food in the stomach?

    a.   Chyme
    b.   Liquid food
    c.   Gastric mucus
    d.   Semiliquid mass

b   66(K)   13.   Which of the following is a characteristic of the appendix?

    a.   It ferments fiber
    b.   It stores lymph cells
    c.   It slows down peristalsis
    d.   It stores preformed stools

c   66-67(K)   14.   Which of the following is <u>NOT</u> a sphincter muscle?

    a.   Anus
    b.   Cardiac
    c.   Duodenum
    d.   Ileocecal valve

a   66(K)   15.   What is mastication?

       a.   The act of chewing
       b.   The act of swallowing
       c.   The wave-like contraction of the intestines
       d.   The wave-like contraction of the esophagus

d   68-69(K)   16.   Which of the following is a feature of the muscular actions of digestion?

       a.   Persistalasis begins first in the stomach upon the initiation of the swallowing reflex
       b.   The colon has the thickest and strongest muscles of the GI organs to withstand the pressure of stool evaluation
       c.   The jejumun has a third layer of diagonal muscles to enhance contraction and relaxation phases for enhanced digestion
       d.   Segmentation in the intestines allows periodic squeezing along its length resulting in momentary reversal of the movement of intestinal contents

a   68(K)   17.   What is meant by the term "motility" in reference to the GI tract?

       a.   The efficiency of peristalsis
       b.   The efficiency of lymph transport
       c.   The speed of gastric digestive juice release
       d.   The speed of pancreatic digestive juice release

a   69(K)   18.   Among the GI tract organs, which has the strongest muscles?

       a.   Stomach
       b.   Small intestine
       c.   Large intestine
       d.   Cardiac sphincter

d   69(K)   19.   Which of the following is a function of sphincter muscles?

       a.   Control peristalsis
       b.   Grind large food particles
       c.   Secrete digestive juices into the GI tract
       d.   Control the passage of food through the GI tract

a   69-70(K)   20.   Which of the following body organs does <u>NOT</u> secrete digestive enzymes?

    a.   Liver
    b.   Stomach
    c.   Pancreas
    d.   Salivary glands

b   69(K)   21.   What is reflux?

    a.   Hard, dry, stools
    b.   Backward flow of chyme
    c.   Soft, poorly formed stools
    d.   The mixture of bile and pancreatic juice

d   70(K)   22.   What is the function of mucus in the stomach?

    a.   Emulsifies fats
    b.   Neutralizes stomach acid
    c.   Activates pepsinogen to pepsin
    d.   Protects stomach cells from gastric juices

d   70(K)   23.   What is a function of hydrochloric acid in the stomach?

    a.   Absorbs water
    b.   Inhibits peristalsis
    c.   Neutralizes the food mass
    d.   Creates an optimum acidity

b   70(K)   24.   What substance protects the stomach lining from damage due to digestive juices?

    a.   Water
    b.   Mucus
    c.   Pepsinogen
    d.   Dietary fats

a   70(K)   25.   Which of the following best describes the normal pH of the stomach?

    a.   Very acidic
    b.   Slightly acidic
    c.   Neutral
    d.   Slightly alkaline

d   70(A)   26.   Why is there little or no digestion of starch in the stomach?

a.   Mucus inhibits starch breakdown
b.   Stomach enzymes are dysfunctional
c.   Starch should not be eaten with protein
d.   Salivary enzyme does not work in an acid environment

a   70(A)   27.   What is the fate of any enzymes that are present in the foods we eat?

a.   Hydrolyzed in the GI tract
b.   Absorbed intact by the stomach
c.   Absorbed intact by the small intestine
d.   Passed through the GI tract and excreted in the stool

c   70(K)   28.   Which part of the GI tract contains highly acidic digestive juices?

a.   Colon
b.   Ileum
c.   Stomach
d.   Duodenum

a   70(K)   29.   Important functions of hydrochloric acid in digestion/absorption include all the following EXCEPT

a.   it activates pancreatic lipase.
b.   it kills pathogenic organisms.
c.   it activates a proteolytic enzyme.
d.   it promotes hydrolysis of dietary protein.

b   70(K)   30.   What is the substance that protects the stomach walls from digestion?

a.   Turns
b.   Mucus
c.   Pepsin
d.   Hydrochloric acid

a   70(A)   31.   The purpose of bicarbonate in the digestive process is to

a.   raise the pH of chyme.
b.   lower the pH of chyme.
c.   hydrolyze large peptides.
d.   provide a little fizz in your life.

d 70;89-90(K) 32. All of the following are features of stomach acid <u>EXCEPT</u>

  a. its secretion is stimulated by ingestion of regular coffee.
  b. its secretion is stimulated by ingestion of decaffeinated coffee.
  c. it destroys most of the bacteria entering the stomach from food ingestion.
  d. its potentially destructive action on stomach cells is prevented by the presence of bile.

a 70-71(K) 33. Which of the following is <u>NOT</u> a component of pancreatic juice?

  a. Bile
  b. Water
  c. Protease
  d. Sodium bicarbonate

d 70(A) 34. After the pancreatic juices have mixed with chyme in the intestine, which of the following describes the pH of the resulting mixture?

  a. Very acidic
  b. Slightly alkaline
  c. Strongly alkaline
  d. Approximately neutral

b 70-71(K) 35. Which of the following is <u>NOT</u> a component of pancreatic juice?

  a. Lipase
  b. Maltase
  c. Amylase
  d. Bicarbonate

b 70-71(A) 36. Which of the following would <u>NOT</u> be acted upon by pancreatic juice secreted into the intestinal tract?

  a. Fats
  b. Fiber
  c. Proteins
  d. Carbohydrates

a   70-71(K)   37.   What is one function of the gallbladder?

    a. Stores bile
    b. Produces bile
    c. Reabsorbs water and salts
    d. Performs enzymatic digestion

a   70-71(K)   38.   What is the function of bile?

    a. Emulsifies fats
    b. Initiates digestion of protein
    c. Enhances absorption of complex carbohydrates
    d. Protects the stomach and small intestine from the action of hydrochloric acid

c   71-72(A)   39.   Which of the following is NOT a typical component of stools?

    a. Water
    b. Fiber
    c. Starch
    d. Bacteria

b   71-72(A)   40.   What is the primary role of the normal, thriving intestinal bacterial population?

    a. Helps degrade meat and dairy proteins
    b. Helps prevent infectious bacteria from attacking the system
    c. Synthesizes most vitamins which can be absorbed into the body
    d. Synthesizes several amino acids which can be absorbed into the body

d   71-72(K)   41.   Which of the following is known to be produced by small intestinal bacteria?

    a. Mucus
    b. Chyme
    c. Glucose
    d. Vitamins

c   72(K)   42.   Which of the following classes of nutrients requires the least amount of digestion?

    a. Lipids
    b. Proteins
    c. Vitamins
    d. Carbohydrates

b   72(A)   43.   Which of the following nutrients requires the least amount of digestion?

    a. Starch
    b. Calcium
    c. Animal fats
    d. Animal proteins

b   72(K)   44.   Which of the following is generally NOT digested but does stimulate intestinal muscle contractions?

    a. Bile
    b. Fiber
    c. Starch
    d. Amylase

b   72(K)   45.   Which of the following is a significant property of dietary fiber?

    a. Inhibits protease activity
    b. Promotes water retention of stools
    c. Inhibits large intestinal contractions
    d. Promotes vitamin excretion in stools

d   72(A)   46.   An example of an important function of the colon would be its absorption of

    a. bile.
    b. fats.
    c. hormones.
    d. sodium chloride.

a   74-75(K)   47.   What is the name of the projections on the inner surface of the small intestine?

    a. Villi
    b. Cilia
    c. Mesenteric vessels
    d. Vascular projectiles

c   74-75(K)   48.   Which of the following is a function of the intestinal microvilli?

    a. Secretion of bile salts
    b. Secretion of digestive acid
    c. Transport of nutrient molecules
    d. Transport of pancreatic enzymes

c   74(K)   49.   What is the primary site for absorption of nutrients?

a.   Crypt
b.   Villus
c.   Microvillus
d.   Macrovillus

c   74-75(K)   50.   Which of the following are found on the microvilli and function to break apart small nutrients into the final products of digestion?

a.   Mucus
b.   Micelles
c.   Enzymes
d.   Hormones

b   76(K)   51.   Absorption of nutrients by intestinal cells occurs by all of the following mechanisms EXCEPT

a.   diffusion.
b.   transmigration.
c   active transport.
d.   facilitated diffusion.

a   76(A)   52.   To assist the process of digestion and absorption, it is usually best to

a.   combine different food types to enhance the absorption process.
b.   avoid eating meat and fruit at the same meal to prevent competition.
c.   eat several snacks per day so the system is not overwhelmed.
d.   take enzyme pills or powder periodically so the system can rest and rejuvenate.

a   76-77(A)   53.   What is the first vessel to receive absorbed water-soluble vitamins?

a.   Portal vein
b.   Hepatic vein
c.   Mesenteric vein
d.   Mesenteric artery

b   77-78(K)   54.   Blood leaving the digestive system goes by way of a vein to the

     a.   heart.
     b.   liver.
     c.   lungs.
     d.   kidneys.

a   76-77(A)   55.   When nutrients are transported from intestinal epithelial cells to the vascular system, what organ is first to receive them?

     a.   Liver
     b.   Heart
     c.   Lungs
     d.   Kidneys

a   78(A)   56.   When alcohol and barbiturates are ingested, they are absorbed from the gastrointestinal tract and transported first to the

     a.   liver.
     b.   heart.
     c.   spleen.
     d.   kidneys.

a   79(K)   57.   Which of the following products of digestion is NOT normally released directly into the bloodstream?

     a.   Fats
     b.   Minerals
     c.   Vitamin C
     d.   Carbohydrates

c   79(K)   58.   Immediately after absorption, what circulatory system carries the fat soluble vitamins and large fats?

     a.   Vascular
     b.   Mesenteric
     c.   Lymphatic
     d.   Enterohepatic

c   79(K)   59.   Which of the following conducts lymph into the vascular system?

     a.   Villi
     b.   Mesentery
     c.   Subclavian vein
     d.   Common bile duct

a   79(K)   60.   Which of the following is a feature of the lymphatic system?

     a.   It carries fats away from the intestines
     b.   It contains a fluid with a composition similar to pancreatic fluid
     c.   It circulates via a one-way pump at the junction to the subclavian vein
     d.   It serves to transport fat-soluble and water-soluble vitamins to the vascular system

b   79(K)   61.   What is the first major organ to receive nutrients that are absorbed into the lymph?

     a.   Liver
     b.   Heart
     c.   Spleen
     d.   Pancreas

b   80(K)   62.   What is the normal pH of the stomach?

     a.   0.25-0.50
     b.   1.5-1.7
     c.   7.0-7.5
     d.   9.5-9.75

a   80(K)   63.   Which of the following regulates the pH of the stomach?

     a.   Gastrin
     b.   Insulin
     c.   Secretin
     d.   Cholecystokinin

b   80(A)   64.   Which of the following substances functions to control the release of hydrochloric acid to prevent excessive acidity?

     a.   Fiber
     b.   Gastrin
     c.   Secretin
     d.   Bicarbonate

a   80-81(A)   65.   All of the following are important enterogastrome hormones EXCEPT

     a.   pepsin.
     b.   secretion,
     c.   cholecystokinin,
     d.   gastric-inhibitory peptide.

a   81(A)   66. Which of the following nutrients requires the greatest amount of digestion?

      a. Fats
      b. Water
      c. Minerals
      d. Carbohydrates

b   81(K)   67. Which of the following stimulates the pancreas to release bicarbonate-rich juice?

      a. Gastrin
      b. Secretin
      c. Glucagon
      d. Gastric-inhibitory peptide

d   81(K)   68. The presence of fat in the intestines stimulates cells of the intestinal wall to release

      a. lipase.
      b. gastrin.
      c. secretin.
      d. cholecystokinin.

b   81(K)   69. Which of the following is associated with the presence of fat in the GI tract?

      a. Inhibition of mucosal enzyme activities
      b. Slowing of the process of digestion and absorption
      c. Inhibition of thiamin, riboflavin, and niacin absorption
      d. Stimulation and hastening of digestion and absorption

c   801K)   70. What substance controls the release of bile into the small intestines?

      a. Gastrin
      b. Secretin
      c. Cholecystokinin
      d. Gastric-inhibitory peptide

d   81(A)   71. What is the very first thing you should do if you suspect someone is choking on food?

      a. Perform the Heimlich maneuver
      b. Strike the person sharply on the back
      c. Attempt to dislodge the food with your fingers
      d. Ask the person to make sounds from the throat

b 85(A) 72. Choking occurs when a piece of food becomes firmly lodged in the

  a. larynx.
  b. trachea.
  c. epiglottis.
  d. esophagus.

c 85(K) 73. Which of the following results from reverse peristalsis?

  a. Gas
  b. Choking
  c. Vomiting
  d. Diarrhea

a 87(A) 74. Chronic diarrhea may result in which of the following?

  a. Dehydration
  b. Constipation
  c. Peptic ulcers
  d. Heimlich's disease

a 86-87(K) 75. The Heimlich maneuver may be helpful in conditions associated with

  a. choking.
  b. vomiting.
  c. heartburn.
  d. constipation.

a 88(A) 76. People are said to be constipated when they experience

  a. painful or difficult bowel movements.
  b. more than a day without a bowel movement.
  c. more than three days without a bowel movement.
  d. soft or watery bowel movements with little notice.

b 88-89(A) 77. Therapy for constipation would include all of the following EXCEPT

  a. increasing water intake.
  b. decreasing fiber intake.
  c. increasing physical activity.
  d. responding promptly to the defecation signal.

c   88(A)   78.   Which of the following is most likely to result from insufficient intake of fiber?

        a.   Diarrhea
        b.   Bloating
        c.   Constipation
        d.   Pancreatitis

c   88(K)   79.   Which of the following is a common cause of constipation?

        a.   High-fat diet
        b.   High-carbohydrate diet
        c.   Lack of physical activity
        d.   Excessive mineral oil intake

b   89(A)   80.   Holding the breath for as long as possible is considered an effective treatment for

        a.   colitis.
        b.   hiccups.
        c.   belching.
        d.   gastro-esophogeal reflux.

d   89(A)   81.   People who have frequent regular bouts of heartburn and indigestion most likely have a condition known as

        a.   colitis.
        b.   watery stools.
        c.   lymphatic malabsorption.
        d.   gastro-esophageal reflux.

c   88(A)   82.   All of the following dietary measures are known to help relieve constipation EXCEPT

        a.   eating honey.
        b.   eating prunes.
        c.   eating less fat.
        d.   drinking more water.

d   89(A)   83.   The use of an antacid is indicated primarily for

        a.   excessive gas.
        b.   acid indigestion.
        c.   excessive belching.
        d.   active ulcer in the stomach.

b   90(K)   84. All of the following are major causes of ulcer formation EXCEPT

       a. bacterial infection.
       b. excessive use of antacids.
       c. excessive gastric acid secretion.
       d. use of certain anti-inflammatory medicines.

b   90(A)   85. Which of the following is least likely to aggravate an existing ulcer?

       a. Beer
       b. Raw carrots
       c. Regular coffee
       d. Decaffeinated coffee

d   90(A)   86. The organism *H. pylori* has been identified as one of the major causes of

       a. hiccups.
       b. hemorrhoids.
       c. diverticulosis.
       d. gastric ulcers.

a   90(A)   87. All of the following are important issues in the treatment or management of existing ulcers EXCEPT

       a. diet therapy plays a major role.
       b. alcohol intake should be curtailed.
       c. antibiotics are frequently administered.
       d. anti-inflammatory drug use should be curtailed.

Matching (Answers can be used only once)

D	66	88.	Controls the entry of chyme into the duodenum
O	66	89.	Controls the entry of chyme into the colon
J	66	90.	Prevents food from entering the windpipe when swallowing
H	66	91.	Organ that stores lymph cells
L	71	92.	Enzyme that digests starch
E	69	93.	Substance that helps make or break a chemical bond
R	70	94.	A component of gastric juice
K	70	95.	Organ that releases bile into intestines
A	70	96.	Organ that synthesizes bile
B	74	97.	Fingerlike projection of small intestinal lining
C	75	98.	Type of cell that secrets mucus
Q	76	99.	Absorption mechanism that requires energy
I	76	100.	Absorption mechanism that does not require energy
G	77	101.	Connects an artery to a vein
N	77	102.	Vessels that carries blood from liver to heart
M	77	103.	Vessels that carries blood from GI tract to liver
S	79	104.	Carries fat soluble vitamins
F	81	105.	Hormone that signals release of pancreatic bicarbonate
T	81	106.	Hormone that slows acid output of stomach
P	81	107.	Organ that signals release of bile

A.	Liver	K.	Gallbladder
B.	Villus	L.	Carbohydrase
C.	Goblet	M.	Portal vein
D.	Pylorus	N.	Hepatic vein
E.	Enzyme	O	Ileocecal valve
F.	Secretin	P.	Cholecystokinin
G.	Capillary	Q	Active transport
H.	Appendix	R.	Hydrochloric acid
I.	Diffusion	S.	Lymphatic system
J.	Epiglottis	T.	Gastric inhibitory peptide

Essay Questions

66-68   108. Name and describe the functions of the four major sphincter muscles which divide the GI tract into its principal regions.

66-72   109. Describe the major events of digestion that occur in the mouth, stomach, and small intestines.

70   110. What is the function of hydrochloric acid and why is it necessary in the process of digestion?

67-68;72   111. What is the primary function of the colon? What are the effects on colonic function from insufficient fluid intake, insufficient fiber intake, or intestinal infection?

73-77   112. Describe features of the small intestines that facilitate absorption.

80-81   113. Name and describe the functions of four major hormones involved in digestion/absorption.

CHAPTER 4
THE CARBOHYDRATES: SUGARS, STARCHES, AND FIBERS

Ans   Page

a   93(A)   01.   In which of the following are ample amounts of carbohydrates almost always found?

                         a.   Plant foods
                         b.   Health foods
                         c.   Animal products
                         d.   Protein-rich foods

d   93(K)   02.   What type of nutrient is starch?

                         a.   Fiber
                         b.   Gluten
                         c.   Simple carbohydrate
                         d.   Complex carbohydrate

b   93-94(K)   03.   How many carbon atoms are found in the ring structure of the most common monosaccharides in nutrition?

                         a.   5
                         b.   6
                         c.   8
                         d.   12

a   94(K)   04.   Which of the following is <u>NOT</u> a simple carbohydrate?

                         a.   Starches
                         b.   White sugar
                         c.   Disaccharides
                         d.   Monosaccharides

c   94(K)   05. The types of atoms found in a glucose molecule include all of the following <u>EXCEPT</u>

a.   carbon.
b.   oxygen.
c.   nitrogen.
d.   hydrogen.

c   94-97(K)   06. Typical dietary sources of carbohydrate include all of the following <u>EXCEPT</u>

a.   starch.
b.   maltose.
c.   glycogen.
d.   hemicellulose.

d   94-95(A)   07. Which of the following is <u>NOT</u> a characteristic of glucose?

a.   Monosaccharide
b.   Soluble in water
c.   Part of the sucrose molecule
d.   Sweeter tasting than sucrose

c   94-95(K)   08. What component accounts for the usually sweet taste of fruits?

a.   Fats
b.   Fiber
c.   Simple sugars
d.   Complex carbohydrates

a   96;   09. Milk that has been treated with a commercially available lactase preparation undergoes which of the following changes?
     102-104(A)

a.   Increase in sweetness
b.   Decrease in sweetness
c.   Increase in carbohydrate content
d.   Decrease in carbohydrate content

a   94(K)   10. Which of the following is known as blood sugar or dextrose?

a.   Glucose
b.   Maltose
c.   Sucrose
d.   Fructose

b   94-95(K)   11.   Which of the following is a component of all three dietary disaccharides?

    a.   Sucrose
    b.   Glucose
    c.   Fructose
    d.   Galactose

c   94(K)   12.   Which of the following is known as fruit sugar or levulose?

    a.   Maltose
    b.   Glucose
    c.   Fructose
    d.   Galactose

c   94(K)   13.   What is the sweetest tasting simple carbohydrate in the diet?

    a.   Glucose
    b.   Lactose
    c.   Fructose
    d.   Sucrose

d   95(K)   14.   What is the reaction that links two monsaccharides together?

    a.   Hydrolysis
    b.   Absorption
    c.   Disaccharide
    d.   Condensation

a   96(A)   15.   Which of the following is a byproduct of the condensation of two molecules of glucose?

    a.   Water
    b.   Oxygen
    c.   Hydrogen
    d.   Carbon dioxide

b   95(K)   16.   What is the composition of sucrose?

    a.   Two fructose units
    b.   One glucose and one fructose unit
    c.   One glucose and one galactose unit
    d.   One galactose and one fructose unit

a   95(A)   17.   The chemical reaction by which starch is split into mono-saccharides is termed

     a.   hydrolysis.
     b.   condensation.
     c.   gluconeogenesis.
     d.   homeostatic balancing.

a   95(K)   18.   What is the composition of maltose?

     a.   Two glucose units
     b.   One glucose and one fructose unit
     c.   One glucose and one galactose unit
     d.   One galactose and one fructose unit

d   96(K)   19.   What is the composition of lactose?

     a.   Two glucose units
     b.   Two fructose units
     c.   One glucose and one fructose unit
     d.   One glucose and one galactose unit

a   96(K)   20.   What is the principle carbohydrate of milk?

     a.   Lactose
     b.   Sucrose
     c.   Maltose
     d.   Glycogen

a   96(K)   21.   What is another name for lactose?

     a.   Milk sugar
     b.   Fruit sugar
     c.   Table sugar
     d.   Artificial sugar

b   96(K)   22.   Which of the following sugars is NOT found in plants?

     a.   Glucose
     b.   Lactose
     c.   Sucrose
     d.   Fructose

d   97(K)   23.   What is the name of the animal polysaccharide composed of glucose units?

                          a.   Fiber
                          b.   Enzyme
                          c.   Dextrin
                          d.   Glycogen

a   97(K)   24.   Glycogen is stored mainly in which of the following tissues?

                          a.   Muscle and liver
                          b.   Pancreas and kidneys
                          c.   Stomach and intestine
                          d.   Brain and red blood cells

b   94-98(A)   25.   Which of the following is NOT a rich source of dietary starch?

                          a.   Grains
                          b.   Fruits
                          c.   Tubers
                          d.   Legumes

c   97(K)   26.   Which of the following is a feature of glycogen?

                          a.   Found in plants
                          b.   Important as a dietary nutrient
                          c.   Virtually absent from animal meats
                          d.   Plays an insignificant role in the body

d   97(K)   27.   What is the primary storage form of carbohydrate in the body?

                          a.   Fiber
                          b.   Starch
                          c.   Glucose
                          d.   Glycogen

d   98(K)   28.   What is the staple grain of Canada, the United States, and Europe?

                          a.   Oats
                          b.   Rice
                          c.   Corn
                          d.   Wheat

b   98(K)   29.   What is the predominant grain product in much of South and
                            Central America?

                            a.   Rice
                            b.   Corn
                            c.   Millet
                            d.   Wheat

a   98-99(K)   30.   What are cellulose, pectin, hemicellulose, and lignin?

                            a.   Fibers
                            b.   Starches
                            c.   Sugar alcohols
                            d.   Artificial sweeteners

d   98-99(A)   31.   Which of the following is an example of the difference between
                            the chemical bonds in starch and those in cellulose?

                            a.   Starch bonds are single
                            b.   Starch bonds are fatty acids
                            c.   Cellulose bonds release energy
                            d.   Cellulose bonds are not hydrolyzed by human enzymes

c   98-99(K)   32.   Which of the following fibers is water insoluble?

                            a.   Gums
                            b.   Pectins
                            c.   Cellulose
                            d.   Mucilages

b   98-99(K)   33.   With few exceptions, which of the following characteristics are
                            shared by water-soluble and water-insoluble fibers?

                            a.   Neither can be used as an energy source by the body
                            b.   Both retard absorption of glucose from the intestines
                            c.   Neither has an appreciable affect on intestinal transit time
                            d.   Both lower blood cholesterol levels in people with high
                                 blood cholesterol concentrations

a   98-99(K)   34.   Which of the following plays a major role in the breakdown of
                            certain types of dietary fiber reaching the large intestines?

                            a.   Bacteria
                            b.   Pancreas
                            c.   Colonic cells
                            d.   Small intestinal villus cells

d   98-99;   35.   Which of the following is a characteristic of dietary fiber?
114-115(K)

    a.   Causes diverticulosis
    b.   Usually found in high fat foods
    c.   Raises blood cholesterol levels
    d.   Classified according to solubility in water

d   98-99;   36.   Which of the following contains the LEAST amount of fiber?
116-117(A)

    a.   Apples
    b.   Prunes
    c.   Potatoes
    d.   White rice

a   99(K)   37.   Which of the following is a feature of the pectins?

    a.   They are used to thicken jelly
    b.   They are classified as insoluble fibers
    c.   They are resistant to intestinal bacterial fermentation
    d.   They are found in the small seeds of fruits such as strawberries

c   98-99(K)   38.   Water soluble fibers include all of the following EXCEPT

    a.   gums.
    b.   pectins.
    c.   lignins.
    d.   mucilages.

a   100(K)   39.   Characteristics of dietary phytic acid include all of the following EXCEPT

    a.   it is classified as a fiber.
    b.   it is found in the husks of grains.
    c.   it is synonymous with the term phytate.
    d.   it inhibits absorption of several minerals.

b   100(K)   40.   Which of the following describes the compound phytic acid?

    a.   Product of starch digestion
    b.   Nonnutrient component of plant seeds
    c.   Found in gastric juice and helps to lower pH of chyme
    d.   Found in high concentrations in the blood of people with diabetes

d   100(K)   41.   What is the name of the short chains of glucose units that result from starch breakdown?

     a.   Sucrose
     b.   Lignins
     c.   Pectins
     d   Dextrins

a   100-101(K)   42.   Digestion of starches takes place in the small intestines and also in the

     a.   mouth.
     b.   colon.
     c.   stomach.
     d.   pancreas.

c   100-102(K)   43.   Which of the following enzymes does NOT act on simple sugars?

     a.   Lactase
     b.   Sucrase
     c.   Amylase
     d.   Maltase

d   100-102(K)   44.   What is the primary absorption site for digestible carbo-hydrates?

     a.   Mouth
     b.   Stomach
     c.   Large intestines
     d.   Small intestines

d   102(K)   45.   Where is the location of enzymes that digest dietary sugars?

     a.   Mouth
     b.   Stomach
     c.   Pancreas
     d.   Small intestines

a   102(K)   46.   What is the primary organ that converts fructose to glucose following absorption?

     a.   Liver
     b.   Pancreas
     c.   Skeletal muscle
     d.   Small intestines

b   102(K)   47.   What is the first organ to receive carbohydrates absorbed from
                             the intestine?

                             a.   Heart
                             b.   Liver
                             c.   Pancreas
                             d.   Skeletal muscle

c   102(A)   48.   Which of the following is a feature of resistant starch?

                             a.   It is common in overripe bananas
                             b.   Excessive intake promotes constipation
                             c.   It resists hydrolysis by digestive enzymes
                             d.   It cannot be fermented by large intestinal bacteria

d   103-104(K)   49.   All of the following are symptoms of lactose intolerance
                             EXCEPT

                             a.   nausea.
                             b.   diarrhea.
                             c.   cramping.
                             d.   constipation.

a   103(K)   50.   What percentage of the world's adult population shows good
                             tolerance to lactose ingestion?

                             a.   30
                             b.   55
                             c.   80
                             d.   95

b   103-104(A)   51.   Which of the following would LEAST likely be associated with
                             the development of lactose intolerance?

                             a.   Medicines
                             b.   Milk allergy
                             c.   Prolonged diarrhea
                             d.   Inherited lactase deficiency

c   104(A)   52.   A person diagnosed with milk allergy would be sensitive to the
                             milk's

                             a.   fat.
                             b.   lactose.
                             c.   protein.
                             d.   minerals.

d   104(K)   53.   Among the following population groups, which shows the highest prevalence of lactose intolerance?

      a.   Hispanics
      b.   Caucasians
      c.   Scandinavians
      d.   African Americans

b   103-104(A)   54.   For most of the world's population, what is the effect of aging on the activity of lactase?

      a.   Declines by 30-40%
      b.   Declines by 90-95%
      c.   Increases by 30-40%
      d.   Increases by 90-95%

c   103-104(A)   55.   Which of the following ingredients listed on food labels would be acceptable to the person who is highly intolerant to lactose in the diet?

      a.   Whey
      b.   Casein
      c.   Dextrins
      d.   Milk solids

d   104(K)   56.   Which of the following is a feature of lactose?

      a.   Its digestion begins in the mouth
      b.   It is found in various amounts in most animal foods
      c.   It causes frequent allergies in certain population groups
      d.   It is used as a filler in one out of five prescription drugs

d   104(K)   57.   Among the following foods, which contains the lowest amount of lactose per serving?

      a.   Doughnut
      b.   Ice cream
      c.   Cottage cheese
      d.   American cheese

b   104(A)   58.   Which of the following is a feature of acidophilus milk?

      a.   It is virtually free of lactose
      b.   It contains live bacterial organisms
      c.   Its low pH results in hydrolysis of the lactose
      d.   It is a recommended substitute for people with milk allergy

b   104(K)   59.   Why are hard cheeses lower in lactose than soft cheeses?

a.   The lactose molecules bond to casein.
b.   More lactose is removed during manufacturing
c.   The bacterial culture is selected to degrade more of the lactose
d.   The lactose molecules condense to form a poorly digested oligosaccharide

a   104(K)   60.   Which of the following is a characteristic of yogurt?

a.   Bacteria in the product produce lactase
b.   It is poorly tolerated in lactose-intolerant people
c.   There are only trace amounts of lactose present
d.   The lactose content is about one-half that of milk

a   104(K)   61.   What is the chief reason that many people with lactose-intolerance can nonetheless learn a strategy for consuming foods containing some lactase without suffering any symptoms?

a.   A change occurs in the GI bacteria
b.   Intestinal lactase enzyme can re-appear in adequate amounts
c.   The lactose-containing foods must be eaten only as part of a full meal
d.   The lactose-containing foods must first be heated to 100°C to degrade lactose

d   105(A)   62.   Gluconeogenesis is a term that describes the synthesis of

a.   amino acids from glucose.
b.   lactose from a source of sucrose.
c.   fat from excess carbohydrate intake.
d.   glucose from a noncarbohydrate substance.

b   106(K)   63.   What is the minimum daily amount of dietary carbohydrate necessary to spare body protein from excessive breakdown?

a.   10-25 g
b.   50-100 g
c.   150-175 g
d.   200-400 g

b   106(K)   64.   What is the primary function of insulin?

a. Raises blood glucose levels
b. Lowers blood glucose levels
c. Stimulates glycogen breakdown
d. Stimulates intestinal carbohydrate absorption

b   106-107(A) 65.   Which of the following is a typical response of the body to changes in blood glucose?

a. Blood glucose levels that fall too low signal the release of insulin
b. Blood glucose levels that fall too low signal the release of glucagon
c. Blood glucose levels that rise too high signal the release of glycogen
d. Blood glucose levels that rise too high signal the release of epinephrine

d   106(A)   66.   What is the first organ to respond to an increase in blood glucose concentration?

a. Brain
b. Liver
c. Muscle
d. Pancreas

b   106-107(A) 67.   When blood glucose concentration falls, what pancreatic hormone is secreted to stimulate release of stored glucose?

a. Insulin
b. Glucagon
c. Epinephrine
d. Cholecystokinin

c   106(A)   68.   Which of the following expressions falls within the normal range of blood glucose?

a. 40 mg/dl
b. 75 mg/dl
c. 110 mg/dl
d. 140 mg/dl

b   106(K)   69.   What is a normal range for blood glucose?

      a.   60-80 mg/dl
      b.   80-120 mg/dl
      c.   120-140 mg/dl
      d.   140-180 mg/dl

d   107-105(A) 70.   When you are under physical stress, what hormone is released quickly to stimulate an increase in blood glucose concentration?

      a.   Insulin
      b.   Secretin
      c.   Glucogen
      d.   Epinephrine

d   108(K)   71.   Which of the following is a feature of diabetes?

      a.   Type I diabetes is also known as adult-onset diabetes
      b.   It is believed to be caused by abnormal intake of dietary carbohydrates
      c.   The insulin-dependent type is more common than the noninsulin-dependent type
      d.   Dietary management should focus on total carbohydrate intake rather than the type of carbohydrate consumed

a   108(K)   72.   Which of the following statements describes the glycemic effect of foods?

      a.   A measure of how fast and high the food causes the blood glucose to rise
      b.   The newest, most practical means for planning diets for people with diabetes
      c.   A well-utilized, highly valued mechanism to control the intake of simple sugars
      d.   A measure of the percentage of digestible carbohydrates in relation to total energy content of the food

a   108(A)   73,   Which of the following blood glucose concentration is most consistent with hypoglycemia?

      a.   40 mg/dl
      b.   80 mg/dl
      c.   115 mg/dl
      d.   150 mg/dl

c   108-109   74. In a person with type 2 diabetes, which of the following foods would ordinarily show the LEAST favorable glycemic effect?

    a. Chocolate
    b. Ice cream
    c. Baked potato
    d. Baked beans

a   108(K)   75. Which of the following is a feature of diabetes?

    a. Many people with type 2 diabetes are obese
    b. Most people who have diabetes require insulin therapy
    c. Diabetes results chiefly from excess dietary intake of simple carbohydrates
    d. People with type I diabetes fail to respond to the insulin made by the pancreas

b   111(K)   76. Approximately how many pounds of added sugars are consumed by the average U.S. resident each year?

    a. 25
    b. 65
    c. 105
    d. 190

b   110(A)   77. What is the name of the sweetener consisting of a mixture of glucose and fructose formed by chemical hydrolysis of sucrose?

    a. Molasses
    b. Invert sugar
    c. Turbinado sugar
    d. High-fructose syrup

d   110(K)   78. What is the predominant sweetener used in formulating beverages?

    a. Glucose
    b. Sucrose
    c. Invert sugar
    d. High-fructose corn syrup

a   110(K)   79.   Which of the following sweeteners contains a significant amount of iron?

    a.   Molasses
    b.   Brown sugar
    c.   Maple sugar
    d.   Invert sugar

c   112(A)   80.   Which of the following is best known to result from regular ingestion of sugar?

    a.   Ulcers
    b.   Diabetes
    c.   Dental caries
    d.   Cardiovascular disease

d   112-113(K)   81.   Which of the following is among food intake recommendations for reducing the incidence of dental caries when the diet contains sugary foods?

    a.   Eat sugary foods separate from meals
    b.   Eat dried fruits in place of whole fruits
    c.   Sip a sugary soft drink slowly rather than quickly
    d.   Eat a sugary snack all at one time rather than in parts throughout the day

c   112-113(A)   82.   Which of the following describes a relationship between carbohydrate intake and dental health?

    a.   Starches can not promote the formation of dental caries
    b.   After exposure to a single snack, mouth bacteria produce acid for 50-60 minutes
    c.   Eating a sugary dessert at the beginning of a meal, rather than the end, is less likely to promote dental caries
    d.   Sugar consumed in a soft drink promotes more bacterial fermentation than the same amount of sugar in a doughnut

a   113(K)   83.   Which of the following correlates most strongly with deaths from heart disease?

    a.   Obesity
    b.   High fiber intake
    c.   High sugar intake
    d.   High corn syrup intake

b   113(K)   84.   According to the current dietary recommendations, what is the maximum percentage of total energy intake that sugar should contribute in the diet?

    a.   5
    b.   10
    c.   15
    d.   20

d   114-115(K)   85.   Which of the following is <u>NOT</u> a feature of high-fiber foods?

    a.   Effective in weight control
    b.   Provide feeling of fullness
    c.   Usually lower in fat and simple sugars
    d.   Provide more energy per gram than processed foods

b   114-115(A)   86.   In general, a diet that is modified by substituting complex carbohydrates for pure sugars results in a diet that is higher in

    a.   fat.
    b.   fiber.
    c.   energy.
    d.   refined foods.

c   116(K)   87.   According to most dietary guidelines, what percentage of the day's total energy intake should be furnished by carbohydrates?

    a.   10-15
    b.   30-35
    c.   55-60
    ·d.   90-95

a   116(K)   88.   According to the American Dietetic Association, what is the recommended daily intake of dietary fiber?

    a.   20-35 g
    b.   40-50 g
    c.   55-70 g
    d.   75-100 g

c   116(K)   89.   What is the average daily intake of fiber in the United States?

    a.   1 g
    b.   5 g
    c.   10 g
    d.   25 g

c   116-117(K)   90.   Which of the following provides the most fiber?

       a.   1 orange
       b.   1/2 c. oatmeal
       c.   1/2 c. split peas
       d.   1/2 c. green peas

c   123-127(K)   91.   All of the following are features of artificial sweeteners EXCEPT

       a.   there is a lack of scientific consensus on their benefits for weight reduction.
       b.   there is an Acceptable Daily Intake which provides a wide margin of safety.
       c.   they provide about one-half the energy of carbohydrates plus small amounts of vitamins and minerals.
       d.   if used, the American Dietetics Association advises moderate intake and only in a well-balanced, nutritious diet.

a   123(K)   92.   What is stevia?

       a.   An herb-derived sweetener
       b.   An FDA-approved sugar alcohol
       c.   A poorly digested polysaccharide
       d.   An inhibitor of lactase enzyme activity

d   124-125(K)   93.   Which of the following is a feature of aspartame?

       a.   Its sweetness increases with heat
       b.   It is made up of three amino acids
       c.   It is recommended for people with PKU
       d.   Two of its breakdown products include methanol and formaldehyde

b   124(K)   94.   Among the following approved sweeteners, which has the highest relative sweetness?

       a.   Sacharin
       b.   Sucralose
       c.   Aspartame
       d.   Acesulfame-k

b   125-126(K)   95.   Among the alternative sweeteners available in the United States, which has a structure that intergrates chlorine atoms?

     a. Sacharin
     b. Sucralose
     c. Aspartame
     d. Acesulfame-k

d   127(K)   96.   Which of the following is a general feature of the sugar alcohols?

     a.   They provide less than 1 kcal/g
     b.   They elicit a high glycemic index
     c.   They are rapidly absorbed from the intestines
     d.   They inhibit the growth of caries-causing bacteria

d   127-128(K)   97.   Which of the following is <u>NOT</u> a classification for the food additives mannitol, sorbitol, and xylitol?

     a.   Carbohydrates
     b.   Sugar alcohols
     c.   Sugar replacers
     d.   Artificial sweeteners

c   127(K)   98.   Which of the following is a characteristic of the sugar alcohols?

     a.   Not sweet
     b.   Not metabolized
     c.   Contain kcalories
     d.   Promote dental caries

c   127(K)   99.   When consumed in excess, which of the following is most likely to lead to diarrhea?

     a.   Fiber
     b.   Sucrose
     c.   Sorbitol
     d.   Wheat starch

b   127(K)   100.   What is the approximate energy content of most sugar alcohols?

     a.   0 kcal/g
     b.   2-3 kcal/g
     c.   4 kcal/g
     d.   7 kcal/g

a   127(K)   101.   Which of the following is a characteristic of the sugar alcohols?

    a.   They promote a low glycemic index
    b.   They promote constipation in children
    c.   They are less effective than alternative sweeteners in inhibiting dental caries
    d.   They demonstrate fewer GI side effects than the alternative sweeteners

Matching (Answers can be used only once)

H	95	102.	Disaccharide containing fructose
R	95	103.	Chemical reaction that links two molecules together
O	95	104.	Chemical reaction that splits a larger molecule into smaller molecules
L	97	105.	A complex carbohydrate in muscle
G	97	106.	A complex carbohydrate in legumes
N	98	107.	Structurally similar to starch but resistant to digestion
D	99	108.	A water-soluble fiber
J	99	109.	A water-insoluble fiber
S	102	110.	Site where digestion of disaccharides takes place
F	100	111.	Site where digestion of starch begins
T	102	112.	Site where fibers may be metabolized to short-chain fatty acids
I	104	113.	When digested, yields galactose
M	107	114.	Substance that signals the release of glucose into blood
E	106	115.	Substance that signals removal of glucose from the blood
Q	107	116.	Stress hormone that modulates blood glucose from the blood
B	113	117.	Recommended upper limit of simple carbohydrate intake, expressed in kcal, from a 2,600 kcal diet
C	116	118.	Recommended intake of carbohydrate, in grams, from a 2,600 kcal diet
P	124	119.	Safe sweetener, except for people with PKU
K	127	120.	A sugar alcohol
A	106	121.	Normal blood glucose level, in mg per 100 ml blood

A.	100	K.	Sorbitol
B.	260	L.	Glycogen
C.	380	M.	Glucagon
D.	Pectin	N.	Cellulose
E.	Insulin	O.	Hydrolysis
F.	Mouth	P.	Aspartame
G.	Starch	Q.	Epinephrine
H.	Sucrose	R.	Condensation
I.	Lactose	S.	Small intestine
J.	Lignin	T.	Large intestine

Essay Questions

93-102   122   Compare and contrast the chemical makeup, major food sources, and digestion/absorption of simple and complex carbohydrates.

98-100   123.   Give several examples of soluble and insoluble dietary fibers. List food sources of these fibers. Contrast the physical characteristics and features of these two types of fiber and their effects on gastrointestinal tract function.

99-100;   124.   List and discuss seven benefits of fiber.
114-117

103-124   125.   Discuss the meaning, significance, and features of lactose intolerance.

105-108   126.   Describe the body's mechanisms for controlling blood glucose levels under normal and stress conditions.

108-109   127. Discuss the pros and cons of using the glycemic index in meal planning for people with diabetes.

111-113   128. List four common accusations made against dietary sugar. What is the evidence for and against these accusations?

114-115   129. Discuss the interactions between fiber and bile.

114   130. Discuss the possible reasons that explain why diets rich in complex carbohydrates may lower the risk of heart disease.

111   131. How is fiber thought to exert an influence over cancer of the colon?

115-116   132. What are potential hazards of consuming too much fiber? Give examples of the circumstances, conditions, and forms in which a person might ingest large amounts of fiber.

123-127   133. Discuss the contribution of artificial sweeteners to the diet and their role in weight control.

127   134. Describe the benefits and adverse effects of the common sugar replacers (sugar alcohols).

CHAPTER 5
THE LIPIDS: TRIGLYCERIDES, PHOSPHOLIPIDS, AND STEROLS

Ans   Page

c   130(K)   01.   Approximately what percentage of the lipids in foods are triglycerides?

a. 5
b. 30
c. 95
d. 100

c   130(K)   02.   What is the chemical composition of fats?

a. Hexose polymers
b. Glycogen granules
c. Fatty acids and glycerol
d. Combinations of long chain fatty acids

b   130(A)   03.   A compound composed of carbon, hydrogen, and oxygen with 3 fatty acids attached to a molecule of glycerol would be known as a

a. diglyceride.
b. triglyceride.
c. phospholipid.
d. monoglyceride.

c   130(K)   04.   What compound is composed of 3 fatty acids and glycerol?

     a.   Steroid
     b.   Lecithin
     c.   Triglyceride
     d.   Monoglyceride

c   130(K)   05.   What percentage of stored body fat is in the form of triglycerides?

     a.   2
     b.   50
     c.   78
     d.   99

b   130(K)   06.   What is the simplest fatty acid found in the diet?

     a.   Oleic acid
     b.   Acetic acid
     c.   Linoleic acid
     d.   Palmitic acid

c   130(K)   07.   In which form are most dietary lipids found?

     a.   Sterols
     b.   Glycerols
     c.   Triglycerides
     d.   Monoglycerides

c   131(K)   08.   Which of the following describes a fatty acid that has one double bond?

     a.   Saturated
     b.   Hydrogenated
     c.   Monounsaturated
     d.   Polyunsaturated

b   131-132(K)   09.   Lipids differ in their degree of saturation or unsaturation due to their number of

     a.   amino acids.
     b.   double bonds.
     c.   saccharide units.
     d.   peptide linkages.

b   131(K)   10.   Which type of fatty acid is found in high amounts in olive oil?

　　　　　　　　　　a.   Saturated
　　　　　　　　　　b.   Monounsaturated
　　　　　　　　　　c.   Polyunsaturated
　　　　　　　　　　d.   Partially hydrogenated

b   131-132(A)   11.   Which one of the following compounds is missing 4 or more hydrogen atoms?

　　　　　　　　　　a.   Monounsaturated fatty acid
　　　　　　　　　　b.   Polyunsaturated fatty acid
　　　　　　　　　　c.   Long chain saturated fatty acid
　　　　　　　　　　d.   Short chain saturated fatty acid

b   131(K)   12.   Which of the following is a common dietary saturated fatty acid?

　　　　　　　　　　a.   Oleic acid
　　　　　　　　　　b.   Stearic acid
　　　　　　　　　　c.   Linolenic acid
　　　　　　　　　　d.   Arachidonic acid

b   131(K)   13.   Approximately how many carbons are contained in a medium-chain fatty acid?

　　　　　　　　　　a.   2-4
　　　　　　　　　　b.   6-10
　　　　　　　　　　c.   12-22
　　　　　　　　　　d.   24-26

d   131(A)   14.   Which of the following is a source of medium-chain fatty acids?

　　　　　　　　　　a.   Fish oils
　　　　　　　　　　b.   Beef products
　　　　　　　　　　c.   Vegetable oils
　　　　　　　　　　d.   Dairy products

b   131-132(A)   15.   Which of the following chemical characteristics of fatty acids determines their susceptibility to spoilage by oxygen?

　　　　　　　　　　a.   Chain length
　　　　　　　　　　b.   Number of double bonds
　　　　　　　　　　c.   Position of first saturated bond
　　　　　　　　　　d.   Size of adjacent fatty acids on the triglyceride molecule

c   132(K)   16.   What is the most common polyunsaturated fatty acid in foods?

a. Oleic acid
b. Stearic acid
c. Linoleic acid
d. Linolenic acid

c   132-133(A)   17.   Of the following foods, which has the highest percentage of its fat in saturated form?

a. Butter
b. Soybean
c. Coconut
d. Beef tallow

b   132-133(A)   18.   Of the following foods, which has the highest percentage of its fat in polyunsaturated form?

a. Butter
b. Soybean
c. Coconut
d. Beef tallow

a   132(K)   19.   Which of the following is considered a major source of polyunsaturated fat?

a. Corn oil
b. Palm oil
c. Peanut oil
d. Chicken fat

d   132-134(A)   20.   Characteristics of hydrogenated oils include all of the following EXCEPT

a. they are stored in adipose tissue.
b. they lower HDL and raise LDL cholesterol in the body.
c. some of their fatty acids change shape from cis to trans.
d. products containing them become rancid sooner, contributing to a shorter shelf life.

d   133-134(A)   21.   Which of the following sources would yield the softest lipids at room temperature?

a. Lard
b. Beef
c. Pork
d. Safflower

a   133-134(A)   22.   Which of the following is a feature of polyunsaturated fats?

    a.   Low melting point
    b.   High melting point
    c.   Solid at room temperature
    d.   Solid at refrigerator temperature

a   133-134(A)   23.   All of the following are rich sources of polyunsaturated fatty acids EXCEPT

    a.   palm oil.
    b.   fish oils.
    c.   soybean oil.
    d.   safflower oil.

d   133-134(A)   24.   Which of the following characteristics is shared by olive oil and canola oil?

    a.   Neither is liquid at room temperature
    b.   Neither contains saturated fatty acids
    c.   Both contain high levels of polyunsaturated fatty acids
    d.   Both contain high levels of monounsaturated fatty acids

b   133-134(A)   25.   Which of the following is a factor that determines the hardness of a fat at a given temperature?

    a.   Origin of the fat
    b.   Degree of saturation
    c.   Number of acid groups
    d.   Number of oxygen atoms

a   134(A)   26.   A major cause of rancidity of lipids in foods is exposure to

    a.   heat and oxygen.
    b.   fluorescent lighting.
    c.   freezer temperatures.
    d.   enrichment additives.

c   134(A)   27.   When stored at room temperature in loosely capped containers, which of the following dietary lipids would turn rancid in the shortest time?

    a.   Lard
    b.   Peanut oil
    c.   Soybean oil
    d.   Coconut oil

d   134(A)   28.   All of the following are methods used by food processors to stabilize the lipids in food products <u>EXCEPT</u>

    a.   refrigeration.
    b.   hydrogenation.
    c.   tightly sealed packaging.
    d.   addition of oxidizing chemicals.

d   134(A)   29.   Which of the following would be <u>LEAST</u> effective at preventing oxidation of the polyunsaturated fatty acids in processed foods?

    a.   Refrigeration
    b.   Addition of BHT
    c.   Partial hydrogenation
    d.   Addition of phosphorus

b   134(A)   30.   In the process of fat hydrogenation, hydrogen atoms are added to which part of the molecule?

    a.   Oxygen
    b.   Carbon
    c.   Glycerol
    d.   Other hydrogens

a   134-135(A) 31.   An oil that is partially hydrogenated sometimes changes one or more of its double bond configurations from

    a.   <u>cis</u> to <u>trans</u>.
    b.   solid to liquid.
    c.   covalent to ionic.
    d.   saturated to unsaturated.

d   134-135(K) 32.   Which of the following is descriptive of fatty acid configuration?

    a.   A <u>cis</u>-fatty acid has an extended, linear formation
    b.   A <u>trans</u>-fatty acid has a folded, U-shape formation
    c.   <u>Trans</u>-fatty acids are made only from polyunsaturated fats
    d.   Naturally occurring <u>trans</u>-fatty acids are found in dairy products

d   136(K)   33.   The composition of lecithin could include all of the following EXCEPT

     a.   choline.
     b.   phosphate.
     c.   fatty acids.
     d   magnesium.

d   136-137(A) 34.   Which of the following characteristics are <u>shared</u> by cholesterol and lecithin?

     a.   Both are sterols
     b.   Both are phospholipids
     c.   Both are essential nutrients
     d.   Both are synthesized in the body

d   136(K)   35.   What type of compound is lecithin?

     a.   Bile salt
     b.   Glycolipid
     c.   Lipoprotein
     d.   Phospholipid

d   136-137(A) 36.   Which of the following is <u>NOT</u> a feature of lecithin?

     a.   Widespread in foods
     b.   Found in cell membranes
     c.   Manufactured by the body
     d.   Dietary supplements inhibit fat absorption

d   136;   37.   Each of the following may act as an emulsifier in the intestinal
      139-140 (A)   tract EXCEPT

     a.   lecithin
     b.   bile acids
     c.   bile phospolipids
     d.   pancreatic lipase

c   137-138(A) 38.   Which of the following foods contains cholesterol?

     a.   Corn
     b.   Olives
     c.   Roasted turkey
     d.   Roasted peanuts

c   137(K)   39.   What is the major sterol in the diet?

        a.   Palm oil
        b.   Lecithin
        c.   Cholesterol
        d.   Arachidonic acid

a   137(A)   40.   Which of the following CANNOT be found in plants?

        a.   Cholesterol
        b.   Triglycerides
        c.   Essential fatty acids
        d.   Nonessential fatty acids

a   137-138(A)   41.   Which of the following is a feature of cholesterol?

        a.   Synthesized by the body
        b.   No relation to heart disease
        c.   Recommended intake is zero
        d.   No function in the human body

b   137(A)   42.   Which of the following contains the LEAST cholesterol per serving size?

        a.   Steamed fish
        b.   Steamed corn
        c.   Broiled chicken
        d.   Very lean grilled steak

b   137(K)   43.   Which of the following is a characteristic of cholesterol?

        a.   It is absorbed directly into the blood
        b.   It is a precursor for bile and vitamin D synthesis
        c.   It is not formed in the body when provided by the diet
        d.   It is found in abundance in tropical fats such as palm oil

b   137-138(K)   44.   All of the following compounds may be synthesized from cholesterol EXCEPT

        a.   bile.
        b.   glucose.
        c.   vitamin D.
        d.   sex hormones.

d   137(A)   45.   What is the usual fate of dietary lecithin?

    a.   Unabsorbed and passes out in the feces
    b.   Absorbed intact and incorporated into tissues
    c.   Absorbed intact and broken down by the liver
    d.   Hydrolyzed by the intestinal enzyme lecithinase

a   137-138(K) 46.   Which of the following is a feature of cholesterol?

    a.   Its synthesis in the body is partially regulated by insulin
    b.   Most of the body's cholesterol is found circulating in the bloodstream
    c.   The amount consumed in the diet usually exceeds the amount synthesized in the body
    d.   It can be synthesized in the body from fat or carbohydrate but not from protein

d   137(A)   47.   How much energy is contributed by one gram of lecithin in a food supplement?

    a.   0 kcal
    b.   4 kcal
    c.   7 kcal
    d.   9 kcal

c   137(A)   48.   What is the approximate energy value of one teaspoon of liquid lecithin supplement?

    a.   0 kcal
    b.   2 kcal
    c.   45 kcal
    d.   200 kcal

c   137-138(K) 49.   Which of the following is a feature of cholesterol?

    a.   Good cholesterol is a form of cholesterol found in plant foods
    b.   Bad cholesterol is a form of cholesterol found in plant foods
    c.   Only about 10% of the body's total cholesterol is extracellular
    d.   Exogenous cholesterol absorption is reduced by lecithin supplements

c   138;148(A)   50.   Which of the following is NOT a destination for cholesterol?

    a.   Synthesized into bile
    b.   Excreted in the feces
    c.   Accumulates on walls of veins
    d.   Accumulates on walls of arteries

a   138(K)   51.   What term may be used to describe a substance that is hydrophobic?

    a.   Lipophilic
    b.   Lipophobic
    c.   Glycerophilic
    d.   Glycerophobic

c   138(K)   52.   Which of the following is characteristic of the enzyme lipase?

    a.   Gastric lipase plays a significant role in fat digestion in adults
    b.   Intestinal mucosal lipase is responsible for most dietary fat digestion
    c.   Salivary gland lipase (lingual lipase) plays a significant role in fat digestion in infants
    d.   Pancreatic lipase hydrolyzes most dietary triglycerides completely to glycerol and free fatty acids

c   138-140(K)   53.   What part of the gastrointestinal tract is the predominant site of dietary fat hydrolysis?

    a.   Mouth
    b.   Stomach
    c.   Small intestine
    d.   Large intestine

c   139-140(K)   54.   Which of the following is NOT a feature of the bile acids?

    a.   Stored in the gallbladder
    b.   Synthesized from cholesterol
    c.   Manufactured by the gallbladder
    d.   Released into the intestines whenever fat is present

a   139-140(A)   55.   Bile is known to assist in the absorption of

    a.   fat only.
    b.   all nutrients.
    c.   carbohydrate and fat only.
    d.   carbohydrate, fat, and protein only.

CHAPTER 6
PROTEIN: AMINO ACIDS

Ans   Page

d   168(K)   01.   What element is found in proteins but <u>NOT</u> in carbohydrates
                          and fats?

                          a.   Carbon
                          b.   Oxygen
                          c.   Calcium
                          d.   Nitrogen

d   168(K)   02.   How many different kinds of amino acids make up proteins?

                          a.   8
                          b.   10
                          c.   14
                          d.   20

c   168K)   03.   In comparison to the composition of carbohydrates and fats,
                          which element found in proteins makes then unique?

                          a.   Carbon
                          b.   Oxygen
                          c.   Nitrogen
                          d.   Hydrogen

c   168(K)   04.   All of the following are contained in an amino acid <u>EXCEPT</u>

                          a.   an acid group.
                          b.   an amino group.
                          c.   an aldehyde group.
                          d.   a central carbon atom.

1

a   168(K)   05.   Which of the following is the primary factor that differentiates one amino from another?

a.   The side group
b.   The central carbon atom
c.   The number of oxygen atoms
d.   The number of nitrogen atoms

c   168(A)   06.   Approximately how many different amino acids are used in the synthesis of body proteins?

a.   5
b.   10
c.   20
d.   35

c   168-169(K)   07.   Terms used to classify amino acids in the diet include all of the following EXCEPT

a.   essential.
b.   nonessential.
c.   partially essential.
d.   conditionally essential.

b   169(K)   08.   What is the simplest amino acid?

a.   Valine
b.   Glycine
c.   Alanine
d.   Methionine

a   168-169(K)   09.   Which of the following is NOT an essential amino acid in human nutrition?

a.   Proline
b.   Threonine
c.   Methionine
d.   Tryptophan

b   168(K)   10.   Which of the following elements is found in certain amino acids?

a.   Iron
b.   Sulfur
c.   Calcium
d.   Potassium

b   169(A)   11.   Any of the following can be used by the body for the synthesis of a nonessential amino acid <u>EXCEPT</u>

  a.   a fragment of fat.
  b.   an essential mineral.
  c.   an essential amino acid.
  d.   a fragment of carbohydrate.

b   169(A)   12.   What amino acid is classified as conditionally essential when dietary intake of phenylalamine is insufficient or the body cannot normally metabolize phenylalanine?

  a.   Cysteine
  b.   Tyrosine
  c.   Glutamine
  d.   Isoleucine

b   169(K)   13.   Which of the following is a feature of an essential amino acid?

  a.   It is not necessary in the diet
  b.   It must be supplied by the diet
  c.   It can be made from fat in the body
  d.   It can be made from glucose in the body

b   169(K)   14.   What is the composition of a tripeptide?

  a.   One amino acid with three carbons
  b.   Three amino acids bonded together
  c.   One amino acid with three acid groups
  d.   Three small protein chains bonded together

d   169(A)   15.   What type of reaction is required to bind two molecules of glycine together and release a molecule of water?

  a.   Hydrolysis
  b.   Deamination
  c.   Denaturation
  d.   Condensation

a   168(K)   16.   When two amino acids are chemically joined together, the resulting structure is called a

  a.   dipeptide.
  b.   diglyceride.
  c.   polypeptide.
  d.   polysaccharide.

c   169-170(K)   17.   What is meant by the amino acid sequence of a protein?

    a.   Number of side chains in the protein
    b.   Folding arrangement of the peptide chain
    c.   Order of appearance of amino acids in the peptide chain
    d.   Order of appearance of only the essential amino acids in the protein

b   169-170(A)   18.   In comparison to the well-defined structure of starch, which of the following is the most important factor that allows for the synthesis of thousands of different proteins?

    a.   Number of cell ribosomes
    b.   Number of different amino acids
    c.   Availability of amino acids containing sulfur
    d.   Availability of amino acids containing hydroxyl groups

c   171-172(K)   19.   What is the process by which heat or acidity disrupts the normal shape of a protein chain?

    a.   Digestion
    b.   Condensation
    c.   Denaturation
    d.   Hydrogenation

c   171   20.   The application of heat or acid to a protein which causes its shape to change is known as

    a.   stiffening.
    b.   condensation.
    c.   denaturation.
    d.   destabilization.

b   171(A)   21.   What is the process that results in the hardening of an egg when it is exposed to heat?

    a.   Solidification
    b.   Denaturation
    c.   Condensation
    d.   Protein interaction

b   171-172(A)   22.   Upon eating a hamburger, in what organ is the hydrolysis of its proteins initiated?

    a.   Mouth
    b.   Stomach
    c.   Small intestine
    d.   Large intestine

a   171-172(A)   23.   In what organ is pepsin active?

    a.   Stomach
    b.   Pancreas
    c.   Small intestine
    d.   Large intestine

a   171-172(A)   24.   What digestive enzyme would be most affected in people who are unable to produce hydrochloric acid?

    a.   Pepsin
    b.   Transaminase
    c.   Pancreatic protease
    d.   Intestinal peptidase

c   171(K)   25.   What is the name given to the inactive form of a protein splitting enzyme in the stomach?

    a.   Peptidase
    b.   Propepsin
    c.   Pepsinogen
    d.   Propeptidase

b   171-172(A)   26.   Which of the following describes the structure of pepsin?

    a.   Lipid
    b.   Protein
    c.   Nucleic acid
    c.   Carbohydrate

a   171-172(A)   27.   What percentage of dietary protein is hydrolyzed in the mouth?

    a.   0
    b.   5-10
    c.   15-20
    d.   25-30

d   172-173(A)   28.   After digestion of proteins, what products are absorbed into the circulation?

a.   Free amino acids only
b.   Free amino acids and oligopeptides
c.   Free amino acids and dipeptides only
d.   Free amino acids, dipeptides and tripeptides only

a   172(K)   29.   Protein hydrolyzing enzymes are commonly known as

a.   proteases.
b.   hydrolyzers.
c.   prodigestins.
d.   denaturases.

a   173(A)   30.   What is the usual fate of orally ingested enzyme supplements?

a.   Digested by gastrointestinal proteases
b.   Rapidly degraded by salivary secretions
c.   Mostly absorbed in original form from stomach
d.   Completely absorbed in original form from jejunum

a   173(A)   31.   Of the following sources of amino acids, which would show the highest absorption in normal, healthy people?

a.   Whole proteins
b.   Raw protein foods
c.   Predigested proteins
d.   Mixture of free amino acids

d   173;176(K)   32.   Which of the following statements is NOT characteristic of enzymes?

a.   They are all catalysts
b.   They have a protein structure
c.   They can be destroyed by heat
d.   They are involved in synthesis reactions only

a   173-175(K)   33.   Which of the following describes a process in protein synthesis?

    a.   The code to make a protein is carried by a strand of messenger RNA
    b.   The final step in completing the protein is carried out in the mitochondria
    c.   The function of transfer RNA is to assist in absorption of amino acids into the cell
    d.   The DNA binds to ribosomes and directs uptake of specific amino acids to form the peptide chain

a   172(K)   34.   The function of a protease is to

    a.   hydrolyze proteins.
    b.   synthesize proteins.
    c.   hydrolyze ribosomes.
    d.   synthesize ribosomes.

d   175(K)   35.   A common genetic variation in the structure of hemoglobin causes the disease

    a.   diabetes.
    b.   marasmus.
    c.   kwashiorkor.
    d.   sickle-cell anemia.

b   176(K)   36.   What is the structure of an enzyme?

    a.   Lipid
    b.   Protein
    c.   Nucleic acid
    d.   Carbohydrate

c   176(K)   37.   What protein is intimately involved in the formation of scar tissue in wound healing?

    a.   Albumin
    b.   Thrombin
    c.   Collagen
    d.   Hydroxyproline

c   176(A)   38.   What type of protein would the body make to heal a wound?

    a.   Ferritin
    b.   Albumin
    c.   Collagen
    d.   Hemoglobin

b   176-177(K)   39.   Which of the following is a characteristic of hormones?

    a.   Coordinate visual response
    b.   Act as messenger molecules
    c.   Capable of inactivating bacteria
    d.   Act as buffers in the bloodstream

a   177-178(A)   40.   What is the relationship between body proteins and water?

    a.   Proteins attract water
    b.   Water attracts proteins
    c.   Water degrades proteins
    d.   Proteins form polymers of water

b   177-178(K)   41.   What function does a buffer perform?

    a.   Helps emulsify fats
    b.   Helps maintain a constant pH
    c.   Facilitates chemical reactions
    d.   Helps protect against plaque buildup

a   177-178(K)   42.   Tissue swelling that results from water that accumulates between cells is known as

    a.   edema.
    b.   acidosis.
    c.   alkalosis.
    d.   extravascularization.

a   178(K)   43.   Which of the following does NOT function as a transport protein?

    a.   Collagen
    b.   Transferrin
    c.   Hemoglobin
    d.   Lipoproteins

b   178(A)   44.   Proteins, because they attract hydrogen ions, can act as

    a.   acids.
    b.   buffers.
    c.   enzymes.
    d.   antibodies.

a   178(K)   45.   Which of the following processes is regulated primarily by the buffering action of proteins?

    a.   pH balance
    b.   Fluid balance
    c.   Blood clotting
    d.   Synthesis of visual pigments

d   178-179((K)   46.   Which of the following are proteins that inactivate foreign bacteria and viruses?

    a.   Enzymes
    b.   Collagen
    c.   Hormones
    d.   Antibodies

c   178-179(K)   47.   Which of the following proteins inactivates foreign bacteria and viruses?

    a.   Enzymes
    b.   Hormones
    c.   Antibodies
    d.   Lipoproteins

c   178-179(K)   48.   Which of the following describes the structure of an antibody?

    a.   Tripeptide
    b.   Small nucleic acid
    c.   Huge protein molecule
    d.   Large peptide molecule

b   179(K)   49.   Which of the following is involved in the clotting of blood?

    a.   Opsin
    b.   Fibrin
    c.   Collagen
    d.   Transferrin

d   180(K)   50.   The body's amino acid pool consists of

    a.   essential amino acids only.
    b.   endogenous amino acids only.
    c.   nonessential amino acids only.
    d.   both essential and nonessential amino acids.

d   181(K)   51.   What amino acid is used to synthesize the important neurotransmitter serotonin and the vitamin niacin?

    a.   Glycine
    b.   Tyrosine
    c.   Methionine
    d.   Tryptophan

d   181(A)   52.   Protein-sparing in the body is best achieved under which of the following circumstances?

    a.   Ingesting proteins of plant origin only
    b.   Ingesting proteins of animal origin only
    c.   Ingesting mixed protein sources on alternate days
    d.   Ingesting adequate levels of carbohydrate and fat

a   181(A)   53.   Which of the following are precursors of urea synthesis?

    a.   All amino acids
    b.   Animal proteins only
    c.   Essential amino acids only
    d.   Nonessential amino acids only

d   179(A)   54.   How many grams of nitrogen are contained in a 2,500 kcal diet that provides 15% of the energy as protein?

    a.   2.5
    b.   5
    c.   10
    d.   15

b   180(A)   55.   Which of the following may be used to determine protein utilization?

    a.   Calorimetry
    b.   Nitrogen balance
    c.   Supplementary value
    d.   Basal metabolic rate

c   180(A)   56.   When nitrogen taken into the body exceeds nitrogen losses, we say the person is in

    a.   a healthy state.
    b.   nitrogen equilibrium.
    c.   positive nitrogen balance.
    d.   negative nitrogen balance.

b   180(K)   57.   Which of the following defines protein turnover?

a.   The sum of protein in food and the body
b.   The sum of protein synthesis and degradation
c.   The amount of protein absorbed from the diet
d.   The amount of protein used to synthesize glucose

a   180(A)   58.   Which of the following describes the state of nitrogen balance for a normal, healthy 35-year-old person who weighs 60 kg and consumes a diet that provides 75 g of protein and adequate energy?

a.   Equilibrium
b.   Positive balance
c.   Negative balance
d.   Endogenous balance

d   180(A)   59.   What is the nitrogen balance of a person who consumed a 3,500 kilocalorie diet containing 10% <u>protein</u> and excreted a total of 12 grams of <u>nitrogen</u>?

a.   0 g
b.   -3 g
c.   -1 g
d.   +2 g

c   180(A)   60.   Which of the following would describe the state of nitrogen balance of a person who ingested 16 g of food nitrogen and lost 19 g of nitrogen?

a.   Equilibrium
b.   Positive balance
c.   Negative balance
d.   Exogenous balance

c   180(A)   61.   What would be the usual state of nitrogen balance for healthy infants, children, and pregnant women?

a.   Equilibrium
b.   Metabolic
c.   Positive
d.   Negative

a   181(A)   62.   Which of the following illustrates a deamination reaction?

    a.   Removal of the amino group from an amino acid
    b.   Separation of an amino acid from a peptide chain
    c.   Addition of an amino group to form a new amino acid
    d.   Addition of an amino acid to form a larger peptide chain

d   181(A)   63.   Which of the following compounds does NOT contain nitrogen?

    a.   Urea
    b.   Enzymes
    c.   Ammonia
    d.   Cholesterol

b   181(A)   64.   What is the fate of excess intake of dietary protein?

    a.   After absorption, the liver will store the extra amino acids
    b.   After absorption, the extra amino acids will be rapidly degraded
    c.   Digestion will be decreased by 30-60%, resulting in less absorption
    d.   After absorption, extra proteins will be synthesized and stored for use when protein intake returns to normal

b   182(A)   65.   Which of the following could NOT be a limiting amino acid in the diet?

    a.   Lysine
    b.   Glycine
    c.   Threonine
    d.   Tryptophan

b   182(A)   66.   If the diet is lacking an essential amino acid, what will be the course of action?

    a.   Body cells will synthesize it
    b.   Protein synthesis will be limited
    c.   Health will not be affected as long as other nutrients are adequate
    d.   Proteins will be made but they will lack that particular amino acid

c   182(A)   67.   Which of the following is <u>NOT</u> considered to be a source of complete protein in human nutrition?

    a.   Soy
    b.   Egg
    c.   Corn
    d.   Fish

b   182-183(K) 68.   What is the chief factor that governs the quality of a food protein?

    a.   Fat content
    b.   Essential amino acid content
    c.   Complex carbohydrate content
    d.   Nonessential amino acid content

c   182(K)   69.   What is a "limiting" amino acid in a protein?

    a.   A nonessential amino acid present in high amounts which inhibits protein synthesis
    b.   An amino acid of the wrong structure to be utilized for protein synthesis efficiently
    c.   An essential amino acid present in insufficient quantity for body protein synthesis to take place
    d.   An amino acid that limits the absorption of other essential amino acids by competing with them for transport sites within the GI tract

c   182(K)   70.   Which of the following animal-derived proteins is classified as an incomplete protein?

    a.   Fish
    b.   Cheese
    c.   Gelatin
    d.   Turkey

b   182(K)   71.   What is protein mutual supplementation?

    a.   A dietary program involving consumption of vegetable and animal proteins on alternating days
    b.   A strategy of combining plant proteins in the same meal to improve the balance of essential amino acids
    c.   A technique developed specifically for the elderly which involves optimizing protein intake to energy intake
    d.   A body process involving synthesis of crucial proteins from amino acids made available by breakdown of storage proteins

a   182(A)   72.   In general, the protein quality in grains would be most improved by the addition of

a. lysine.
b. tryptophan.
c. methionine.
d. glutamic acid.

c   183(A)   73.   Relative to animal proteins, which of the following amino acids is present in lesser amounts in proteins of legumes?

a. lysine.
b. tryptophan.
c. methionine.
d. glutamic acid.

a   183(A)   74.   Which of the following is related to the quality of a food protein?

a. Essential amino acid balance
b. Nonessential amino acid balance
c. Total amino acids per gram of food
d. Quantity of nonessential amino acids that can be converted to glucose

a   183(A)   75.   Which of the following food proteins has the best assortment of essential amino acids for the human body?

a. Egg
b. Fish
c. Corn
d. Rice

a   183(K)   76.   In the study of protein nutrition, what is the term given to the amount of amino acids absorbed as a percentage of the amount of protein consumed?

a. Digestibility
b. Completeness
c. Biological Value
d. Comparative Equivalence

c   183-184(K)   77.   Which of the following is <u>NOT</u> a common measure of protein quality?

a.   Chemical score
b.   Biological value
c.   Metabolic utilization
d.   Protein efficiency ratio

b   183-184(K)   78.   Which of the following is a common measure of protein quality?

a.   Metabolic value
b.   Biological value
c.   Protein excretion score
d.   Protein complementation index

d   184(K)   79.   What protein quality measure is used to assess the protein in foods for the Daily Value percentages seen on food labels?

a.   Biological value
b.   Amino acid scoring
c.   Net protein utilization efficiency ratio
d.   Protein-digestibility-corrected amino acid score

a   184-185(K)   80.   Which of the following is a feature of malnutrition?

a.   Dysentery is a common occurrence and leads to diarrhea and nutrient depletion
b.   Intestinal villi grow slightly larger to provide additional absorptive surfaces for nutrients
c.   Digestive enzyme production increases in order to extract as much of the ingested nutrients as possible
d.   Infections are uncommon due to insufficient availability of nutrients in the body to support growth of bacteria and viruses

d   184(K)   81.   On food labels, what measure is used to assess the quality of the proteins for people over one year of age?

a.   Biological value
b.   Net protein utilization
c.   Protein efficiency ratio
d.   Protein digestibility-corrected amino acid score

b   185-186(K)   82.   Which of the following is <u>NOT</u> a characteristic of marasmus?

    a.   Results in a low resistance to disease
    b.   Affects brain development only minimally
    c.   Occurs most commonly in children aged 6 to 18 months
    d.   Results in little or no fat under the skin to insulate against cold

b   186(A)   83.   Which of the following conditions is associated with edema?

    a.   Excessive use of certain drugs which causes high excretion of water and amino acids
    b.   Below-normal concentration of blood protein which causes fluid to leak from the blood vessels
    c.   Above-normal concentration of blood protein which causes fluid to leak from the blood vessels
    d.   Excessive protein in the diet leading to increased retention of fluid, especially in the extravascular spaces

b   186(A)   84.   What term describes the following quote: "The evil spirit that infects the first child when the second child is born"?

    a.   Marasmus
    b.   Kwashiorkor
    c.   Psychomalnutrition
    d.   Postbirth malnutrition

d   186(A)   85.   What is the most likely explanation for the fatty liver that develops from protein deficiency?

    a.   Increased uptake of circulating fats
    b.   Increased absorption of dietary fats
    c.   Inability of adipose tissue to remove circulating fats
    d.   Inability of the liver to synthesize lipoproteins for fat export

d   186(A)   86.   Which of the following would you <u>NOT</u> expect to see in a person with kwashiorkor?

    a.   Edema
    b.   Dysentery
    c.   Increased infection rate
    d.   increased physical activity

c   186(A)   87.   Which of the following is associated with the presence of tissue edema in kwashiorkor?

a.   Inadequate intake of water
b.   Excessive intake of dietary protein
c.   Low concentration of blood protein
d.   High concentration of blood protein

d   186(K)   88.   Which of the following is a feature of kwashiorkor?

a.   It makes the child appear grossly dehydrated
b.   It usually occurs prior to the onset of marasmus
c.   It is usually found in communities where marasmus is present
d.   It may be precipitated in the undernourished child who consumes moldy grain

c   187(K)   89.   Excessive amounts of homocysteine in the blood are thought to increase the risk for

a.   cancer.
b.   diabetes.
c.   heart disease.
d.   protein-energy malnutrition.

d   187(A)   90.   What is the usual initial therapy for the treatment of kwashiorkor?

a.   Fat replacement
b.   Energy replacement
c.   Protein replacement
d.   Fluid balance restoration

c   187(K)   91.   Which of the following is a feature of homocysteine?

a.   It is found only in animal foods
b.   It is a risk factor for osteoporosis
c.   It is increased in the blood of coffee drinkers
d.   It is increased in the blood of vitamin C-deficient people

b   188(K)   92.   Which of the following describes a relationship between protein intake and calcium metabolism?

    a.   Calcium <u>excretion</u> falls with increasing intake of animal-derived proteins
    b.   Calcium <u>excretion</u> rises with increasing intake of animal-derived proteins
    c.   Calcium <u>absorption</u> declines with higher intakes of plant-derived proteins
    d.   Calcium <u>absorption</u> increases with higher intakes of animal-derived proteins

c   189(A)   93.   According to recommendations in the report <u>Diet</u> <u>and</u> <u>Health</u>, what would be the highest safe level of protein intake for a 60 kg adult?

    a.   48 g
    b.   60 g
    c.   96 g
    d.   120 g

a   189(A)   94.   Which of the following is a feature of the protein RDA?

    a.   The recommendations are generous
    b.   It is highest proportionately for adult males
    c.   It is established at 8 grams per kilogram of ideal body weight
    d.   An assumption is made that dietary protein is from animal sources only

a   188(K)   95.   Which of the following is a known consequence of excess protein intake in animals or human beings?

    a.   Increased excretion of water
    b.   Decreased excretion of calcium
    c.   Decreased size of the liver and kidneys
    d.   Increased protein storage by the liver and kidneys

b   188-190(K)   96.   What would be the primary principle of wise diet planning as related to protein nutrition?

    a.   Variety
    b.   Moderation
    c.   Nutrient density
    d.   Calorie control

c   189(A)   97.   What is the RDA for protein for a 48 kg woman?

    a.   24 g
    b.   34 g
    c.   38 g
    d.   40 g

c   189(K)   98.   All of the following assumptions are made by the committee in setting the RDA for protein <u>EXCEPT</u>

    a.   adequate kcalories will be consumed.
    b.   protein eaten will be of mixed quality.
    c.   the fat content of the diet will be high.
    d.   other nutrients in the diet will be adequate.

c   189(A)   99.   If proteins needs are expressed per kilogram of body weight, which of the following describes the requirements of infants?

    a.   Less than adults
    b.   Similar to adults
    c.   Greater than adults
    d.   Less than adolescents

c   189(A)   100.   What is the percentage of total energy derived from protein in a diet containing 50 grams of protein and 2,000 kcal?

    a.   2.5
    b.   5
    c.   10
    d.   20

b   189(A)   101.   If a man consumes 65 grams of protein and a total of 2,700 kcal per day, approximately what percentage of energy would be derived from protein?

    a.   7
    b.   10
    c.   14
    d.   20

c   189(A)   102.   Which of the following is an assumption made in the formulation of the RDA for protein?

    a.   Dietary protein is of high quality only
    b.   Dietary protein is of animal origin only
    c.   Dietary carbohydrate and fat intakes are adequate
    d.   Dietary protein should represent 12% of total energy

d   190(A)   103.   According to the Daily Food Guide, an adult who consumes
                              the minimum recommended number of servings of each food
                              group would obtain the RDA level of protein for a body weight
                              of about

                              a.   75 lbs.
                              b.   110 lbs.
                              c.   160 lbs.
                              d.   200 lbs.

c   191-192(K)   104.   What amino acid has been linked to the development of the
                              rare blood disorder eosinophilia myalgia in people who took it
                              as a supplement?

                              a.   Glycine
                              b.   Arginine
                              c.   Tryptophan
                              d.   Phenylalanine

c   199-200(A)   105.   All of the following are advantages of vegetarian diets
                              EXCEPT

                              a.   fat content is lower.
                              b.   fiber content is higher.
                              c.   vitamin B_{12} intake is higher.
                              d.   vitamins A and C are found in liberal quantities.

b   197-199(A)   106.   All of the following are documented benefits for people
                              practicing vegetarianism EXCEPT

                              a.   better digestive function.
                              b.   lower rates of osteoporosis.
                              c.   lower blood cholesterol levels.
                              d.   lower rates of certain kinds of cancer.

d   198(A)   107.   Which of the following are allowed in the diet of a
                              lactovegetarian?

                              a.   Plant foods only
                              b.   Eggs and plant foods only
                              c.   Meat, eggs, and plant foods only
                              d.   Milk products and plant foods only

b   198(A)   108.   Which of the following ingredients found on a food label is a protein?

    a.   BHT
    b.   Tofu
    c.   Corn starch
    d.   Diglycerides

a   200(K)   109.   Studies reveal that many vegetarian women have intakes of vitamins and mineral that exceed the RDA except for

    a.   iron.
    b.   calcium.
    c.   folic acid.
    d.   vitamin A.

d   200(K)   110.   In general, a newborn infant is able to thrive during the early months by ingesting only breast milk and a source of

    a.   iron.
    b.   calcium.
    c.   vitamin C.
    d.   vitamin D.

b   200-201(K)   111.   What is the primary reason for the observation that vegan children are shorter and weigh less than meat-eating children?

    a.   Deficiency of vitamin D
    b.   Insufficient energy intake
    c.   Inherited growth disorders
    d.   Deficiencies of calcium and iron

Matching (Answers can be used only once)

F	169	112.	A dietary nonessential amino acid
I	169	113.	A conditionally essential amino acid
G	170	114.	A small protein
Q	171	115.	A large protein that carries oxygen
R	171	116.	Substances repelled by water
K	171	117.	The result of protein exposed to severe heat
C	172	118.	An active protease
L	174	119.	A cell structure where protein synthesis takes place
J	176	120.	A connective tissue protein
M	176	121.	A protein catalyst
P	178	122.	Fluid situated between cells
T	177	123.	Fluid within blood vessels
O	180	124.	A condition that favors positive nitrogen balance
H	180	125.	A condition that favors negative nitrogen balance
B	181	126.	A product of amino acid breakdown
E	182	127.	A dietary protein lacking tryptophan
A	182	128.	A good quality protein source
D	182	129.	A typical limiting amino acid
N	186	130.	A cancer-causing substance found on contaminated grains
S	187	131.	An amino acid associated with heart disease

A.	Soy		K.	Denatured
B.	Urea		L.	Ribosome
C.	Pepsin		M.	Enzyme
D.	Lysine		N.	Aflatoxin
E.	Gelatin		O.	Pregnancy
F.	Alanine		P.	Intercellular
G.	Insulin		Q.	Hemoglobin
H.	Infection		R.	Hydrophobic
I.	Tyrosine		S.	Homocysteine
J.	Collagen		T.	Intravascular

Essay Questions

168-169   132. Explain the differences among amino acids that are classified as essential, nonessential, or conditionally essential.

173-175;   133. Describe the processes involved in cellular protein synthesis.
183-184   How would synthesis be affected by intake of an otherwise adequate diet which is very low in glycine or low in tryptophan? How would synthesis be affected by a diet that is low in energy?

175   134. Explain the manner by which a gene becomes expressed to direct the synthesis of a protein.

180   135. What is meant by nitrogen balance and how are nitrogen balance studies conducted?

183-184   136. Compare and contrast the characteristics of the common protein quality evaluation methods.

183   137. Explain the rationale for the establishment of a new standard of reference protein for the measurement of protein quality. Why is this new standard considered to be superior to that of egg protein?

184-186   138. Compare and contrast kwashiorkor and marasmus.

187-188   139. Explain the proposed relationship between:

                     A. Body homocysteine levels and heart disease.

                     B. Protein intake and calcium metabolism

187-188;   140. A. What are the possible consequences of consuming too
191   much protein?

                     B. What are the hazards of consuming amino acid supplements?

191 141. List population groups for which amino acid dietary supplements are especially inappropriate.

197-201 142. List the advantages of a vegetarian diet. What nutrient requirements are more difficult to meet on this diet, and what precautions are needed to prevent insufficient intakes in the child and in the adult?

CHAPTER 7
METABOLISM: TRANSFORMATIONS AND INTERACTIONS

Ans   Page

b   204(K)   01.   Which of the following describes the sum of all chemical reactions that go on in living cells?

a. Digestion
b. Metabolism
c. Absorption
d. Catabolism

a   205(A)   02.   What term is specific to reactions in which simple compounds are combined into more complex molecules?

a. Anabolic
b. Catabolic
c. Ergogenic
d. Gluconeogenic

c   205(A)   03.   Which of the following reactions is an example of an anabolic reaction?

a. Formation of pyruvate from glucose
b. Formation of carbon dioxide from citric acid
c. Formation of cholesterol from acetyl-CoA molecules
d. Formation of acetyl-CoA molecules from cholesterol

c   205(A)   04. The formation of glycogen by the liver cell is an example of

a. oxidation.
b. glycolysis.
c. anabolism.
d. catabolism.

a   205(K)   05. Which of the following is a feature of catabolic reactions?

a. Involve release of energy
b. Occur only in mitochondria
c. Involve consumption of energy
d. Occur only during loss of body weight

b   205(A)   06. Which of the following is an example of a catabolic reaction?

a. Formation of glucose from glycerol
b. Formation of urea from an amino acid
c. Formation of albumin from amino acids
d. Formation of palmitic acid from acetate

a   205(K)   07. What is the major energy carrier molecule in most cells?

a. ATP
b. Glucose
c. Pyruvate
d. A kcalorie

c   205-206(A)   08. Which of the following metabolic reactions occurs when a cell
                         uses energy?

a. ATP gains a phosphate group and becomes ADP
b. ADP gains a phosphate group and becomes ATP
c. ATP releases a phosphate group and becomes ADP
d. ADP releases a phosphate group and becomes ATP

b   207(K)   09. Which of the following defines a coenzyme?

a. A unit consisting of an enzyme bound to reactants plus
    ATP
b. A small organic molecule required for the functioning of
    an enzyme
c. The small, active part of an enzyme that binds to the
    organic reactants
d. An inactive enzyme that becomes functional upon contact
    with specific cofactors

c   208(K)   10. All of the following are among the functions of the liver EXCEPT

    a. synthesis of urea.
    b. formation of lymph.
    c. production of red blood cells.
    d. conversion of fructose to glucose.

c   209(K)   11. Glycolysis is the conversion of

    a. glycogen to fat.
    b. glycogen to protein.
    c. glucose to pyruvate.
    d. glucose to glycogen.

b   209(K)   12. The series of reactions involving the conversion of glucose to pyruvate is known as

    a. pyrolysis.
    b. glycolysis.
    c. beta-oxidation.
    d. coupled reaction.

a   209-211(K)   13. Which of the following is NOT an aspect of glycolysis?

    a. It is irreversible
    b. It generates ATP
    c. It occurs in the absence of oxygen
    d. It generates two molecules of pyruvate

b   209(A)   14. An aerobic reaction is one that requires

    a. alcohol.
    b. oxygen.
    c. nitrogen.
    d. ammonia.

a   211(K)   15. Which of the following can NOT be formed from acetyl-CoA molecules?

    a. Glucose
    b. Cholesterol
    c. Stearic acid
    d. Carbon dioxide

d   211-214(A)   16.   Which of the following can NOT be formed from pyruvate in human beings?

   a.   Glucose
   b.   Fructose
   c.   Lactic acid
   d.   Linoleic acid

a   210(K)   17.   The Cori cycle involves the interconversion of

   a.   lactic acid and glucose.
   b.   glucose and amino acids.
   c.   pyruvate and citric acids.
   d.   fatty acids and acetyl-CoA.

c   210(A)   18.   When a person is performing intense physical exercise and begins to feel fatigue and a stinging or burning pain in the muscles, it is most likely due to the muscle's accumulation of

   a.   ammonia.
   b.   citric acid.
   c.   lactic acid.
   d.   pyruvic acid.

c   211-212(A)   19.   Which of the following is a possible fate of acetyl CoA?

   a.   Degradation to urea
   b.   Synthesis to glycerol
   c.   Synthesis to fatty acids
   d.   Degradation to ammonia

c   212(A)   20.   What is the first product of fatty acid catabolism?

   a.   Glycerol
   b.   Pyruvate
   c.   Acetyl CoA
   d.   Triglycerides

d   212-213(A)   21.   Which of the following nutrients can be made from compounds composed of 2-carbon skeletons?

   a.   Glucose
   b.   Fructose
   c.   Glycogen
   d.   Fatty acids

b 211-214(A) 22. Which of the following dietary components <u>CANNOT</u> be used to synthesize and store glycogen?

    a. Lactose
    b. Animal fats
    c. Wheat starch
    d. Plant protein

a 211-212(K) 23. In a triglyceride that contains 54 carbon atoms, how many can become part of glucose?

    a. 3
    b. 9
    c. 54
    d. 108

b 211-214(K) 24. Which of the following compounds <u>CANNOT</u> be formed from fatty acids?

    a. Ketones
    b. Glucose
    c. Acetyl CoA
    d. Carbon dioxide

a 211-214(A) 25. Production of excessive amounts of acetyl-CoA molecules leads to the synthesis of

    a. fatty acids only.
    b. fatty acids and glucose only.
    c. fatty acids and fructose only.
    d. fatty acids, glucose, and amino acids.

d 214(K) 26. Approximately what percentage of triglycerides <u>CANNOT</u> be converted to glucose?

    a. 70
    b. 80
    c. 90
    d. 95

c 211-214(A) 27. Which of the following <u>CANNOT</u> be used to make body proteins?

    a. Glucose
    b. Glycerol
    c. Fatty acids
    d. Amino acids

d 216(A) 28. What is the immediate fate of excess dietary protein in the body?

    a. Stored
    b. Reduced
    c. Oxidized
    d. Deaminated

a 217(A) 29. After digestion and absorption, an amino acid not used to build protein will first be subjected to

    a. removal of its amino group.
    b. removal of its carboxyl group.
    c. hydrolysis of its peptide bond.
    d. condensation of its peptide bond.

c 216-217(A) 30. If the carbohydrate content of the diet is insufficient to meet the body's needs for glucose, which of the following can be converted to glucose?

    a. Fatty acids
    b. Acetyl-CoA
    c. Amino acids
    d. Carbon dioxide

b 217-218(A) 31. Which of the following leads to the production of urea?

    a. Oxidation of glucose
    b. Oxidation of amino acids
    c. Incomplete oxidation of fatty acids
    d. Synthesis of protein from amino acids

d 216(A) 32. When protein consumption is in excess of body needs and energy needs are met, the excess amino acids are metabolized and the energy in the molecules is

    a. stored as fat only.
    b. excreted in the feces.
    c. stored as amino acids only.
    d. stored as glycogen and fat.

c 217(K) 33. What is the process whereby an amino group is combined with a keto acid to form an amino acid?

    a. Deamination
    b. Ureagenesis
    c. Transamination
    d. Ammoniogenesis

a   217-218(K)   34. In the metabolism of amino acids for energy, what is the fate of the amino group?

a. Excreted as urea
b. Burned for energy
c. Stored in the liver
d. Converted to glucose

a   217-218(A)   35. Which of the following is NOT a possible fate of metabolized glucose?

a. Urea
b. Acetyl CoA
c. Amino acids
d. Muscle glycogen

c   217-219(A)   36. Which of the following products is NOT generated via TCA cycle or electron transport chain?

a. Water
b. Energy
c. Ammonia
d. Carbon dioxide

a   218(K)   37. The body's need for water increases on a diet high in

a. protein.
b. carbohydrate.
c. saturated fat.
d. unsaturated fat.

a   218(A)   38. What is the most likely cause for a person to have abnormally high blood ammonia levels?

a. Liver dysfunction
b. Kidney dysfunction
c. Protein intake of twice the RDA
d. Protein intake of one-tenth the RDA

b   218(A)   39. What is the most likely reason for having an abnormally high blood urea level?

a. Liver dysfunction
b. Kidney dysfunction
c. Protein intake of twice the RDA
d. Protein intake of one-tenth the RDA

c   218(A)   40.   Which of the following is the most likely side effect of a high-protein, low-carbohydrate diet?

a.   Edema
b.   Diarrhea
c.   Dehydration
d.   Nitrogen toxicity

d   219(A)   41.   When energy-yielding nutrients are consumed in excess, which one(s) can lead to storage of fat?

a.   Fat only
b.   Carbohydrate only
c.   Fat and carbohydrate only
d.   Fat, carbohydrate, and protein

a   219-220(K)   42.   In addition to energy, what are the principal end products of cellular oxidation of carbohydrates?

a.   Water and carbon dioxide
b.   Carbon, hydrogen, and urea
c.   Indigestible fiber and nitrogen
d.   Monosaccharides and amino acids

d   211-214;   43.   What are the products from the complete oxidation of fatty
       219-220(K)   acids?

a.   Urea and acetone
b.   Fatty acids and glycerol
c.   Carbon, hydrogen, and oxygen
d.   Water, carbon dioxide, and energy

b   209-211;   44.   Which of the following outlines the overall sequence of events
       219-220(A)   in the complete oxidation of glucose?

a.   Cori cycle, TCA cycle, glycolysis
b.   Glycolysis, TCA cycle, electron transport chain
c.   Electron transport chain, TCA cycle, Cori cycle
d.   TCA cycle, electron transport chain, glycolysis

b   220(K)   45. Which of the following accounts for the higher energy density of a fatty acid compared with the other energy-yielding nutrients?

a. Fatty acids have a lower percentage of hydrogen-carbon bonds
b. Fatty acids have a greater percentage of hydrogen-carbon bonds
c. Other energy-yielding nutrients have a lower percentage of oxygen-carbon bonds
d. Other energy-yielding nutrients undergo fewer metabolic reactions thereby lowering the energy yield

d   220-221(A)   46. The number of ATP's that can be produced from a molecule of protein, fat, or carbohydrate is generally related to the number of atoms of

a. carbon.
b. oxygen.
c. nitrogen.
d. hydrogen.

b   223(K)   47. All of the following are features of the metabolism of surplus dietary carbohydrate in human beings EXCEPT

a. excess glucose suppresses fat oxidation.
b. excess glucose is oxidized only very slowly.
c. excess glucose is first used to fill glycogen reserves.
d. conversion of excess glucose to fat occurs only to a very limited extent.

a   223(K)   48. Which of the following is a feature of the metabolism of surplus dietary fat?

a. Excess fat is almost all stored
b. Excess fat promotes increased fat oxidation
c. Excess fat spares breakdown of body proteins
d. Conversion of excess fat to storage fat is inefficient

a   224-225(A)   49. After the first day or so of fasting, which of the following is most depleted in the body?

a. Glycogen
b. Fatty acids
c. Amino acids
d. Triglycerides

d   225(A)   50. If a normal person expends 1500 kcal while at rest, approximately how many are used by the brain?

    a.   40
    b.   100
    c.   200
    d.   300

a   225(K)   51. During the first few days of a fast, what energy source provides about 90% of the <u>glucose</u> needed to fuel the body?

    a.   Protein
    b.   Ketones
    c.   Glycogen
    d.   Triglycerides

a   225(A)   52. How soon would death occur from starvation if the body was unable to shift to a state of ketosis?

    a.   Within 3 weeks
    b.   Less than 2 weeks
    c.   Between 5 and 6 weeks
    d.   Between 2 and 3 months

d   225(K)   53. Which of the following is classified as a ketone body?

    a.   Sorbitol
    b.   Pyruvate
    c.   Acetyl-CoA
    d.   Acetoacetate

a   225-226(A)   54. Which of the following is used to supply some of the fuel needed by the brain only after the body has been fasting for a while?

    a.   Ketones
    b.   Glycerol
    c.   Fatty acids
    d.   Amino acids

b   225-226(K)   55. How are ketones formed?

    a.   Condensing of lactic acid molecules
    b.   Condensing of acetyl CoA molecules
    c.   Hydrolysis of excess glycerol fragments
    d.   Hydrolysis of excess pyruvate fragments

a   225-226(A)   56. Which of the following is a feature of ketosis?

        a.   Occurs when fats are partially oxidized
        b.   Occurs from lack of protein in the diet
        c.   Results from excess acetoacetate in the diet
        d.   Results from excess carbohydrate in the diet

d   225-226(A)   57. Which of the following dietary nutrients would most rapidly reverse a state of ketosis in a starving person?

        a.   Fat
        b.   Protein
        c.   Amino acids
        d.   Carbohydrate

a   225(K)   58. Which of the following is a characteristic of ketosis?

        a.   It may lead to a lowering of blood pH
        b.   It leads to increased appetite in most individuals
        c.   It may be alleviated quickly by ingestion of some dietary fat
        d.   It is a necessary physiological adjustment for maximum weight loss

b   226(A)   59. All of the following are general features of starvation in people EXCEPT

        a.   a decrease in metabolic rate.
        b.   a decrease in mental alertness.
        c.   a decrease in immune function.
        d.   a decrease in body temperature.

d   225-226(A)   60. Which of the following are consequences of low-carbohydrate diets?

        a.   Increases in bowel movements
        b.   Minimal losses of muscle and high losses of fat
        c.   Increases in energy level of body and mental alertness
        d.   High losses of water and protein and lower losses of fat

c   230(A)   61. What is the percentage of ethanol in 120-proof scotch whiskey?

        a.   5
        b.   30
        c.   60
        d.   95

c   230-231(K)   62. One average-sized can of beer contains about the same amount of alcohol as

    a. ½ ounce of rum.
    b. ½ quart of wine.
    c. 1 ounce of vodka.
    d. 1 quart of wine cooler.

c   230-232(K)   63. Which of the following statements is <u>NOT</u> characteristic of alcohol metabolism?

    a. There are gender differences in the rate of breakdown
    b. The average person needs about 3 hours to metabolize two drinks
    c. Alcohol is metabolized by muscle and brain cells as well as by the liver
    d. The amount of alcohol in the breath is proportional to the amount in the blood

a   230(A)   64. Which of the following defines a moderate level of alcohol intake per day for the average-sized woman?

    a. Up to 1 drink
    b. Up to 2 drinks
    c. Up to 3 drinks
    d. Up to 5 drinks

b   230(K)   65. Which of the following defines a moderate level of alcohol intake per day for the average-sized man?

    a. Up to 1 drink
    b. Up to 2 drinks
    c. Up to 3 drinks
    d. Up to 5 drinks

c   231(K)   66. The metabolism of alcohol begins in the

    a. liver.
    b. brain.
    c. stomach.
    d. intestines.

b   231(A)   67. What organ is first to absorb the alcohol after taking a drink?

    a. Colon
    b. Stomach
    c. Jejunum
    d. Duodenum

a 231(K) 68. Which of the following is characteristic of alcohol absorption?

    a. It is increased about 20% on an empty stomach
    b. It is increased from the GI tract by high-fat snacks
    c. It is increased from the GI tract by carbohydrate snacks
    d. It is lower in women than men of the same body weight

b 232-233(K) 69. What is the primary organ that oxidizes alcohol for fuel?

    a. Brain
    b. Liver
    c. Pancreas
    d. Digestive tract

d 231(A) 70. Which of the following is/are best suited for slowing alcohol absorption?

    a. Not eating
    b. Protein snacks
    c. Caffeine drinks
    d. Carbohydrate snacks

c 232(K) 71. Which of the following plays a major role in regulating the elimination of alcohol from the body?

    a. Lung respiratory rate
    b. Kidney antidiuretic hormone
    c. Liver alcohol dehydrogenase
    d. Brain acetaldehyde dehydrogenase

d 233(K) 72. What is the sequence of stages that brings about advanced liver disease caused by chronic alcohol toxicity?

    a. Fibrosis, gout, cirrhosis
    b. Fibrosis, cirrhosis, fat depletion
    c. Cirrhosis, fat accumulation, fibrosis
    d. Fat accumulation, fibrosis, cirrhosis

b 233(K) 73. Excess alcohol intake leads to a reduction in the synthesis rate of

    a. liver fat.
    b. liver glucose.
    c. ketone bodies.
    d. acetyl CoA molecules.

d   233(K)   74.   What is MEOS?

a.   An advanced liver disorder
b.   A drug that inhibits alcohol absorption
c.   A waste product of alcohol metabolism
d.   A system of enzymes that oxidizes alcohol and drugs

a   235(K)   75.   What <u>minimum</u> concentration of alcohol in the blood is usually fatal?

a.   0.5%
b.   1%
c.   5%
d.   50%

a   235-236(A)   76.   Chronic excess alcohol intake leads to all of the following effects on folate <u>EXCEPT</u>

a.   the intestines recycle more folate.
b.   the liver releases more folate into the blood.
c.   the kidney excretes more folate via the urine.
d.   the intestines absorb less folate from the diet.

a   235-236(K)   77.   Which of the following is a feature of ethanol metabolism?

a.   It increases gastric acid output
b.   It decreases activity of the MEOS
c.   It decreases secretion of gastric histamine
d.   It increases secretion of antidiuretic hormone

c   235(A)   78.   Approximately how many kcal from <u>ethanol</u> are contained in one standard alcoholic drink?

a. 25
b. 50
c. 100
d. 200

d   237(K)   79.   What percentage of all traffic fatalities involve alcohol?

a. 5
b. 12
c. 22
d. 38

Matching (Answers can be used only once)

S	205	80.	Example of an anabolic reaction
R	205	81.	Example of a catabolic reaction
F	207	82.	A protein that accelerates a chemical reaction
J	207	83.	A small non-protein organic substance that promotes optimal activity of an enzyme
O	209	84.	A product of glycolysis
N	209	85.	The oxidation product of pyruvate
L	210	86.	A product of pyruvate metabolism when oxygen is limiting
K	210	87.	A recycling process of converting lactic acid to glucose
T	211	88.	An irreversible reaction
H	211	89.	The part of a triglyceride that is convertible to glucose
I	217	90.	A product of deamination
P	217	91.	An enzyme involved in synthesis of amino acids
B	218	92.	The principal nitrogen-containing waste product
D	220	93.	Waste product of the electron transport chain
G	223	94.	A storage form of carbohydrate
E	225	95.	The major energy fuel for the central nervous system
M	236	96.	A ketone
C	233	97.	A system for metabolizing drugs and alcohol
Q	231	98.	An enzyme with activity levels related to a person's sex
A	232	99.	A coenzyme required for metabolism of alcohol

A.	NAD	K.	Cori cycle
B.	Urea	L.	Lactic acid
C.	MEOS	M.	Acetoacetate
D.	Water	N.	Acetyl-CoA
E.	Glucose	O.	Pyruvic acid
F.	Enzyme	P.	Transaminase
G.	Glycogen	Q.	Alcohol dehydrogenase
H.	Glycerol	R.	Synthesis of pyruvate from glycogen
I.	Ammonia	S.	Synthesis of cholesterol from acetate
J.	Coenzyme	T.	Synthesis of acetyl-CoA from glucose

Essay Questions

204-208   100. Compare and contrast the various ways in which the body uses carbohydrate, fat, and amino acids.

208-211   101. What are the major differences between aerobic and anaerobic metabolism? Give an example of an aerobic reaction and an anaerobic reaction.

218-219   102. What is urea? How and where is it synthesized and how is it removed from the body?

224-227   103. Discuss ways in which the body's metabolism adapts to conditions of fasting/starvation. How do these adaptations affect the rate of weight loss when dieting?

214-216;   104. Explain the roles of protein and fat as nutrients for
221-227   gluconeogenesis. What are the circumstances that favor low and high rates of gluconeogenesis?

221-223   105. Describe interactions among the energy nutrients when each is consumed in excess.

225-226   106. What is ketosis and how can it be identified? What conditions typically induce a state of ketosis? What are the adverse effects of this abnormality?

232-233;   107. Discuss ways in which alcohol interferes with metabolism of
235-237   proteins, fats, carbohydrates, vitamins, minerals, and water.

233;235-237 108. Describe the two major pathways for metabolism of alcohol in the liver. How does the liver adapt when forced to metabolize high quantities of alcohol on a daily basis?

230-232   109. Compare and contrast the metabolism of alcohol in men versus women.

235-236   110. Describe the effects of excess alcohol intake on folate utilization.

237   111. List 6 common myths concerning alcohol use and discuss ways to dispel them.

CHAPTER 8
ENERGY BALANCE AND BODY COMPOSITION

Ans   Page

c   241(A)   01.   What is the recommended rate of weight loss per week for a
                          250-pound obese individual?

                          a.   1 lb
                          b.   5 lbs
                          c.   1 % of body weight
                          d.   5 % of body weight

d   241(A)   02.   What would be the approximate weight gain of a person who
                          consumes an excess of 500 kcal daily for one month?

                          a.   0.5 lb
                          b.   2 lbs
                          c.   3 lbs
                          d.   4 lbs

a   241(K)   03.   What is considered to be a safe rate of maximum weight loss
                          on a long term basis for most overweight people?

                          a.   0.5-2 1bs/week
                          b.   3-4 lbs/week
                          c.   5% body weight per month
                          d.   10% body weight per month

d   241(A)   04.   Approximately what percentage of weight loss during starvation is lean body mass?

    a. 0
    b. 20
    c. 35
    d. 50

c   241(A)   05.   In an adult who gains 20 pounds of excess body weight, about how much of this is lean tissue?

    a. 0 lbs
    b. 2 lbs
    c. 5 lbs
    d. 10 lbs

b   241(A)   06.   When an adult gains an extra 10 pounds of body weight, approximately how much of this weight is fat?

    a. 5 lbs
    b. 7.5 lbs
    c. 9.5 lbs
    d. 10 lbs

c   242(K)   07.   What instrument is used to measure the energy content of foods?

    a. Energy chamber
    b. Exothermic meter
    c. Bomb calorimeter
    d. Combustion chamber

a   242-243(K)   08.   Which of the following identifies a specific food intake behavior?

    a. The absence of appetite is called anorexia
    b. A physiological need to eat is called satiety
    c. A pleasurable desire for food is called hunger
    d. An intense feeling of hunger is called insatiable nervosa

d   242(A)   09.   Which of the following describes an association between energy measurement and foods?

    a.   Indirect calorimetry cannot be used to determine the energy value of alcohol
    b.   A bomb calorimeter measures the amount of oxygen released when a food is oxidized
    c.   Direct calorimetry and indirect calorimetry of the same food rarely give the similar values
    d.   The physiological fuel value of a food is almost always lower than the energy value of that food as determined by bomb calorimetry

c   243(A)   10.   After consuming a very large meal, the desire to eat a slice of chocolate cake is an example of behavior known as

    a.   satiety.
    b.   hunger.
    c.   appetite.
    d.   pigging out.

a   243(A)   11.   What are the effects on fat digestion (hydrolysis) and absorption after a person switches to a high-fat diet?

    a.   Both digestion and absorption efficiencies are increased
    b.   Both digestion and absorption efficiencies are decreased
    c.   Digestion efficiency is increased but absorption is not affected
    d.   Absorption efficiency is increased but digestion is not affected

d   243(A)   12.   An emotionally insecure person might eat for all of the following reasons EXCEPT

    a.   to relieve boredom.
    b.   to ward off depression.
    c.   in preference to socializing.
    d.   to satisfy energy needs only.

b   243-244(K)   13.   External cues that may cause an obese person to respond helplessly to food typically include all of the following EXCEPT

    a.   TV commercials.
    b.   outdoor exercises.
    c.   availability of food.
    d.   "time of day" patterns.

c   244-245(K)   14.   What is the most satiating macronutrient?

     a.   Fat
     b.   Water
     c.   Protein
     d.   Carbohydrate

a   244-245(A)   15.   Among the following, which has the greatest power to suppress hunger?

     a.   Apples
     b.   Peanuts
     c.   Doughnuts
     d.   Potato chips

d   245(K)   16.   The brain chemical neuropeptide Y is known to specifically enhance the craving for

     a.   fat.
     b.   salt
     c.   protein.
     d.   carbohydrate.

c   246(K)   17.   Which of the following describes the process of thermogenesis?

     a.   Burning of fat
     b.   Synthesis of fat
     c.   Generation of heat
     d.   Generation of water

c   246(K)   18.   What method is used to measure the amount of heat given off by the body?

     a.   Bomb calorimetry
     b.   Basal calorimetry
     c.   Direct calorimetry
     d.   Indirect calorimetry

a   246(K)   19.   Which of the following is used to calculate the amount of energy expended by the body?

     a.   Oxygen consumed
     b.   Total air exchanged
     c.   Intestinal gas expelled
     d.   Carbon dioxide consumed

c   246(A)   20.   What fraction of the day's energy expenditure of the average person is represented by the basal metabolism?

      a.   about 1/10
      b.   up to 1/2
      c.   about 2/3
      d.   over 9/10

c   246-247(K)   21.   Which of the following is a feature of the basal metabolic rate (BMR)?

      a.   Fever decreases the BMR
      b.   Fasting increases the BMR
      c.   Pregnancy increases the BMR
      d.   Females have higher BMR's than males on a body weight basis

b   246(K)   22.   For every decade beyond the age of 30, what is the percentage decrease in the need for kcalories?

      a.   2
      b.   5
      c.   10
      d.   15

c   246-247(K)   23.   Among the following groups, which has the highest metabolic rate?

      a.   Females
      b.   Older individuals
      c.   Younger individuals
      d.   People with smaller surface areas

d   246-247(K)   24.   What is the major factor that determines metabolic rate?

      a.   Age
      b.   Gender
      c.   Amount of fat tissue
      d.   Amount of lean body tissue

a   246-237(K)   25.   Which of the following does NOT decrease the metabolic rate?

      a.   Fever
      b.   Injury
      c.   Fasting
      d.   Malnutrition

c 246(A) 26. If a normal 30 year-old woman has a daily energy expenditure of 2,200 kcal, what would be her expected output when she reaches 60 years of age?

  a. 1210 kcal
  b. 1450 kcal
  c. 1885 kcal
  d. 2275 kcal

d 246-247(A) 27. If a dancer and a typist are the same height and have the exact same body build, the dancer will be heavier because she has

  a. more body fat.
  b. stronger bones.
  c. stronger muscles.
  d. more muscle mass.

c 247(K) 28. What is the main explanation for the difference in basal metabolic rates between males and females of the same body weight?

  a. Males are usually taller than females
  b. Females have lower levels of thyroid hormones
  c. Males have a higher percentage of lean body mass
  d. Females have a lower percentage of adipose tissue

a 247-250(A) 29. If a normal 60 kg person has a resting energy expenditure of 1300 kcal/day, about how many extra kcal are needed to sustain 4 hours of studying?

  a. 50
  b. 120
  c. 260
  d. 400

b 247-248(A) 30. What is the approximate value for the thermic effect of a 2,500 kcal diet?

  a. 25 kcal
  b. 250 kcal
  c. 400 kcal
  d. 500 kcal

d   249(A)   31.   What is the term that describes the increase in energy expenditure that occurs in a person who fractures a leg?

      a.   Febrile hyperthermia
      b.   Physical hyperthermia
      c.   Specific thermogenesis
      d.   Adaptive thermogenesis

a   249(K)   32.   To estimate the basal metabolic rates of individuals, which of the following was used in the equations by the Committee on Dietary Allowances?

      a.   Weight
      b.   Surface area
      c.   Activity level
      d.   Fat-fold thickness

d   249(A)   33.   How does the metabolic rate of males compare with that of females of the same body weight?

      a.   About 3% lower
      b.   About 3% higher
      c.   About 10% lower
      d.   About 10% higher

b   249-250(A)   34.   If a 60 kg woman expends 750 kcal in her daily activities, approximately how many kcal are needed to maintain energy equilibrium?

      a.   1950
      b.   2250
      c.   2400
      d.   2600

c   250(A)   35.   What is the approximate basal metabolism of a 110-pound woman?

      a.   850 kcal/day
      b.   960 kcal/day
      c.   1080 kcal/day
      d.   1240 kcal/day

c   251K)   36.   Which of the following describes a feature of body weight standards?

a.   Current weight-for-height tables specify recommendations by age and sex
b.   Weight-for-height tables for adults have been the same for at least 15 years
c.   The weight-for-height tables are used less frequently than the body mass index
d.   Weight-for-height tables and body mass index have been blended to yield a more precise measure known as the Minimal Health Risk classification

a   251(A)   37.   An index of a person's weight in relation to height is called

a.   body mass index.
b.   height to weight index.
c.   ideal body weight index.
d.   desirable body weight index.

a   251(K)   38.   Which of the following is a feature of the body mass index?

a.   It correlates with disease risks
b.   It decreases by 1 unit for every 10 years of life
c.   It provides an estimate of the fat level of the body
d.   It is defined as the person's height divided by the square of the weight

a   251(A)   39.   What is the approximate body mass index of a woman who is 5'5" and 125 lbs?

a.   21
b.   26
c.   31
d.   36

d   251-252(K)   40.   Which of the following is a characteristic associated with using weight measures to assess risk of disease?

a.   They are expensive to perform
b.   They are complicated to perform
c.   They fail to quantitate total body fat
d.   They are subject to gross inaccuracies

d   251-252(K)   41.   All of the following are features of using weight measures to assess risk of disease <u>EXCEPT</u>

     a.   they are inexpensive.
     b.   they are very accurate.
     c.   they are easy to perform.
     d.   they provide information on body composition.

b   252-253(K)   42.   What is the range of body fat content for normal weight women?

     a.   9-17%
     b.   20-30%
     c.   33-37%
     d.   38-44%

b   252-253(K)   43.   What is the range of body fat content for normal weight men?

     a.   5-10%
     b.   12-20%
     c.   22-30%
     d.   32-40%

d   251-252(K)   44.   Which of the following is a disadvantage of using weight measures for the assessment of disease risk?

     a.   Cost
     b.   Accuracy
     c.   Complexity
     d.   Limited amount of body composition data

c   253(A)   45.   Which of the following is <u>NOT</u> a known side effect of having insufficient fat stores?

     a.   Infertility
     b.   Clinical depression
     c.   Elevated body temperature
     d.   Abnormal hunger regulation

b   253(A)   46.   What is the weight classification assigned both to young women with 30% body fat and young men with 20% body fat?

     a.   Obese
     b.   Normal
     c.   Mildly overweight
     d.   Slightly underweight

b   254-255(K)   47.   In what region of the body is the storage of excess body fat associated with highest risks for cardiovascular disease and diabetes?

a.   Neck
b.   Abdomen
c.   Hips and thighs
d.   Arms and shoulders

b   254(K)   48.   Which of the following defines central obesity?

a.   Accumulation of fat during the mid-years of life
b.   Storage of excess fat around the central part of the body
c.   Overfatness due to a large number of interacting behavioral problems
d.   Overfatness due to reliance on high fat foods as a central part of the diet

c   254-255(A)   49.   Research in obese people seems to show that there is no increase in the risks for strokes and hypertension provided that the excess body fat is distributed around the

a.   stomach.
b.   arms and chest.
c.   hips and thighs.
d.   neck and shoulders.

c   255(K)   50.   A high risk of weight-related health problems is seen in women whose waist circumference begins to exceed

a.   24 inches.
b.   28 inches.
c.   35 inches.
d.   42 inches.

d   254-255(K)   51.   Which of the following is a characteristic of excess body fat that is distributed primarily around the abdomen?

a.   It is related directly to exercise
b.   Its presence lowers the risk for diabetes
c.   It is less common in women past menopause
d.   It is associated with increased mortality for both sexes

a   255-256(K)   52.   Which of the following is <u>NOT</u> a feature of the fatfold test?

    a.   It is usually self-administered
    b.   It correlates with risk of heart disease
    c.   It provides a direct estimate of the amount of body fat
    d.   It is considered a practical diagnostic tool for trained users

b   255-256(K)   53.   Which of the following is a feature of fatfold <u>assessment</u> techniques?

    a.   The device to measure fatfold thickness is called a lipidometer
    b.   The folds of fat increase in size in proportion to the gain in body fat
    c.   Measures taken from upper-body sites are more precise than those from the lower-body sites
    d.   The principles are based on the assumption that subcutaneous fat mass represents about 20% of total body fat

a   255(K)   54.   The known health risks for being underweight include all of the following <u>EXCEPT</u>

    a.   diabetes.
    b.   infertility in women.
    c.   giving birth to unhealthy infants.
    d.   increased cancer-induced wasting.

b   255(K)   55.   A high risk of weight related health problems is seen in men whose waist circumference begins to exceed

    a.   34 inches
    b.   40 inches.
    c.   45 inches.
    d.   52 inches.

b   257(K)   56.   Which of the following describes an association between body weight and mortality?

    a.   Obesity is the fourth leading cause of premature death
    b.   Overweight men who are physically fit have a lower mortality risk than normal-weight, unfit men
    c.   Normal-weight men who are physically unfit have a similar mortality risk versus normal-weight fit men
    d.   The amount of weight gain in adulthood that is not associated with increased mortality is 20 pounds or less

d   257(K)   57.   All of the following are an association between type 2 diabetes and body fat <u>EXCEPT</u>

a.   people with the disease often have central obesity rather than lower-body obesity.
b.   a woman who gains 12 pounds since age 18 has double the risk of developing the disease.
c.   an obese person is 3 times more likely to develop the disease than is a nonobese individual.
d.   overweight people with the disease who lose weight show only minimal improvement in glucose tolerance and insulin resistance.

d   257(K)   58.   The risks for dying prematurely are doubled when the body mass index first rises above

a.   27.
b.   30.
c.   32.
d.   35.

b   263-265(A)   59.   Current dietary trends in fat and/or energy intake for adult Americans include all of the following <u>EXCEPT</u>

a.   our actual fat intake has increased by 4 g per day.
b.   our recommended fat intake is 25 g per 1,000 kcal.
c.   our average daily energy intake has risen by 200 kcal.
d.   our fat intake has decreased from 36% to 34% of daily energy intake.

c   264-265(A)   60.   All of the following are features of high-protein diets <u>EXCEPT</u>

a.   they have a high satiety index.
b.   they advise dieters to not count kcal.
c.   they provide for long-term weight maintenance.
d.   they typically recommend intakes of 800 to 1200 kcal/day.

d   264-266(K)   61.   The dieter's typical responses to a high-protein diet include all of the following <u>EXCEPT</u>

a.   a state of ketosis.
b.   a loss of appetite.
c.   a loss of glycogen.
d.   a slow re-gain of the lost weight.

d   264-265(K)   62.   Adverse side effects of typical low-carbohydrate diets include all of the following EXCEPT

a.   fatigue.
b.   nausea.
c.   constipation.
d.   high blood pressure.

a   264-265(A)   63.   What is the primary reason for the weight loss seen on common high protein diets?

a.   Low energy intake
b.   A fall in the rate of de novo lipogenesis
c.   Liberal intake of low glycemic index foods
d.   Low blood insulin levels which favors fat oxidation

Matching (Answers can be used only once)

G	241	64.	Approximate number of kcal in 2 lbs of body fat
Q	242	65.	Technique used to measure the amount of heat given off when a food burns
R	242	66.	Technique used to measure the amount of oxygen consumed when a food burns
D	242	67.	Amount of kcal required to raise 1,000 g of water 50°C
L	243	68.	A psychological desire to eat
J	242	69.	A physiological need to eat
I	243	70.	A feeling of fullness after eating
N	243	71.	Eating in response to arousal
M	243	72.	Eating in response to the time of day
P	246	73.	Energy needed to maintain the body at rest
B	246	74.	The percentage decline in basal metabolism per decade of adult life
H	247	75.	A factor that lowers basal metabolism
K	247	76.	A factor that raises basal metabolism
F	250	77.	Approximate total number of kcal expended over 2 days by a 120 lb college-aged woman engaged in light activity
O	247	78.	Term that describes the energy needed to process food
S	249	79.	Changes in energy expenditure consequent to changes in environment
E	247	80.	The amount of kcal in a 1,000 kcal meal that is expended as specific dynamic activity
A	248	81.	Maximum amount of kcal expended during one minute of studying
T	247	82.	Synonymous with the thermic effect of food
C	251	83.	Body mass index of an adult of 180 lbs and 5 feet 11 inches in height

A.	2	K.	Caffeine
B.	5	L.	Appetite
C.	25	M.	External cue
D.	50	N.	Stress eating
E.	100	O.	Thermic effect
F.	3,800	P.	Basal metabolism
G.	7,000	Q.	Direct calorimetry
H.	Fasting	R.	Indirect calorimetry
I.	Satiety	S.	Specific dynamic effect
J.	Hunger	T.	Adaptive thermogenesis

Essay Questions

241   84.   Discuss the benefits and adverse effects of slow and rapid rates of weight loss in overweight people.

242   85.   Discuss common methods for determining the energy content of foods and energy expenditure of individuals.

242-245   86.   Discuss factors that affect the sensations of hunger and those of appetite.

243-245   87.   Explain the difference between safety and satiation. Give examples of nutrients with a high or low satiating index.

246-247   88.   Define basal metabolic rate and discuss factors that increase and decrease it.

246-249   89.   List the major components that contribute to the body's daily expenditure of energy. Compare the relative contributions of a sedentary person with a marathon runner of the same body weight.

247-249   90.   Explain the meaning and significance of

     a.   The thermic effect of food.

     b.   Adaptive thermogenesis.

251-255   91.   Describe the difficulties in using standard weight-for-height tables to assess people's body weights.

252-253   92.   What factors should be considered for determining the optimal or ideal body fat levels in people or population groups?

254-255   93.   Explain the adverse effects of excess body fat deposited around the abdominal region.

250-256   94.   Briefly explain the following techniques for the estimation of body composition: a) fatfold measures, b) hydrodensitometry, and c) bioelectrical impedance.

255-257   95.   List several health risks associated with being underweight and with being overweight.

263   96.   Explain the connection between fad diets and high-protein diets.

263-266   97.   Discuss the pros and cons of high-protein diets.

CHAPTER 9
WEIGHT CONTROL: OVERWEIGHT AND UNDERWEIGHT

Ans   Page

c   269(K)   01.   What is the rationale for the fat cell theory of obesity?

     a.   Fat cell number increases dramatically after puberty
     b.   Fat cell number in an adult can decrease only by fasting
     c.   Fat cell number increases most readily in late childhood and early puberty
     d.   Weight gain from overeating in adults takes place primarily by increasing the number of fat cells

d   269(K)   02.   According to body mass index values, what fraction of the U.S. adult population is considered overweight?

     a.   1/10
     b.   1/6
     c.   1/3
     d.   1/2

a   269(K)   03.   All of the following describe the behavior of fat cells <u>EXCEPT</u>

     a.   the number decreases when fat is lost from the body.
     b.   the storage capacity for fat depends on both cell number and cell size.
     c.   the number increases at a faster rate in obese children than it does in lean children.
     d.   the number increases several-fold during the growth years and tapers off when adult status is reached.

1

d   269(A)   04.   In the quest for achieving desirable body weight, adults have control over all of the following EXCEPT

a.   diet.
b.   behavior.
c.   physical activity.
d.   adipocyte number.

b   269(K)   05.   Obesity resulting from an increase in the size of fat cells is termed

a.   hyperplastic obesity.
b.   hypertrophic obesity.
c.   idiopenthic leptinemia.
d.   anaplastic hypometabolism.

a   269(K)   06.   Obesity resulting from an increase in the number of fat cells is termed

a.   hyperplastic obesity.
b.   hypertrophic obesity.
c.   idiopenthic leptinemia.
d.   anaplastic hypometabolism.

b   269-270(K) 07.   Which of the following is known to promote fat storage in adipocytes?

a.   Glucagon
b.   Lipoprotein lipase
c.   Cellulite synthetase
d.   Lipoprotein synthetase

b   270(A)   08.   What is the most likely explanation for why women readily store fat around the hips whereas men readily store fat around the abdomen?

a.   Differences in blood insulin levels
b.   Differences in the activity of lipoprotein lipase
c.   Differences in circulating lipid transport proteins
d.   Differences in the activity of lipoprotein synthetase

d   271-257(K)   09.   Which of the following defines the body's set point?

    a.   Minimum weight of a person
    b.   Maximum weight of a person
    c.   Point at which a dieter plateaus and then drops weight quickly
    d.   Point above which the body tends to lose weight and below which it tends to gain weight

a   272(K)   10.   What is the chief factor that determines a person's risk for obesity?

    a.   Heredity
    b.   Environment
    c.   Metabolic rate
    d.   Fat content of diet

c   272-273(K)   11.   Which of the following describes a relationship between leptin and energy balance?

    a.   Fat cell sensitivity to leptin is higher in obese people
    b.   A deficiency of leptin is characteristic of all obese people
    c.   Blood levels of leptin usually correlate directly with body fat
    d.   Major functions of leptin include an increase in hunger and a decrease in metabolic rate

b   272(K)   12.   Which of the following is a feature of leptin?

    a.   It is an enzyme
    b.   It acts primarily on the brain
    c.   It is usually deficient in obese people
    d.   It is secreted by the brain and acts on fat cells

c   273-274(K)   13.   What serves as the body's chief storage site for lipid?

    a.   Yellow fat
    b.   Brown adipose tissue
    c.   White adipose tissue
    d.   High-density lipoproteins

c   275(K)   14.   In comparison with non-obese people, obese people are shown to have a lower

    a.   basal metabolic rate.
    b.   thermic effect of food.
    c   physical activity level.
    d.   metabolic response to exercise.

b 275-276(K) 15. What is considered to be the most important single contributor to the obesity problem in the United States?

a. Overeating
b. Physical inactivity
c. Environmental factors
d. Overabundance of foods

c 275(K) 16. Television watching contributes to obesity for all of the following reasons EXCEPT

a. it promotes inactivity.
b. it promotes between-meal snacking.
c. it replaces time that could be spent eating.
d. it gives high exposure to energy-dense foods featured in the commercial advertisements.

c 272(K) 17. What term has been assigned to the easy access and overabundance of high-fat, high-kcalorie foods in our society?

a. Fast food heaven
b. Death by hamburgers
c. Toxic food environment
d. Fats galore and glorious fats

d 276(K) 18. Approximately what percentage of people who lose weight by dieting fail to maintain the weight loss?

a. 5
b. 25
c. 75
d. 95

a 277-278(K) 19. Which of the following defines weight cycling?

a. A series of weight loss and regain episodes that affects body composition and metabolism
b. An ergonometric device designed to force the user to achieve higher levels of energy expenditure and thus weight loss
c. A safe weight loss program consisting of a 2-week period of dieting and then 1 week off the diet, and a repeat of this cycle until the desired amount of body weight is lost
d. A technique designed by the American Medical Association involving the use of a combination of aerobic activities and light-weight strength conditioning as a safe method of weight loss

d   277-278(K)   20.   Which of the following terms is <u>NOT</u> commonly used to describe the typical situation of an overweight individual who experiences repeated bouts of weight loss and regain, with the gain frequently to a greater body weight than before?

    a.   Yo-yo effect
    b.   Weight cycling
    c.   Ratchet effect
    d.   Elevator effect

a   279(K)   21.   What is the primary action of the substance benzocaine, found in certain candy and gum and used as an over-the-counter weight loss aid?

    a.   It reduces taste sensations
    b.   It inhibits lipoprotein lipase
    c.   It inhibits pancreatic lipase
    d.   It alters circulating leptin concentrations

c   279(K)   22.   What is the primary action of orlistat, a weight loss drug?

    a.   It reduces taste sensation
    b.   It inhibits lipoprotein lipase
    c.   Its inhibits pancreatic lipase
    d.   It alters circulating leptin concentrations

d   279(K)   23.   The drug sibutramine reduces appetite by affecting

    a.   ketone production.
    b.   insulin to glucagon ratio.
    c.   leptin sensitivity of fat cells.
    d.   serotonin utilization in the brain.

c   279(K)   24.   Which of the following is an FDA approved over-the-counter medication for weight loss?

    a.   Leptin
    b.   Ephedrine
    c.   Benzocaine
    d.   Tetrahydrolipostatin

a   279(K)   25.   The prescription drug sibutramine acts by regulating the utilization of

    a.   serotonin.
    b.   blood insulin.
    c.   hormone-sensitive lipase.
    d.   adipocyte lipoprotein lipase.

c 280(K) 26. Fraudulent weight reduction literature refers to visually apparent lumpy forms of body fat as

a. lipomas.
b. lipidosis.
c. cellulite.
d. hyperphagic deposits.

b 281-283(K) 27. All of the following are sensible guidelines for diet plans EXCEPT

a. consume low-fat foods regularly.
b. eat rapidly to avoid prolonged contact with food.
c. adjust energy intake downward as weight loss progresses.
d. include vegetables, fruits, and grains as the mainstay of the diet.

d 281-285(A) 28. What is the best approach to weight loss?

a. Avoid foods containing carbohydrates
b. Eliminate all fats from the diet and decrease water intake
c Greatly increase protein intake to prevent body protein loss
d Reduce daily energy intake and increase energy expenditure

d 281-287(A) 29. Which of the following would NOT be a recommendation of weight-reduction counseling?

a. Reorganize some established behavior patterns
b. Use the exchange system to keep track of energy intake
c. Perform physical exercise to increase energy expenditure
d. Reduce daily energy intake to less than 1000 kcal to overcome the decrease in metabolic rate

c 282-283(K) 30. As a general rule, what minimum number of kcalories per day is necessary to assure nutritional adequacy in an eating plan for reducing body weight?

a. 500
b. 800
c. 1200
d. 1600

c   282(K)   31.   In a weight reduction regimen, the most realistic time frame for losing 10% of initial body weight is

    a.   6 weeks
    b.   3 months
    c.   6 months
    d.   1 year

a   282-283(K)   32.   Which of the following describes the research results of obese women in weight-loss programs?

    a.   They initially expected to lose unrealistic amounts of weight
    b.   They were mostly satisfied with a 15% reduction in weight
    c.   They typically lost about 30% more weight than they predicted
    d.   They expressed far less psychological benefits than expected after losing weight

d   282-284(A)   33.   All of the following are behavior modifications for losing weight EXCEPT

    a.   shopping only when not hungry.
    b.   eating only in one place and in one room.
    c.   participating in activities such as television viewing only when not eating.
    d.   taking smaller portions of food but always eating everything on the plate quickly.

d   283(K)   34.   The feeling of satiety from weight-loss diets is best promoted by diets rich in

    a.   fat.
    b.   water.
    c.   simple carbohydrates.
    d.   complex carbohydrates.

a   284(A)   35. Which of the following describes a connection between physical activity and energy expenditure?

    a. Walking a mile uses about the same energy as running a mile
    b. Walking a mile uses about half as much energy as running a mile
    c. Exercising the leg muscles is effective at burning away fat primarily around the thighs and hips
    d. Exercising the abdominal muscles is effective at burning away fat primarily around the abdomen

c   284-285(K) 36. Features of the adaptive response to regular physical exercise include all of the following EXCEPT

    a. it curbs appetite.
    b. it increases slightly the basal metabolic rate.
    c. it stimulates digestive function in the postexercise period.
    d. it triggers release of lipid from adipocytes from all over the body.

b   284-285(A) 37. An important aid in any weight-loss diet program is to

    a. decrease water intake.
    b. increase physical activity.
    c. speed up thyroid activity with metabolic enhancers.
    d. develop ketosis by maintaining carbohydrate intake as low as possible.

a   284-285(K) 38. Which of the following is a feature of the body's response to engaging in physical activity?

    a. After an intense and vigorous workout, basal metabolism remains elevated for several hours
    b. Lower body fat is more readily lost from vigorous exercises that work primarily the hip and leg muscles
    c. Blood glucose and fatty acid levels are low immediately after working out, but thereafter recover on their own
    d. After an intense workout, most people immediately feel the urge to eat a large carbohydrate meal to replace glycogen stores

b   285-286(A)   39.   An example of a behavior modification technique for weight control is to

a.   feel guilty after you overeat.
b.   keep a record of your eating habits.
c.   always clean your plate when you eat.
d.   have someone watch you to prevent overeating.

a   285-287(A)   40.   To help maximize the long-term success of a person's weight-loss program, which of the following personal attitudes should be encouraged in the individual?

a.   Strongly believing that weight can be lost
b.   Viewing the body realistically as being fat rather than thin
c.   Refraining from expressing overconfidence in ability to lose weight
d.   Accepting that underexercising is a part of the lifestyle of most overweight people

c   300(K)   41.   Which of the following is a characterisitic of people with anorexia nevosa?

a.   Most are aware of their condition and seek treatment
b.   Fewer than 200 women die each year from the disease
c.   In those who are treated, many relapse into abnormal eating patterns.
d.   During initial treatment, metabolism slows and appetite increases but thereafter subsides

c   287 (K)   42.   Which of the following is a feature of energy metabolism in formerly obese people who have lost weight?

a.   Energy expenditure is the same as in people who were never obese
b.   Basal metabolic rates are higher than those during the obese state
c.   Energy requirements are lower than expected for their current body weight
d.   Energy expenditure is the same per kg body weight compared with the obese state

c   288(K)   43.   Since obesity apparently ahs many causes, even in a single individual, the best approach to the condition seems to be

a.   fasting.
b.   medicines.
c.   prevention.
d.   genetic counseling.

c   289-290(A)   44.   Of the following, which is <u>NOT</u> among the recommended strategies for weight gain in an underweight person?

    a.   Behavior modification training
    b.   Increased physical activity, especially strength training
    c   Forced awakening during the night for supplemental meals and snacks
    d.   Consumption of regular meals and snacks that provide high-kcalorie foods in small volumes

d   289-290(A)   45.   Which of the following would <u>NOT</u> be part of a successful program of weight gain in an underweight individual?

    a.   Physical exercise
    b.   Energy-dense foods
    c.   Energy-dense beverages
    d.   Large number of small meals

d   296(K)   46.   Anorexia nervosa is most common in

    a.   male elderly.
    b.   male adolescents.
    c.   female executives.
    d.   female adolescents.

a   296(K)   47.   What term is given to a female athlete who has an eating disorder and develops amenorrhea and osteoporosis?

    a.   Female athlete triad
    b.   Triathlete medical disorder
    c.   High stress tertiary disorder
    d.   Nonadaptable training syndrome

b   300(K)   48.   Approximately what fraction of people treated for anorexia nervosa show reasonable maintenance of their weight gain?

    a.   1/4
    b.   1/2
    c.   4/5
    d.   9/10

d   301(A)   49.   Typical foods chosen by a person with bulimia nervosa during a binge include all of the following <u>EXCEPT</u>

    a.   bread.
    b.   cookies.
    c.   ice cream.
    d.   vegetables.

a   301(K)   50.   What is cathartic?

    a.   A strong laxative
    b.   An antidiarrheal medication
    c.   An over-the-counter weight loss product
    d.   A medication for the treatment of eating disorders

c   301(K)   51.   Which of the following is characteristic of the eating pattern of people with bulimia nervosa?

    a.   Bingeing is frequently done at buffets
    b.   Binge eating usually occurs during the daytime
    c.   Bingeing typically occurs after a period of strict dieting
    d.   A binge eating episode is usually completed within 20 minutes

c   302-303(K)   52.   Diet recommendations for people with bulimia nervosa include all of the following EXCEPT

    a.   eat sitting down.
    b.   include fiber-rich foods.
    c.   eat cold foods to stimulate satiety.
    d.   avoid "finger" foods to minimize overeating.

a   303(K)   53.   What is the primary factor that differentiates bulimia nervosa from binge-eating?

    a.   Purging is rarely practiced in binge-eating disorder
    b.   Higher rates of depression are reported in bulimia nervosa
    c.   More food is consumed at one setting in binge-eating disorders
    d.   Uncontrollable cravings for high-fat foods are seen only in bulimia nervosa

Matching (Answers can be used only once)

T	269	54.	A term that describes an increase in fat cell number in obesity
S	269	55.	A term that describes an increase in fat cell size in obesity
L	274	56.	Type of adipose that primarily stores fat
K	274	57.	Type of adipose that primarily produces heat
G	272	58.	A fat cell hormone
R	269	59.	An enzyme that promotes fat storage
B	276	60.	Percentage of people who maintain their weight loss after dieting
Q	I279	61.	A drug that interferes with serotonin metabolism
H	279	62.	Inhibitor of pancreatic lipase
O	281	63.	A cosmetic surgical procedure
I	280	64.	A fraudulent term to describe lumpy fat
N	279	65.	Inhibitor of taste sensations
F	280	66.	BMI of a clinically severely obese person
A	269	67.	Average weight gain (lb) per year between 25 and 55 years of age
D	282	68.	Recommended maximum rate of weight loss, in pounds per week
E	283	69.	Number of minutes for satiety signal to appear after beginning to eat
C	283	70.	Recommended minimum number of glasses of water to drink on a weight-loss diet
J	284	71.	Cause of an increase of basal metabolic rate
P	277	72.	A synonym for weight cycling
M	279	73.	Substance in some herbs that may cause heart attacks and seizures

A.	0.5	K.	Brown fat
B.	5	L.	White fat
C.	8	M.	Ephedrine
D.	1	N.	Benzocaine
E.	20	O.	Liposuction
F.	40	P.	Ratchet effect
G.	Leptin	Q.	Sibutramine
H.	Orlistat	R.	Lipoprotein lipase
I.	Cellulite	S.	Hypertrophic obesity
J.	Exercise	T.	Hyperplastic obesity

Essay Questions

269-277;   74.   List the major causes of obesity.   Which ones can be
285-287   controlled by dietary manipulations or behavior modification?

269-271;   75.   Explain why the efficiency of conversion to body fat is higher
275   for dietary fat than for carbohydrate and protein. What are the
                   results of research studies concerning the importance of low
                   fat diets in weight-reduction regimes?

270-571   76.   Explain the set point theory of obesity.

272-273   77.   Discuss the role of leptin in the regulation of food intake and
                   energy storage.

273-274   78.   Contrast the metabolic roles of white adipose tissue and brown
                   adipose tissue.

273-274   79.   Explain the significance of uncoupling reactions in energy
                   metabolism.

275   80. Explain the factors involved in the promotion of obesity by high-fat diets.

276-278   81. Describe psychological problems encountered by overweight people in their attempts to lose weight.

277   82. What types of information might be found in a weight-loss consumer "bill of rights"?

277-280   83. List several factors that help identify inappropriate, unsound, and possibly dangerous commercial weight-loss programs.

277-280   84. Explain the attraction of unsound weight-loss procedures and plans to obese people.

278-279   85. Discuss the use and abuse of prescription drugs for the treatment of obesity.

279-280   86.   Discuss the use of herbal products for weight loss.

280-281   87.   List the approaches for lowering body weight by surgery. What are the adverse side effects of these procedures?

282-283   88.   Describe a good weight-reduction diet in relation to energy content, meal size, carbohydrate and fat levels, and water intake.

284-285   89.   Explain the changes in metabolism consequent to a decrease in energy intake. How are these changes modified by regular physical exercise?

284-285   90.   Describe the benefits of regular physical activity as an aid to weight loss dieting.

285-287   91.   Explain the role of behavior modification in weight reduction programs.

288-290 92. Present a sound diet plan for weight gain in the underweight person.

278-303 93. List the adverse side effects of anorexia nervosa and bulimia nervosa. Describe the typical personality traits of individuals with these eating disorders.

272-272 94. Explain the role of behavior modification in weight reduction programs.

303 95. Discuss the characteristics of binge eating disorder. What is known about its treatment?

CHAPTER 10
THE WATER-SOLUBLE VITAMINS: B VITAMINS AND VITAMIN C

a   307;316(K)   01.   Expressions of vitamin quantities in foods and in the body include all of the following <u>EXCEPT</u>

    a.   grams.
    b.   milligrams.
    c.   equivalents.
    d.   micrograms.

c   307-308(K)   02.   What is a precursor?

    a.   A conditionally essential vitamin
    b.   A sign or symptom of a vitamin deficiency disorder
    c.   A substance that is used to synthesize another compound
    d.   A substance that is recycled through the liver and intestines

a   308-309(K)   03.   General characteristics of the water-soluble vitamins include all of the following <u>EXCEPT</u>

    a.   they must be consumed daily.
    b.   toxic levels in the body are rarely found.
    c.   they are absorbed directly into the blood.
    d.   excesses are eliminated from the kidneys.

a   307-309(K)   04.   Which of the following is NOT a general characteristic of the fat-soluble vitamins?

a.   Excesses are eliminated from the kidneys
b.   Absorption is via the lymphatic circulation
c.   Several of them require protein carriers for transport
d.   They can be stored in relatively large amounts in certain body tissues

b   308(A)   05.   Which of the following vitamins would be removed in the production of skim milk?

a.   Thiamin
b.   Vitamin A
c.   Riboflavin
d.   Vitamin B$_{12}$

c   308(A)   06.   Cooking a food in liberal amounts of water is LEAST likely to affect the vitamin content of

a.   folate.
b.   thiamin.
c.   vitamin A.
d.   riboflavin.

b   308(K)   07.   What is the primary excretory route for the water-soluble vitamins?

a.   Bile
b.   Kidney
c.   Intestine
d.   Perspiration

b   308(A)   08.   When vitamin B$_1$ is consumed in excess of needs, how does the body treat the excess?

a.   Not absorbed
b.   Excreted primarily in the urine
c.   Excreted primarily in the feces
d.   Stored in liver, bone, and adipose tissue

d   310(K)   09.   What is the primary function of the B vitamins?

a.   Energy source
b.   Anticoagulation
c.   Antibody stabilization
d.   Coenzyme participation

d   310(A)   10.   Which of the following explains why B vitamin deficiencies lead to lack of energy?

a.   B vitamins are a source of kilocalories
b.   Absorption of carbohydrates and fats is decreased
c.   Oxygen for energy metabolism cannot be transported to the cells
d.   Coenzymes needed for energy metabolism are produced in insufficient amounts

c   310(K)   11.   Which of the following describes the basic function of a coenzyme?

a.   Attaches to RNA to assist in the synthesis of an enzyme
b.   Attaches to cell membranes to assist in uptake of an enzyme
c.   Attaches to an enzyme and allows a chemical reaction to take place
d.   Attaches to an enzyme which allows for transport of the enzyme through the circulation

c   310-311(A)   12.   Which of the following functions has a requirement for thiamin?

a.   Blood coagulation
b.   Formation of red blood cells
c.   Energy release from energy-yielding nutrients
d.   Formation of epithelial cell mucopolysaccharides

d   310-311(K)   13.   What is the primary chemical reaction in which thiamin participates as its coenzyme?

a.   Transfers amine groups in the synthesis of amino acids
b.   Transfers hydrogen atoms in the synthesis of erythrocytes
c.   Assists in addition of methyl groups to compounds involved in energy metabolism
d.   Assists in removal of one carbon units from compounds involved in energy metabolism

b   310-311(K)   14.   Which of the following is the coenzyme form of thiamin?

a.   Thiaminacide
b.   Thiamin pyrophosphate
c.   Thiamin adenine dinucleotide
d.   Thiamin flavin mononucleotide

b   311(K)   15.   Beriberi results from a deficiency of

      a.   niacin.
      b.   thiamin.
      c.   vitamin C.
      d.   vitamin B_{12}.

b   311(K)   16.   The need for which of the following vitamins is generally related directly to the amount of energy expended?

      a.   Folate
      b.   Thiamin
      c.   Vitamin C
      d.   Vitamin B_6

b   311-312(K)   17.   Which of the following is a property of thiamin nutrition?

      a.   Participates in activation of prothrombin
      b.   Poor sources include seafood and cheeses
      c.   Significant amounts are found in leafy vegetables
      d.   Deficiency results in cheilosis and marked dermatitis

b   311(A)   18.   Which of the following diets is most likely to lead to beriberi?

      a.   Low intakes of whole grains
      b.   High intakes of polished rice
      c.   High intakes of unrefined rice
      d.   Low intakes of enriched grains

b   311(A)   19.   The Wernicke-Korsakoff syndrome which is often observed in poorly nourished alcohol abusers, is known to respond to supplements of

      a.   folacin.
      b.   thiamin.
      c.   vitamin C.
      d.   vitamin B_{12}.

a   311-312(A)   20.   Which of the following provides muscle tissue with the highest concentration of thiamin?

      a.   Pig
      b.   Fish
      c.   Steer
      d.   Chicken

a   311-312(K)   21.   Which of the following provides the most thiamin per serving size?

    a.   Ham
    b.   Squash
    c.   Whole milk
    d.   Whole-grain breads

b   311-312(A)   22.   Of the following, which is the richest food source of thiamin?

    a.   Milk
    b.   Pork
    c.   Lettuce
    d.   Refined rice

a   313(K)   23.   Which of the following is a characteristic of thiamin stability in relation to cooking method?

    a.   Microwaving the food conserves much of the thiamin
    b.   Prolonged heating of the food has little, if any, effect on the thiamin
    c.   Boiling the food tends to conserve thiamin by forming a stable, hydrated complex
    d.   Steaming the food can lead to substantial thiamin loss due to the high heat needed to form the steam

d   313(K)   24.   Which of the following food groups ordinarily contains the highest amount of vitamins when expressed per kcalorie?

    a.   Dairy
    b.   Meats
    c.   Fruits
    d.   Vegetables

d   314(K)   25.   Riboflavin in its coenzyme form functions in the transfer of

    a.   methyl groups.
    b.   1-carbon units.
    c.   2-carbon units.
    d.   hydrogen atoms.

c   314(K)   26.   Which of the following vitamins is involved substantially in energy transformation reactions?

    a.   Biotin
    b.   Cobalamin
    c.   Riboflavin
    d.   Pyridoxine

d   314;316(K)   27.   Which of the following is indicative of a dietary deficiency of riboflavin?

    a.   Beriberi
    b.   Diarrhea
    c.   Keratomalacia
    d.   Inflamed eyelids

a   314(A)   28.   Of the following commonly eaten foods, which makes the greatest contribution to riboflavin intake?

    a.   Milk
    b.   Potatoes
    c.   Orange juice
    d.   Peanut butter

c   314(A)   29.   Milk and milk products provide liberal amounts of which of the following vitamins?

    a.   Folate
    b.   Biotin
    c.   Riboflavin
    d.   Pantothenic acid

d   314(A)   30.   Riboflavin needs are more difficult to meet when the diet is low in

    a.   meats.
    b.   grains.
    c.   vegetables.
    d.   dairy foods.

d   314(K)   31.   Riboflavin is most easily destroyed when exposed to

    a.   heat.
    b.   acid.
    c.   alkali.
    d.   ultraviolet light.

b   314(A)   32.   What type of container is best for protecting the riboflavin content of milk?

    a.   Airtight
    b.   Cardboard
    c.   Transparent glass
    d.   Translucent plastic

a   314;316(K)   33.   Which of the following is a property of riboflavin in nutrition?

    a.   Stability to heat is good
    b.   Deficiency leads to beriberi
    c.   Requirements are proportional to body weight
    d.   Significant amounts are found in citrus products

c   314;316(K)   34.   The signs and symptoms of riboflavin deficiency are known collectively as

    a.   pellagra.
    b.   antiflavonosis.
    c.   ariboflavinosis.
    d.   flavin adenine dinucleosis.

c   314;316(K)   35.   A deficiency of what vitamin produces a characteristic cracking and redness at the corners of the mouth?

    a.   Biotin
    b.   Niacin
    c.   Riboflavin
    d.   Ascorbic acid

c   316(A)   36.   When the diet contains an adequate amount of protein, what amino acid can be used by the body to synthesize niacin?

    a.   Lysine
    b.   Valine
    c.   Tryptophan
    d.   Phenylalanine

d   316(K)   37.   Which of the following is a property of niacin in nutrition?

    a.   It is susceptible to destruction in foods exposed to light
    b.   It participates primarily in reactions involving amino acids
    c.   It is soluble in both water and lipids depending upon its chemical form
    d.   It can be synthesized in the body from the essential amino acid tryptophan

b   316(A)   38.   Which of the following properties is shared by niacin and riboflavin coenzymes?

    a.   Unstable to irradiation
    b.   Transfer of hydrogen atoms
    c.   Transfer of carboxyl groups
    d.   Unstable to metal cooking utensils

a   316-317(A)   39.   A diet low in protein and in which corn is a principal food has been found to cause a deficiency of what vitamin?

     a.   Niacin
     b.   Thiamin
     c.   Vitamin C
     d.   Vitamin B_{12}

b   316-317(K)   40.   What vitamin deficiency disease appeared in people who had subsisted on a diet high in corn and low in protein?

     a.   Scurvy
     b.   Pellagra
     c.   Wet beriberi
     d.   Pernicious anemia

d   316(K)   41.   Which of the following is NOT among the common signs of pellagra?

     a.   Dementia
     b.   Diarrhea
     c.   Dermatitis
     d.   Demineralization

b   316(K)   42.   A general niacin deficiency is known to be manifested in abnormalities of all of the following organs/systems EXCEPT

     a.   skin.
     b.   skeletal.
     c.   nervous system.
     d.   gastrointestinal tract.

b   316(A)   43.   Which of the following substances is found in corn and is known to contribute to the development of pellagra?

     a.   Avidin
     b.   Leucine
     c.   Phytates
     d.   Phenylalanine

a   316;319(A)   44.   Which of the following nutrients functions to prevent the appearance of a bilateral, symmetrical dermatitis, primarily on areas exposed to the sun?

     a.   Niacin
     b.   Choline
     c.   Inositol
     d.   Riboflavin

c   316-317(A)   45.   A typical diet of a 50 kg woman provides the RDA level of protein plus 6 mg of niacin. The protein contains an average of 1% tryptophan and 2% tyrosine. Approximately how many niacin equivalents are contributed by the diet?

    a.   2
    b.   5
    c.   13
    d.   20

a   317(A)   46.   What is the term that identifies the characteristic cutaneous tingling sensations and reddening of the skin after ingesting a pharmacologic dose of nicotinic acid?

    a.   Niacin flush
    b.   NAD dermatitis
    c.   Niacin erythremia
    d.   Bilateral symmetrical dermatitis

c   317(A)   47.   Which of the following overt side effect(s) is likely to appear after a person ingests a high quantity of nicotinic acid?

    a.   Constipation
    b.   Mental confusion
    c.   Painful, tingling, itching sensation
    d.   Hair loss, bloating, and photophobia

b   317(K)   48.   Which of the following is a feature of niacin nutrition?

    a.   Low doses may lead to kidney stones
    b.   High doses may lower blood cholesterol
    c.   Low doses may lead to heartburn and low blood pressure
    d.   High doses may elevate red blood cell count in mildly anemic individuals

a   317(A)   49.   When taken in large doses, which of the following vitamins is associated with liver injury and peptic ulcers?

    a.   Niacin
    b.   Thiamin
    c.   Vitamin B_6
    d.   Vitamin B_{12}

d   317(K)   50.   Large doses of nicotinic acid are known to result in all of the following EXCEPT

a.   liver injury.
b.   peptic ulcer disease.
c.   dilation of capillaries.
d.   disappearance of learning disorders in children.

b   316-317(A)   51.   Approximately how many niacin equivalents would be provided from the protein in the diet of a 130 lb person ingesting the RDA amount of protein?

a.   4
b.   8
c.   12
d.   16

d   319-320(K)   52.   Features of biotin in nutrition include all of the following EXCEPT

a.   it functions in the breakdown of amino acids and fatty acids.
b.   it functions as a carrier of carbon dioxide in energy metabolism.
c.   a deficiency can be induced by ingesting large quantities of raw egg whites.
d.   a deficiency can be induced by ingesting large amounts of thiamin and folic acid which interfere with its absorption.

a   319;331(K)   53.   Among the following compounds that serve as coenzymes in metabolism, which is considered a vitamin for human beings?

a.   Biotin
b.   Inositol
c.   Lipoic acid
d.   Orotic acid

a   319(K)   54.   Which of the following foods contains a protein that decreases bioavailability of biotin?

a.   Raw eggs
b.   Aged wine
c.   Aged cheese
d.   Raw cauliflower

b   319(K)   55.   A protein that binds with biotin (thus inhibiting absorption) is found in which food?

     a.   Aged cheese
     b.   Raw egg whites
     c.   Whole wheat bread
     d.   Unhomogenized milk

d   319-320(K)   56.   Biotin can be synthesized by

     a.   avidin.
     b.   the skin.
     c.   the liver.
     d.   intestinal bacteria.

b   319-320(K)   57.   Which of the following vitamins is known to be synthesized by intestinal bacteria?

     a.   Folate
     b.   Biotin
     c.   Cyanocobalamin
     d.   Pantothenic acid

d   320(K)   58.   What vitamin forms a part of coenzyme A?

     a.   Biotin
     b.   Folate
     c.   Riboflavin
     d.   Pantothenic acid

c   321(K)   59.   What vitamin is involved intensively in amino acid metabolism?

     a.   Biotin
     b.   Vitamin A
     c.   Vitamin B_6
     d.   Riboflavin

b   321-322(A)   60.   Which of the following is <u>NOT</u> a characteristic of vitamin B_6 in nutrition?

     a.   It is stored in muscle tissue
     b.   It is required in amounts proportional to energy expenditure
     c.   It can lead to irreversible nerve damage when taken in large doses
     d.   It functions, in part, in the synthesis of glycine and glutamic acid

d   321-322(K)   61. All of the following are features of vitamin B6 metabolism EXCEPT

    a. a deficiency or toxicity leads to depression.
    b. its destruction and excretion are promoted by alcohol intake.
    c. it functions primarily as the coenzyme pyridoxal phosphate.
    d. it enhances physical performance when supplied at a level of I mg/g of dietary protein.

d   321(K)   62. What vitamin has been taken in large amounts by women in hopes of combatting the symptoms of pre-menstrual syndrome?

    a. Thiamin
    b. Inositol
    c. Cobalamin
    d. Vitamin B6

a   321-322(K)   63. Which of the following statements confirms our knowledge of water-soluble vitamin toxicity?

    a. Toxicity symptoms for vitamin B6 can be severe and irreversible
    b. Toxicity symptoms for vitamin C include constipation and hyperactivity
    c. Toxicities of the B-vitamins occur almost as often from foods as from supplements
    d. Toxicity of niacin has been reported in body builders taking large amounts of amino acid supplements

d   322-323(A)   64. On a per-kcalorie basis, which of the following foods is richest in vitamin B6?

    a. Meats
    b. Fruits
    c. Legumes
    d. Vegetables

a   322;331(K)   65. Which of the following is an essential nutrient for human beings?

    a. Folate
    b. Inositol
    c. Methoxatin
    d. Lipoic acid

CHAPTER 10, THE WATER-SOLUBLE VITAMINS: B VITAMINS AND VITAMIN C

b   322;324(K)   66.   All of the following are properties of folate in nutrition <u>EXCEPT</u>

        a.   it is needed for proper functioning of vitamin B_{12}.
        b.   it functions primarily in the transfer of amino groups.
        c.   the coenzyme of folate requires vitamin B_{12} to function properly.
        d.   it requires enzymes on the intestinal mucosa to enhance its absorption from most foods.

a   322;324;(A)   67.   Which of the following activities is shared by vitamin B_{12} and
     328   folate?

        a.   Both are required for nucleic acid synthesis
        b.   Both require intrinsic factors for their release from food proteins
        c.   Both are found in significant amounts in green leafy vegetables
        d.   Both are considered problem nutrients for strict vegetarians

a   322;324(K)   68.   Which of the following vitamins is usually found in a form that is bound to one or more glutamic acid molecules in food?

        a.   Folate
        b.   Thiamin
        c.   Vitamin B_6
        d.   Ascorbic acid

a   324(A)   69.   A person with a disorder that limits absorption of bile is at increased risk for deficiency of

        a.   folate.
        b.   niacin.
        c.   riboflavin.
        d.   ascorbic acid.

b   324(A)   70.   What is the most likely explanation for the impaired functioning of the GI tract resulting from folate deficiency?

    a.   Since folate is required for bile synthesis, folate deficiency results in insufficient bile production, thereby promoting fat malabsorption and diarrhea
    b.   Since folate functions, in large part, in the process of cell renewal, a deficiency slows mucosal cell replacement, thereby resulting in decreased GI functioning
    c.   The anemia of folate deficiency results in decreased oxygen supply to body tissues, with the intestines being particularly affected because of their high metabolic activity
    d.   Since folate functions, in part, in the synthesis of pancreatic digestive enzymes, a deficiency leads to decreased enzymatic capacity in the intestines, thereby resulting in malabsorption

c   324(K)   71.   Approximately what percentage of dietary folate is bioavailable?

    a.   10
    b.   25
    c.   50
    d.   80

a   322;324(A)   72.   What vitamin is involved mainly with the replacement of red blood cells and digestive tract cells?

    a.   Folate
    b.   Niacin
    c.   Thiamin
    d.   Riboflavin

d   324(K)   73.   The percent bioavailability of a folate supplement taken on an empty stomach is

    a.   5
    b.   25
    c.   50
    d.   100

a 324(K) 74. Which of the following vitamins undergoes significant enterohepatic circulation?

a. Folate
b. Niacin
c. Thiamin
d. Pyridoxine

b 325(A) 75. Research has shown that the risk for neural tube defects is lowered by taking supplements of

a. niacin.
b. folate.
c. vitamin C.
d. vitamin B$_{12}$.

d 325(K) 76. Which of the following is a type of neural tube defect?

a. Scurvy
b. Beriberi
c. Pellagra
d. Spina bifida

b 326K) 77. Which of the following is known to significantly affect the body's folate status?

a. Sedentary lifestyle
b. Some anticancer drugs
c. Insufficient fiber intake
d. Some antituberculosis drugs

b 326(A) 78. Physiological stresses such as blood loss, burns, measles, and cancer are known particularly to increase the risk of deficiency for

a. biotin.
b. folate.
c. riboflavin.
d. pantothenic acid.

d 326(K) 79. Which of the following is associated with a deficiency of folate?

a. Hemolysis
b. Hypoxemia
c. Hemolytic anemia
d. Large-cell type anemia

c 326(K) 80. Which of the following substances is known to adversely affect folate utilization?

    a. Insulin
    b. Calcium supplements
    c. Heavy use of antacids
    d. Vitamin B_{12} supplements

d 326-327(K) 81. Which of the following foods is highest in folate?

    a. Meats
    b. Starches
    c. Dairy products
    d. Green leafy vegetables

d 326;328(K) 82. Which of the following is representative of folate availability in foods?

    a. Good sources are dairy products and meats
    b. Poor sources are fruit juices and vegetable juices
    c. Only about 10% of the amount in foods is bioavailable
    d. Much of the vitamin is unstable to ordinary cooking and storage conditions

a 326(K) 83. Among all the vitamins, which is believed to be most vulnerable to interactions with drugs?

    a. Folate
    b. Niacin
    c. Vitamin B_6
    d. Vitamin B_{12}

b 326(K) 84. Folate deficiency has been reported in infants fed

    a. soy milk.
    b. goat's milk.
    c. chicken liver.
    d. infant formula.

d 328(A) 85. What is the RDA for folate for a woman weighing 132 pounds?

    a. 180 µg
    b. 220 µg
    c. 242 µg
    d. 400 µg

c   328(K)   86.   Which of the following is required for the absorption of dietary vitamin B_{12}?

       a.   Bile
       b.   Lipase
       c.   Intrinsic factor
       d.   Carboxypeptidase

b   328-329(A)   87.   A similar type of anemia is produced when there is a deficiency of either

       a.   riboflavin or niacin.
       b.   vitamin B_{12} or folate.
       c.   thiamin or riboflavin.
       d.   vitamin B_6 or vitamin B_{12}.

b   328(K)   88.   What is the function of intrinsic factor in vitamin B_{12} absorption?

       a.   It catalyzes release of the vitamin from its protein-bound form
       b.   It attaches to the vitamin thereby allowing absorption from the intestines
       c.   It acts as a storage protein for the vitamin within the intestinal epithelial cells
       d.   It acts as a cofactor for mucosal enzymes involved in absorption of the vitamin

a   328(K)   89.   Which of the following is a property of vitamin B_{12}?

       a.   It is efficiently recycled by the body
       b.   It is necessary for protection from pinpoint hemorrhages
       c.   It requires attachment to fatty acids for transport in the circulation
       d.   It is absorbed from the stomach with the aid of a special binding protein

c   328-329(A)   90.   What is the most likely reason for the development of a vitamin B_{12} deficiency?

       a.   Inadequate intake
       b.   Increased excretion
       c.   Inadequate absorption
       d.   Increased losses in food preparation

d   328-329(A)   91.   Among the following water-soluble vitamins, a secondary deficiency would most likely be seen for

    a.   biotin.
    b.   thiamin.
    c.   vitamin C.
    d.   vitamin B_{12}.

a   329(A)   92.   What is the most common treatment for pernicious anemia caused by inadequate absorption?

    a.   Injection of cobalamin
    b.   Topical administration of liver extract
    c.   Oral supplements of B-vitamin complex
    d.   A diet high in liver and green leafy vegetables

d   329(A)   93.   If a person refrained from ingesting any of the water-soluble vitamins, deficiency symptoms would appear last for

    a.   folate.
    b.   vitamin C.
    c.   vitamin B_1.
    d.   vitamin B_{12}.

b   329(A)   94.   Why are vegetarians at risk of developing vitamin B_{12} deficiency?

    a.   Vegetarian diets inhibit absorption of the vitamin
    b.   Vegetarian diets provide insufficient amounts of the vitamin
    c.   High fiber content of vegetarian diets causes decreased storage by the liver
    d.   High fiber content of vegetarian diets causes increased excretion of the vitamin

d   329(A)   95.   Normally, the body's storage and re-utilization of vitamin B_{12} prevents a primary or secondary deficiency from occurring until after about

    a.   several days.
    b.   three weeks.
    c.   three months.
    d.   three years.

d   329(A)   96.   In a person who loses the ability to absorb vitamin B_{12}, approximately what period of time could elapse before deficiency signs develop?

       a.   One month
       b.   Six months
       c.   One year
       d.   Three years

c   329(A)   97.   The absorption of which of the following vitamins is most affected by the disorder atrophic gastritis?

       a.   Choline.
       b.   Vitamin C
       c.   Vitamin B_{12}
       d.   Pantothenic acid

b   329(K)   98.   Pernicious anemia results from a combination of lack of intrinsic factor and

       a.   ariboflavonosis.
       b.   atrophic gastritis.
       c.   pancreatic vitaminases
       d.   pharmacologic intakes of folate

a   330(A)   99.   Of the following foods, which would be the only source of vitamin B_{12}?

       a.   Hot dog
       b.   Pecan pie
       c.   Cauliflower
       d.   Blueberry muffin

a   331(K)   100.   Which of the following is known to perform an essential function in the human body?

       a.   Inositol
       b.   Ubiquinone
       c.   Pangamic acid
       d.   Para-aminobenzoic acid

b   331(K)   101.   Which of the following is classified as a conditionally essential nutrient?

       a.   PABA
       b.   Choline
       c.   Inositol
       d.   Ubiquinone

b 331(K) 102. Which of the following acids is <u>NOT</u> known to be required in the diet of human beings?

    a. Folic acid
    b. Lipoic acid
    c. Ascorbic acid
    d. Pantothenic acid

a 331(K) 103. Which of the following is probably required in the diet of human beings?

    a. Choline
    b. Inositol
    c. Lipoic acid
    d. Pangamic acid

b 331(K) 104. Which of the following is <u>NOT</u> known to be a vitamin for human beings?

    a. Cobalamin
    b. Ubiquinone
    c. Pyridoxine
    d. Pantothenic acid

c 332(K) 105. Which of the following vitamins has an RDA?

    a. Biotin
    b. Choline
    c. Cobalamin
    d. Pantothenic acid

a 332;335(A) 106. Which of the following characteristics is shared by vitamins B_6, B_{12}, C and folate?

    a. Prevention of anemia
    b. Required for glycolysis
    c. Required in microgram quantities
    d. Found in citrus products and legumes

b 334-335(K) 107. Which of the following is frequently affected by deficiencies of the B vitamins?

    a. Bones
    b. Tongue
    c. Eyesight
    d. Hair and nails

b   334(A)   108.   Which of the following is an overt sign of a possible B vitamin deficiency?

    a.   Anemia
    b.   Smooth tongue
    c.   Abnormal liver function
    d.   Abnormal heart function

b   336(K)   109.   In what capacity does vitamin C function?

    a.   Coenzyme for energy release
    b.   Cofactor in collagen formation
    c.   Cofactor with calcium in blood coagulation
    d.   Coenzyme in the formation of red blood cells

d   336(K)   110.   Which of the following is a general function of vitamin C?

    a.   Antiviral agent
    b.   Antifungal agent
    c.   Anticancer agent
    d.   Antioxidant agent

c   336-337(K)   111.   The protein that requires ascorbic acid for its formation is

    a.   keratin.
    b.   albumin.
    c.   collagen.
    d.   hydroxyproline.

c   337(A)   112.   Under which of the following circumstances have intakes of vitamin C above the RDA been shown to NOT be of any benefit?

    a.   Infections
    b.   Major surgery
    c.   Psychological stress
    d.   Oral contraceptive use

b   337(A)   113. Which of the following represents the results of well-controlled studies of vitamin C supplementation on the resistance to, and recovery from, colds?

    a. There was a reduction in the duration of colds by 50% on the average
    b. There was only a minor effect on reducing the number and severity of colds
    c. There was a significant reduction in the duration of colds only in people who consumed at least one gram a day
    d. There was a significant reduction in the number of colds only in people who consumed more than three grams per day

a   337(A)   114. Why might vitamin C supplements be beneficial in treating the common cold?

    a. It deactivates histamine
    b. It destroys intestinal pathogens
    c. It reduces episodes of sneezing
    d. It alters hypothalamic control of body temperature

c   337(K)   115. Which of the following vitamins is known to deactivate histamine, a substance that causes nasal congestion?

    a. Niacin
    b. Vitamin E
    c. Vitamin C
    d. Vitamin B-12

a   337(A)   116. What is the minimum amount of ascorbic acid that will prevent the appearance of scorbutic symptoms in human beings?

    a. 10 mg
    b. 30 mg
    c. 50 mg
    d. 60 mg

a   338(K)   117. Which of the following is an early sign of vitamin C deficiency?

    a. Bleeding gums
    b. Pernicious anemia
    c. Appearance of a cold
    d. Hysteria and depression

d   338(K)   118. Which of the following symptoms is indicative of a deficiency of vitamin C?

    a.   Hair loss
    b.   Muscle spasms
    c.   Bilateral symmetrical dermatitis
    d.   Subcutaneous pinpoint hemorrhages

c   339(A)   119. What term is used to describe the outcome of a diagnostic test that apparently shows that you have mononucleosis when in reality you do not?

    a.   True positive
    b.   True negative
    c.   False positive
    d.   False negative

d   339(A)   120. Which of the following is a possible withdrawal symptom from chronic vitamin C megadoses?

    a.   Diarrhea
    b.   Metallic taste
    c.   GI discomfort
    d.   Bleeding gums

c   339;341(A)   121. All of the following are consequences of ingesting excess vitamin C supplements <u>EXCEPT</u>

    a.   they frequently cause diarrhea.
    b.   they appear safe at levels up to 300 mg/day.
    c.   they enhance the action of anticlotting medications.
    d.   they interfere with laboratory urine tests for the diagnosis of diabetes.

c   339(K)   122. Which of the following foods provides ample amounts of vitamin C?

    a.   Milk group
    b.   Meat group
    c.   Fruit group
    d.   Bread-cereal group

a   339-341(A)   123.   Which of these meals is lacking in vitamin C?

    a.   Roast beef, carrots, noodles, and tea
    b.   Hot dog, cabbage, french fries, and milk
    c.   Roast beef, broccoli, noodles, and coffee
    d.   Spaghetti with tomato sauce, meatball, garlic bread, and red wine

c   339(K)   124.   Which of the following food groups is a rich source of vitamin C?

    a.   Milk group
    b.   Meat group
    c.   Fruit group
    d.   Bread-cereal group

c   339-341(A)   125.   Which of the following would be a very good source of vitamin C for the lacto-ovo-vegetarian?

    a.   Milk
    b.   Eggs
    c.   Broccoli
    d.   Whole-grain bread

c   339-341(A)   126.   Which of the following would be the poorest dietary source of vitamin C?

    a.   Liver
    b.   Potatoes
    c.   Whole grains
    d.   Cruciferous vegetables

d   339(A)   127.   People with a certain genetic predisposition would be at high risk for serious iron toxicity from taking pharmacologic amounts of the vitamin

    a.   niacin.
    b.   retinol.
    c.   cobalamin.
    d.   ascorbic acid.

a   340-341(K)   128. What food makes a significant contribution to vitamin C intakes in the U.S. population despite the modest vitamin C concentration?

     a.   Potatoes
     b.   Organ meats
     c.   Breaded fish
     d.   Whole-grain cereals

c   342-348(A)   129. Which of the following statements is representative of vitamin supplementation practices?

     a.   Most people who take supplements consume a poor diet
     b.   Most people should take supplements daily because of the great difficulty in obtaining the needed amounts from food
     c.   People who have low energy intakes or are pregnant are at risk for developing deficiencies and may benefit from supplementation
     d.   People should take supplements daily because nutrition surveys in the U.S. and Canada have detected deficiencies in some population groups

a   347-350(A)   130. Groups of people who are at risk for developing marginal deficiencies and may benefit from taking vitamin supplements include all of the following EXCEPT

     a.   athletes.
     b.   food faddists.
     c.   pregnant or lactating women.
     d.   people with low energy intakes, such as habitual dieters and the elderly.

b   347(K)   131. Approximately what percentage of people take daily multi-nutrient supplements?

     a.   5
     b.   20
     c.   50
     e.   80

c   349(A)   132. All of the following are known to occur from a mild iron overdose <u>EXCEPT</u>

      a.   nausea.
      b.   GI distress.
      c.   black tongue.
      d.   black diarrhea.

c   349(K)   133. In the United States, what is the adult RDA for vitamin C?

      a.   10-20 mg
      b.   50-60 mg
      c.   75-90 mg
      d.   100-135 mg

d   348-350(K)   134. The known dangers of taking vitamin supplements include all of the following <u>EXCEPT</u>

      a.   vitamin toxicity.
      b.   the taker may ignore warning signs of a disease.
      c.   the taker may feel a false sense of security and consume a poor diet.
      d.   pathogenic bacterial overgrowth of the large intestines leading to increased risk of infection.

Matching (Answers can be used only once)

J	311	135.	Name of thiamin deficiency disease
A	311	136.	A food unusually rich in thiamin
L	316	137.	Deficiency of this vitamin leads to cracks and redness at corners of the mouth
S	314	138.	Exposure to this leads to destruction of riboflavin
C	314	139.	A food source that supplies a substantial amount of people's riboflavin intake
O	316	140.	Used for synthesis of niacin
B	316	141.	Overconsumption of this food has resulted in pellagra
F	317	142.	High doses are known to lower blood cholesterol
E	319	143.	Deficiency of this vitamin is induced by feeding raw egg whites
T	320	144	This vitamin is required for synthesis of acetyl-CoA
M	322	145.	Toxicity from this vitamin is known to cause irreversible nerve damage
D	325	146.	Prevention of neural tube defects is related to increased intake of this substance by pregnant women
H	326	147.	One of the first symptoms of folate deficiency
N	328	148.	Required to maintain nerve fiber sheath
R	328	149.	Required for absorption of vitamin B_{12}
G	331	150.	A conditionally essential nutrient
Q	336	151.	The antiscorbutic factor
I	336	152.	Vitamin C is required for the synthesis of this substance
P	339	153.	Excess intakes of vitamin C increases the risk for this disorder
K	339	154.	A concentrated source of vitamin C

A.	Ham	K.	Broccoli
B.	Corn	L.	Riboflavin
C.	Dairy	M.	Vitamin B_6
D.	Folate	N.	Vitamin B_{12}
E.	Biotin	O.	Tryptophan
F.	Niacin	P.	Iron overload
G.	Choline	Q.	Ascorbic acid
H.	Anemia	R.	Intrinsic factor
I.	Collagen	S.	Ultraviolet light
J.	Beriberi	T.	Pantothenic acid

Essay Questions

317;321-322; 155. Under what circumstances can water-soluble vitamins be
334;339;   toxic? Cite several examples.
349-350

325-326   156. Discuss the expected benefits of folate supplementation of
                     flour. What are the possible adverse effects of this
                     practice?

329-330   157. Discuss the interrelationships of folate and vitamin B_{12} in the
                     diagnosis and treatment of large-cell type anemia.

328-330   158. Define intrinsic factor and discuss its relationship to vitamin
                     B_{12} absorption. What other factors are associated with
                     vitamin B_{12} absorption? What is the most common cause of
                     vitamin B_{12} deficiency and how is vitamin B_{12} deficiency
                     treated under this condition?

330   159. Why might vegans have a normal vitamin B_{12} status?

332-333   160.   Discuss the roles of the B vitamins in energy metabolism.

334   161.   Discuss similarities in the deficiency symptoms of the B vitamins.

334   162.   What is meant by the expression: vitamins are like horseshoe nails?

335-337   163.   Explain the modes of action of vitamin C.

337-338   164.   Under what conditions and for what reasons would intakes of vitamin C above the RDA be desirable?

337   165.   In what ways have vitamin C supplements been shown to affect nasal congestion?

339   166.   Discuss how megadoses of vitamin C could possibly lead to symptoms of scurvy.

339   167.   Describe the hazards of excessive vitamin C intake.

339   168.   What is meant by false positive and false negative medical tests as influenced by vitamin supplements?

347-350   169.   List several arguments for and against the regular use of vitamin supplements.

351   170.   For people who require a dietary multinutrient supplement, what are the guidelines regarding the form of the supplement?

351-352   171.   Explain the major aspects of the Dietary Supplement Health and Education Act of 1994.

CHAPTER 11
THE FAT-SOLUBLE VITAMINS: A, D, E, AND K

Ans   Page

c   355(A)   01.   Which of the following is <u>NOT</u> among the features of the fat-soluble vitamins?

                       a.   Require bile for absorption
                       b.   Found in the fat and oily parts of foods
                       c.   Transported permanently to the liver and adipose tissue
                       d.   Pose a greater risk for developing a toxicity than water-soluble vitamins

c   355(K)   02.   What is the major carrier of the fat-soluble vitamins from the intestinal epithelial cell to the circulation?

                       a.   Albumin
                       b.   Cholesterol
                       c.   Chylomicrons
                       d.   Liposoluble binding proteins

d   355(K)   03.   Which of the following is <u>NOT</u> a fat-soluble vitamin?

                       a.   Retinol
                       b.   Tocopherol
                       c.   Phylloquinone
                       d.   Cyanocobalamin

a 355-358(A) 04. As far as is known, vitamin A does <u>NOT</u> play an important role in which of the following processes?

a. Blood clotting
b. Growth of bones and teeth
c. Synthesis of visual pigment
d. Maintaining mucous membranes

c 355(K) 05. Which of the following is a property of the fat-soluble vitamins?

a. Most of them are synthesized by intestinal bacteria
b. Intestinal transport occurs by way of the portal circulation
c. Deficiency symptoms may take years to develop on a poor diet
d. Toxicity risk is higher for vitamins E and K than for other fat soluble vitamins

c 355(K) 06. Which of the following is responsible for transporting vitamin A from the liver to other tissues?

a. Albumin
b. Rhodopsin
c. Retinol-binding protein
d. Transcarotenoid protein

c 355(K) 07. How many different forms of vitamin A are active in the body?

a. 1
b. 2
c. 3
d. 5

d 355(K) 08. All of the following are forms of vitamin A <u>EXCEPT</u>

a. retinol.
b. retinal.
c. retinoic acid.
d. retinoquinone.

d 355(A) 09. If the diet contains precursor vitamin A, which of the following tissues can use it to form vitamin A?

a. Eyes
b. Kidneys
c. Adipose cells
d. Intestinal cells

c   356(K)   10.   Which of the following is the name of the vitamin A compound that is active in the visual response?

    a.   Opsin
    b.   Keratin
    c.   Retinal
    d.   Carotene

a   356(K)   11.   Which of the following describes an event in the visual response process?

    a.   Light energy strikes the retina and excites pigments to release retinal
    b.   Light energy strikes the cornea and excites pigments to release retinoic acid
    c.   Visual pigments deep in the brain are excited by light transmitted through the retina
    d.   Epithelial cells on the surface of the eye respond to light energy by transmitting opsin molecules along nerve pathways to the brain

d   357(A)   12.   Which of the following functions of vitamin A accounts for most of the body's need for the vitamin?

    a.   Promoting good night vision
    b.   Assisting in immune reactions
    c.   Promoting the growth of bones
    d.   Maintaining mucous membranes

d   357-358(K)   13.   Which of the following describes the primary function of vitamin A in bone health?

    a.   It stimulates uptake of calcium from the intestines
    b.   It promotes synthesis of specific bone proteins involved in the mineralization process
    c.   It inhibits oxidation of bone mucopolysaccharides thereby preserving bone crystal integrity and promoting growth
    d.   It signals the release of enzymes that degrade certain regions of the bone thereby allowing the elongation process to occur

a   358(A)   14.   Which of the following functions is shared by beta-carotene and vitamin E?

    a.   Inhibition of oxidation
    b.   Prevention of keratinization
    c.   Prevention of hemolytic anemia
    d.   Inhibition of bone calcium loss

d   358(K)   15.   Approximately what percent of the body's vitamin A stores are found in the liver?

a.   20
b.   50
c.   70
d.   90

a   358(K)   16.   What tissue contains the majority of the body's store of vitamin A?

a.   Liver
b.   Adipose
c.   Retinal cells
d.   Intestinal mucosal cells

d   358(K)   17.   Which of the following substances is converted to vitamin A in the body?

a.   Cholesterol
b.   Chlorophyll
c.   Xanthophyll
d.   Beta-carotene

d   358(K)   18.   Which of the following food substances can be converted to vitamin A in the body?

a.   Tryptophan
b.   Chlorophyll
c.   Xanthophyll
d.   Beta-carotene

d   358-359(A)   19.   Vitamin A supplements are helpful in treating which of the following conditions?

a.   Acne
b.   Rickets
c.   Osteomalacia
d.   Night blindness

c   358(A)   20.   The effects of vitamin A deficiency are most severe in what population group?

a.   Adults
b.   Elderly
c.   Newborns
d.   Adolescents

d   358(K)   21.   If a normal, healthy adult were to begin consuming a vitamin A poor diet, approximately how much time would pass before the first deficiency symptoms would appear?

  a.   2 weeks
  b.   1 to 2 months
  c.   6 months
  d.   1 to 2 years

b   358(K)   22.   Studies in developing countries have demonstrated that the mortality rate of children with measles can be significantly reduced by providing supplements of

  a.   iron.
  b.   vitamin A.
  c.   folic acid.
  d.   phylloquinone.

c   359(A)   23.   Which of the following is most likely to occur from a prolonged dietary deficiency of vitamin A?

  a.   Osteomalacia
  b.   Osteoporosis
  c.   Xerophthalmia
  d.   Prolonged blood-clotting time

c   359(K)   24.   Keratinization is the result of

  a.   toxicity of vitamin A.
  b.   toxicity of vitamin D.
  c.   deficiency of vitamin A.
  d.   deficiency of vitamin D.

b   359-360(A)   25.   Which of the following is likely to induce vitamin A toxicity in adults?

  a.   Eating liver more than once a week
  b.   Consuming high-dose vitamin A supplements
  c.   Drinking 2 quarts of vitamin A-fortified milk daily
  d.   Consuming too many dark green and deep orange vegetables

d   359;360;(A)   26.   Which of the following poses the greatest health risk when consumed in large amounts?

     a.   Wheat germ
     b.   Desiccated liver
     c.   Nutritional yeast
     d.   Vitamin A and D supplements

c   359-360(A)   27.   Which of the following is the most likely side effect for a person who regularly consumes large quantities of carrots or carrot juice?

     a.   Bone pain
     b.   Dermatitis
     c.   Skin yellowing
     d.   Vitamin A toxicity

c   359-360(A)   28.   In which of the following individuals would vitamin A toxicity be most likely to occur?

     a.   Adolescent women
     b.   Overweight adults
     c.   Those taking vitamin A supplements
     d.   Those consuming more than 100 g of carrots daily

c   359(A)   29.   To decrease risk for vitamin A toxicity-related birth defects, it is suggested that pregnant women limit vitamin A supplements to less than

     a.   5,000 RE.
     b.   10,000 RE.
     c.   3 times RDA.
     d.   10 times RDA.

b   360(K)   30.   On the average, one retinol equivalent is equal to about how many international units?

     a.   3
     b.   5
     c.   8
     d.   10

b   360-362(A)   31.   All of the following are good sources of vitamin A EXCEPT

     a.   liver.
     b.   pears.
     c.   apricots.
     d.   sweet potatoes.

b   360-362(K)   32.   Which of the following foods is a very good source of vitamin A?

    a.   Corn
    b.   Pumpkin pie
    c.   Baked potato
    d.   Whole-grain bread

a   360-362(A)   33.   Which of the following provides the least amount of precursor vitamin A?

    a.   Corn
    b.   Spinach
    c.   Carrots
    d.   Cantaloupe

d   360(K)   34.   Which of the following is a feature of Accutane?

    a.   It is effective in treating rickets
    b.   It is less toxic than pure vitamin A
    c.   It is known to be effective in treating mild but not severe acne
    d.   It is known to cause birth defects when used by pregnant women

a   362(A)   35.   Which of the following disorders is associated with a deficiency of either vitamin A or folic acid?

    a.   Anemia
    b.   Nyctalopia
    c.   Hemorrhaging
    d.   Osteomalacia

b   362(K)   36.   Which of the following is a characteristic of vitamin A and foods?

    a.   Fast foods are generally considered good sources of vitamin A
    b.   A regular intake of chicken liver is known to induce toxicity in children
    c.   Xanthophylls in certain vegetables can be converted to active vitamin A in the liver
    d.   Chlorophyll in vegetables can be converted to active vitamin A in the intestinal cells

c   362(K)   37.   The adult RDA for vitamin A is approximately

    a.   400 mg.
    b.   1,000 mg.
    c.   1,000 retinol equivalents.
    d.   5,000 retinol equivalents.

d   363(A)   38.   Which of the following can be used by the body to synthesize vitamin D?

    a.   Bone
    b.   Carotene
    c.   Tryptophan
    d.   Exposure to sunlight

c   363-364(A)   39.   In what tissues must a molecule of vitamin D be chemically altered to yield a compound that is fully active?

    a.   Liver only
    b.   Kidney only
    c.   Liver and kidney
    d.   Liver and intestines

b   364;366(K)   40.   All of the following are other names for vitamin D EXCEPT

    a.   calciferol.
    b.   calcitonin.
    c.   cholecalciferol.
    d.   dihydroxy vitamin D.

d   364(K)   41.   What is the main function(s) of vitamin D?

    a.   Promotes secretion of calcitonin
    b.   Promotes synthesis of 7-dehydrocholesterol
    c.   Promotes synthesis of carotenoids and controls absorption of fat soluble vitamins
    d.   Promotes calcium and phosphorus absorption and promotes calcium mobilization from bone

a   364(K)   42.   Which of the following compounds is known to function like a hormone?

    a.   Vitamin D
    b.   Vitamin K
    c.   Phylloquinone
    d.   Alpha-tocopherol

b   364(A)   43.   In what system would the effects of a vitamin D deficiency be most readily observed?

        a.   Nervous
        b.   Skeletal
        c.   Muscular
        d.   Circulatory

a   364(K)   44.   Which of the following symptoms would indicate a vitamin D deficiency?

        a.   Bowed legs
        b.   Rupture of red blood cells
        c.   Frequent respiratory infections
        d.   Abnormally high blood calcium level

a   364(A)   45.   Which of the following conditions or diseases are known to be caused by a deficiency of the same nutrient?

        a.   Osteomalacia and rickets
        b.   Xerophthalmia and breath pentane release
        c.   Kwashiorkor and fibrocystic breast disease
        d.   Hemolytic anemia and large-cell type anemia

b   364(K)   46.   What is the name of the vitamin D-deficiency disease in adults?

        a.   Rickets
        b.   Osteomalacia
        c.   Keratomalacia
        d.   Hyperkeratosis

d   364-366(K)   47.   All of the following are characteristics of vitamin D nutrition EXCEPT

        a.   deficient intake may lead to altered bone composition.
        b.   excessive intake may lead to mineral deposits in the kidneys.
        c.   fortified milk is the major dietary source in the U.S. population.
        d.   the requirement is increased in most people who are exposed to the sun.

c   364-365(A)   48.   The risk for vitamin D deficiency increases with advancing age for all of the following reasons <u>EXCEPT</u>

    a.   exposure to sunlight is reduced.
    b.   older people decrease milk intake.
    c.   absorption of dietary vitamin D declines.
    d.   the kidneys are less efficient at activating vitamin D.

d   365-366(K)   49.   Which of the following is a feature of vitamin D synthesis?

    a.   Tanning lamps and tanning booths do not stimulate vitamin D synthesis
    b.   Suncreens with sunburn protection factors of 2 and above prevent synthesis of vitamin D
    c.   The ultraviolet rays of the sun are able to easily pierce heavy clouds and smog to promote vitamin D synthesis
    d.   Dark skinned people require longer sunlight exposure than light-skinned people to synthesize equivalent amounts of vitamin D

c   365(A)   50.   Which of the following is a feature of vitamin D?

    a.   Toxicity from vitamin D may result from overexposure to the sun
    b.   Requirements are much higher in the elderly due to degenerative bone diseases
    c.   Fortification of milk with the vitamin is common in order to provide people with a reliable source
    d.   Absorption from most food sources is very poor, necessitating the addition of liberal quantities to grain products

d   365(A)   51.   Which of the following may result from excessive intakes of vitamin D by adults?

    a.   Increased bone density
    b.   Increased bone calcification
    c.   Deformity of leg bones, ribs, and skull
    d.   Mineral deposits in soft tissues such as the kidney

a   365(A)   52.   Which of the following conditions is known to lead to formation of mineral deposits in the blood vessels and kidney?

    a.   Excessive intake of vitamin D
    b.   Inadequate intake of vitamin D
    c.   Excessive intake of tocopherols
    d.   Inadequate intake of tocopherols

b   365(A)   53.   Which of the following is the most reliable source of vitamin D in the diet?

    a.   Meat
    b.   Fortified milk
    c.   Fruits and vegetables
    d.   Enriched breads and cereals

a   365(A)   54.   Which of the following enables much of the world's population to maintain adequate vitamin D status?

    a.   Outdoor exposure of the skin to sunlight
    b.   Wide availability of low-cost fish products
    c.   Wide availability of food assistance programs
    d.   World Health Organization distribution of vitamin D capsules

c   367(K)   55.   What is the Adequate Intake level for vitamin D in individuals around 20 years of age?

    a.   5 µg
    b.   8 µg
    c.   10 µg
    d.   14 µg

c   368(K)   56.   The main function of vitamin E in the body is to act as a(n)

    a.   coenzyme.
    b.   peroxide.
    c.   antioxidant.
    d.   free radical.

d   368(A)   57.   There is some evidence for benefits from vitamin E supplements in all of the following groups EXCEPT

    a.   premature infants.
    b.   people exposed to air pollution.
    c.   women with fibrocystic breast disease.
    d.   people with problems of sexual impotence.

d   368(K)   58.   Which of the following disorders may result from vitamin E deficiency in people?

    a.   Rickets
    b.   Xerophthalmia
    c.   Muscular dystrophy
    d.   Erythrocyte hemolysis

c 368-369(A) 59. Which of the following is a feature of vitamin E?

    a. Functions as a hormone-like substance
    b. Toxicity symptoms include bone abnormalities
    c. Deficiencies occur from inability to absorb dietary lipids
    d. Important food sources include enriched breads and pasta

d 368(A) 60. Which of the following conditions may benefit from vitamin E therapy?

    a. Diabetes
    b. Pernicious anemia
    c. Muscular dystrophy
    d. Intermittent claudication

c 370;372;(K) 61. The process of bone remodeling is known to be dependent on
    367;363   all of the fat-soluble vitamins EXCEPT

    a. vitamin A.
    b. vitamin K.
    c. vitamin E.
    d. vitamin D.

b 369(A) 62. What is the reason that vitamin E deficiencies are rarely observed in human beings?

    a. The vitamin is not essential
    b. The vitamin is so widespread in foods
    c. Most people take vitamin E supplements
    d. The vitamin can be synthesized by the body

b 369(A) 63. Increasing the amount of polyunsaturated fats in the diet increases the need for vitamin

    a. A.
    b. E.
    c. K.
    d. D.

c 369-370(K) 64. Which of the following are major sources of vitamin E in the diet?

    a. Meats
    b. Citrus fruits
    c. Vegetable oils
    d. Milk and dairy products

d   369-370(A)   65.   Among the following, which contains the highest concentration of vitamin E?

    a.   Butter
    b.   Carrots
    c.   Milk fat
    d.   Corn oil

a   369-370(K)   66.   Which of the following is a property of the tocopherols?

    a.   Easily destroyed by air and oxygen
    b.   Act as precursors for the menaquinones
    c.   May dissolve from foods into cooking water
    d.   Absorbed from the intestines into the portal circulation

a   370(K)   67.   In what chief capacity does vitamin K function?

    a.   Blood clotting
    b.   Energy metabolism
    c.   Calcium utilization
    d.   Epithelial tissue renewal

d   370-371(K)   68.   What is prothrombin?

    a.   A storage protein for vitamin K
    b.   A transport protein for vitamin E
    c.   A protein needed for bone formation
    d.   A protein needed for blood clot formation

a   370-371(K)   69.   Which of the following is a feature of vitamin K?

    a.   It participates in synthesis of a bone protein
    b.   Large amounts can be stored in adipose tissue
    c.   Good food sources are legumes and raw fruits
    d.   Intestinal bacterial synthesis provides over 90% of the body's need for most people

c   370(K)   70.   Which of the following is known to require vitamin K for its synthesis?

    a.   Albumin
    b.   GI mucosa
    c.   Prothrombin
    d.   Mucopolysaccharides

b   371(A)   71.   Of the following, which would most readily induce a vitamin K
                           deficiency?

                           a.   Achlorhydria
                           b.   Antibiotic therapy
                           c.   Presence of oxalic acid in food
                           d.   Insufficient intake of green leafy vegetables

c   371(K)   72.   What population group has the highest risk for vitamin K
                           deficiency?

                           a.   Adults
                           b.   Elderly
                           c.   Newborns
                           d.   Teenagers

d   371-372(A)   73.   What type of foods should be controlled in individuals taking
                           anticoagulant medicines?

                           a.   Cold water fish
                           b.   Processed soups
                           c.   Enriched breads
                           d.   Green leafy vegetables

c   371(A)   74.   What vitamin is routinely given as a single dose to newborns?

                           a.   Vitamin A
                           b.   Vitamin E
                           c.   Vitamin K
                           d.   Vitamin B_{12}

a   371-372(A)   75.   Knowing the role of vitamin K in the body, in what organ would
                           you expect to find it in large quantities?

                           a.   Liver
                           b.   Pancreas
                           c.   Gallbladder
                           d.   Small intestine

d   372(A)   76.   All of the following are features of vitamin K in nutrition
                           EXCEPT

                           a.   infants frequently require a supplement at birth.
                           b.   good food sources are plants of the cabbage family.
                           c.   risk of deficiency is increased in people taking antibiotics
                                for prolonged periods.
                           d.   gut microflora synthesis supplies sufficient amounts to

meet the needs of most healthy adults.

c   372(K)   77.   Which of the following vitamins is synthesized by intestinal bacteria?

a.   A
b.   E
c.   K
d.   D

a   377(K)   78.   What is a free radical?

a.   A highly reactive, unstable molecule because it contains unpaired electrons
b.   An antioxidant substance that prevents accumulation of cell-damaging oxides
c.   A substance in food that interacts with nutrients to decrease their utilization
d.   A nutrient in excess of body needs that the body is free to degrade with no consequence

b   377(K)   79.   Which of the following is a characteristic of free radicals?

a.   They are destroyed by cigarette smoking
b.   They arise from normal metabolic reactions
c.   They typically stop chain reactions associated with the production of peroxides
d.   They are known to accumulate even in the presence of abundant antioxidant nutrients

a   379(K)   80.   Which of the following features are shared by vitamins C and E?

a.   Both function as antioxidants
b.   Both require bile for absorption
c.   Neither participates in protein synthesis
d.   Neither is affected by the processing of foods

c   379(K)   81.   What is the role of vitamin E in the metabolism of free radicals?

a.   Carrier
b.   Promoter
c.   Eliminator
d.   Synthesizer

b   379(K)   82.   What is lycopene?

    a. An antioxidant found in abundance in legumes
    b. An antioxidant found in abundance in tomatoes
    c. A prooxidant substance with activity higher than iron
    d. A cancer-causing substance that is neutralized by phyto-chemicals

Matching (Answers can be used only once)

T	355	83.	Transport protein of vitamin A
F	358	84.	Promotes bone dismantling prior to bone elongation
N	359	85.	Condition that results from severe vitamin A deficiency
C	359	86.	The protein of hair and nails
A	360	87.	Severe inflammation of skin follicles and oil producing glands
E	360	88.	Pigment in carrots and pumpkins
B	364	89.	Vitamin D deficiency disease in children
I	364	90.	Precursor for vitamin D synthesis
L	364	91.	Vitamin D deficiency disease in adults
M	365	92.	Term denoting high blood calcium
G	368	93.	May be beneficial for treating fibrocystic breast disease
R	368	94.	Vitamin E deficiency disorder in premature infants
K	371	95.	Use of this increases risk for vitamin K deficiency
H	370	96.	Substance that promotes synthesis of prothrombin
J	370	97.	Another term for blood clotting
Q	369	98.	Typical food source of vitamin E
D	371	99.	Serious condition associated with yellow discoloration of the skin
O	371	100.	Substance that prevents the clotting of the blood
P	371	101.	Catalyzes the conversion of prothrombin to thrombin
S	372	102.	Food source of vitamin K

A.	Acne	K.	Antibiotics
B.	Rickets	L.	Osteomalacia
C.	Keratin	M.	Hypercalcemia
D.	Jaundice	N.	Xerophthalmia
E.	Carotene	O.	Anticoagulant
F.	Vitamin A	P.	Thromboplastin
G.	Vitamin E	Q.	Vegetable oils
H.	Vitamin K	R.	Erythrocyte hemolysis
I.	Cholesterol	S.	Green leafy vegetables
J.	Coagulation	T.	Retinol-binding protein

Essay Questions

355-357;   **103.**   Explain why vitamin A and vitamin D may function as
363-364   hormones rather than as vitamins.

356-357   **104.**   Explain the mechanism associated with the function of vitamin
A in the visual response.

358-359   **105.**   Why is the eye especially vulnerable to vitamin A degradation
at night?

358-359   **106.**   Distinguish between the roles of vitamin A in preventing night
blindness and permanent blindness.

359   **107.**   Why are children more likely than others to be affected by
vitamin A toxicity?

363-364   108.   Describe how the body can synthesize active vitamin D with the help of sunlight.

363-364   109.   How does vitamin D function to raise blood levels of calcium and phosphorus?

364-365;   110.   Compare and contrast the characteristics of the two
367   deficiency diseases osteomalacia and rickets.

368-370   111.   Describe the known functions of vitamin E and false claims of vitamin E supplementation.

371   112.   Discuss the conditions under which deficiencies of vitamin K are most likely to occur.

379-380   113.   Discuss the role of antioxidant nutrients in the prevention of degenerative diseases.

379-383   114.   Discuss the pros and cons of taking antioxidant supplements.

379-380   115.   Discuss the potential applications of phytochemicals in disease prevention.

377-378   116.   Discuss the beneficial effects and adverse effects of free radicals.

379-380   117.   Discuss the similarities between vitamins C and E in defending against heart disease.

CHAPTER 12
WATER AND THE MAJOR MINERALS

Ans   Page

b   387(K)   01.   Which of the following is <u>NOT</u> a function of water in the body?

                                a.   Lubricant
                                b.   Source of energy
                                c.   Component of compounds
                                d.   Participant in chemical reactions

b   387(K)   02.   Which of the following contributes most to the weight of the human body?

                                a.   Iron
                                b.   Water
                                c.   Protein
                                d.   Calcium

d   387-388(K)   03.   Which of the following body structures helps to regulate thirst?

                                a.   Brain stem
                                b.   Cerebellum
                                c.   Optic nerve
                                d.   Hypothalamus

d   387-388(K)   04.   Which of the following is a feature of water?

a.   Not a vital nutrient
b.   Not found in beverages
c.   Oxidized to yield energy
d.   Generated from oxidation of energy nutrients

b   387(K)   05.   Among the following groups, which has the highest percentage of body water?

a.   Elderly
b.   Children
c.   Obese people
d.   Female adolescents

b   387(K)   06.   Where is interstitial water found?

a.   Within cells
b.   Between cells
c.   Within the lungs
d.   Within blood vessels

c   388-389(K)   07.   The average daily loss of water via the kidneys, lungs, feces, and skin approximates

a.   0 to 0.5 liter.
b.   0.5 to 1.5 liters.
c.   1.5 to 2.5 liters.
d.   3.0 to 4.0 liters.

c   388(K)   08.   What is the minimum amount of water excreted each day as urine that is needed to carry away the body's waste products?

a.   100 ml
b.   250 ml
c.   500 ml
d.   1,000 ml

a   388-389(K)   09.   Which of the following is a feature of water and health?

a.   Water intoxciation can result in death
b.   Water losses from the body are highest through the feces
c.   Chronic high intakes increase the risk for bladder cancer
d.   Caffeinated beverages are approved sources for meeting daily fluid needs

d 389(A) 10. What is the appropriate water intake for a 65 kg adult with an energy expenditure of 2,500 kcal?

      a. 250 to 500 ml
      b. 650 to 1300 ml
      c. 1,000 ml
      d. 2,500 to 3,250 ml

d 389(K) 11. What pituitary hormone regulates kidney retention of water?

      a. Thyroxine
      b. Cortisone
      c. Epinephrine
      d. Antidiuretic hormone

c 389(A) 12. What organ provides the major control for homeostasis of body fluids?

      a. Liver
      b. Heart
      c. Kidneys
      d. Skeletal muscle

a 389-390(A) 13. Factors that are effective in regulating the body's water balance include all of the following EXCEPT

      a. adrenaline.
      b. aldosterone.
      c. angiotensin.
      d. antidiuretic hormone.

a 390(A) 14. What is the function of renin?

      a. Activates angiotensin
      b. Activates antidiuretic hormone
      c. Stimulates the thirst mechanism
      d. Stimulates water absorption from the GI tract

b 390-391(K) 15. Aldosterone and renin each function to promote

      a. electrolyte balance.
      b. retention of sodium.
      c. excretion of calcium.
      d. constriction of blood vessels.

b   391(K)   16.   Ions that carry a positive charge are called

    a.   anions.
    b.   cations.
    c.   mineralytes.
    d.   valence ions.

d   391-392(A)   17.   All of the following are properties of electrolytes <u>EXCEPT</u>

    a.   they attract water.
    b.   they are charged particles.
    c.   they carry electrical current.
    d.   they include fat-soluble as well as water soluble particles.

a   391-392(A)   18.   Which of the following describes a way to make an electrolyte solution?

    a.   Dissolve a teaspoon of salt in a glass of water
    b.   Vigorously shake a mixture of corn oil and water
    c.   Dissolve a pinch of corn starch in a glass of water
    d.   Vigorously shake a pinch of table sugar in warm water

a   392(K)   19.   What is the major extracellular cation?

    a.   Sodium
    b.   Sulfate
    c.   Protein
    d.   Potassium

d   392(K)   20.   What is the major intracellular cation?

    a.   Sodium
    b.   Calcium
    c.   Phosphate
    d.   Potassium

d   392(K)   21.   What is the major extracellular anion?

    a.   Sodium
    b.   Lactate
    c.   Sulfate
    d.   Chloride

c   392(K)   22.   What is the major intracellular anion?

         a.   Protein
         b.   Sodium
         c.   Phosphate
         d.   Bicarbonate

c   392-393(K)   23.   What is the term for the pressure that develops when two solutions of varying concentrations are separated by a membrane?

         a.   Hypotension
         b.   Hypertension
         c.   Osmotic pressure
         d.   Hypertonic pressure

b   392-393(K)   24.   What is the force that moves water into a space where a solute is more concentrated?

         a.   Buffer action
         b.   Osmotic pressure
         c.   Permeable selectivity
         d.   Electrolyte imbalance

b   393-394(K)   25.   What is the sodium-potassium pump?

         a.   A cell membrane enzyme that uses energy to pump sodium into the cell
         b.   A cell membrane enzyme that uses energy to pump sodium out of the cell
         c.   A mechanism present throughout interstitial fluid for draining sodium from the circulation
         d.   A mechanism present in the kidneys that exchanges sodium with lactic acid in order to regulate organic acid concentration

c   394(K)   26.   What organ is the chief regulator of the body's acid-base balance?

         a.   Skin
         b.   Liver
         c.   Kidneys
         d.   Stomach

a   394(A)   27.   When a person loses fluid by sweating or bleeding, what minerals are lost in greatest quantity?

    a. Sodium and chloride
    b. Bicarbonate and sulfate
    c. Calcium and magnesium
    d. Potassium and phosphate

d   394(A)   28.   All of the following are typical ingredients in an oral rehydration therapy formula EXCEPT

    a. salt.
    b. water.
    c. sugar.
    d. protein.

b   394-395(K)   29.   All of the following are common participants in the regulation of body fluid pH EXCEPT

    a. proteins.
    b. oxalic acid.
    c. bicarbonate.
    d. carbonic acid.

a   397-398(A)   30.   In a normal individual with a daily requirement of 500 mg sodium, what would be the sodium balance after an intake of 10 g of common salt?

    a. Equilibrium
    b. Slight positive balance
    c. Strong positive balance
    d. Moderate positive balance

c   397-398(A)   31.   Normally, what is the relationship of the amount of sodium excreted to the amount ingested that day?

    a. Sodium intake is higher
    b. Sodium excretion is higher
    c. Sodium intake and excretion are equal
    d. Sodium excretion is unrelated to intake

a   398-400(K)   32.   Which of the following is a feature of sodium nutrition?

    a.   It has no RDA because diets rarely lack sodium
    b.   It has no RDA because the kidneys are highly efficient at regulating sodium balance
    c.   The RDA is 3 g, an amount that has been shown to have little or no effect on blood pressure
    d.   The RDA is only 500 mg because the body possesses an unusually efficient retention mechanism

b   398(K)   33.   What is another term for hypertension?

    a.   High blood sodium
    b.   High blood pressure
    c.   Excessive mental stress
    d.   Excessive muscular contraction

c   398(A)   34.   How much sodium is contained in a fast-food deluxe hamburger that lists a salt content of 2.5 g?

    a.   100 mg
    b.   125 mg
    c.   1,000 mg
    d.   2,500 mg

a   398(A)   35.   What is the greatest single source of sodium in the diet?

    a.   Processed foods
    b.   Unprocessed foods
    c.   Natural salt content of foods
    d.   Salt added during cooking and at the table

b   398(K)   36.   Which of the following is a feature of sodium and health?

    a.   Salt sensitivity is generally low in African-Americans
    b.   High sodium intake is known to promote calcium excretion
    c.   High sodium intake over many years leads to hypertension in most people
    d.   Sodium alone and sodium in salt have nearly equivalent effects on blood pressure

b   399(K)   37.   Which of the following is a general characteristic of minerals in processed foods?

   a.   Instant chocolate pudding is a low sodium food
   b.   Salted peanuts contain less sodium than cornflakes on a gram basis
   c.   Processed foods contribute less than half of the sodium in our diets
   d.   Processed foods contain more sodium and more potassium than their less-processed counterparts

b   399(K)   38.   Hyponatremia refers to low blood concentration of

   a.   renin.
   b.   sodium.
   c.   chloride.
   d.   aldosterone.

b   400-401(K)   39.   Which of the following is a major function of chloride?

   a.   Participates in wound healing
   b.   Helps maintain gastric acidity
   c.   Acts as principal intracellular electrolyte
   d.   Protects bone structures against degeneration

c   400-401(K)   40.   All of the following are characteristics of chloride in nutrition EXCEPT

   a.   deficiencies are extremely rare.
   b.   intake is related, in large part, to sodium intake.
   c.   the RDA has recently been set at 10 mg/kg body weight.
   d.   it is necessary for maintaining electrolyte balance of body fluids.

c   401-402(K)   41.   Which of the following is the primary function of potassium?

   a.   Participates in wound healing
   b.   Helps maintain gastric acidity
   c.   Acts as principal intracellular electrolyte
   d.   Protects bone structures against degeneration

c   401(K)   42.   What is the cause of most electrolyte imbalances?

   a.   Sodium excess
   b.   Calcium deficiency
   c.   Potassium deficiency
   d.   Magnesium deficiency

b   401(K)   43.   Which of the following is a feature of potassium?

a.   It is unrelated to blood pressure
b.   Liberal intake may correct hypertension
c.   Major dietary sources are processed foods
d.   Deficiencies are usually the result of deficient intakes

a   402(A)   44.   Which of the following is NOT among the common food sources of potassium?

a.   Cheese
b.   Potatoes
c.   Dried fruits
d.   Orange juice

a   401-402(A)   45.   All of the following are features of potassium in nutrition EXCEPT

a.   processed foods are a major source.
b.   high intakes may protect against stroke.
c.   per serving size, legumes are a rich source.
d.   per serving size, bananas are a rich source.

d   401-402(K)   46.   Which of the following is NOT a feature of potassium deficiency?

a.   Prolonged vomiting and dehydration are known to lead to deficiencies
b.   Deficiencies occur due to excessive losses rather than to insufficient intakes
c.   Chronic use of certain diuretics and laxatives is known to lead to deficiencies
d.   Dietary deficiencies are common due to availability of only a few good food sources

a   401;403(A)   47.   Which of the following is a feature of potassium supplements?

a.   Can cause toxicity
b.   Should always be taken with diuretics
c.   Necessary in treatment of low blood pressure
d.   Absorption of the mineral decreases markedly as intake increases

b   402-403(A)   48.   Which of the following people are at known risk for potassium depletion?

a.   Athletes who are body-builders
b.   Those who use diuretics regularly
c.   Construction workers in cold climates
d.   Those who consume insufficient amounts of salted foods

b   403(K)   49.   Which of the following is an early symptom of potassium deficiency?

a.   Extreme thirst
b.   Muscle weakness
c.   Profound sweating
d.   Lowered blood pressure

b   403(A)   50.   Almost all (99%) of the calcium in the body is used to

a.   provide energy for cells.
b.   provide rigidity for the bones and teeth.
c.   regulate the transmission of nerve impulses.
d.   maintain the blood level of calcium within very narrow limits.

a   403-404(A)   51.   As far as is known, which of the following is NOT a process that directly involves calcium?

a.   pH regulation
b.   Blood clotting
c.   Nerve transmission
d.   Maintenance of heart beat

b   403(K)   52.   What is hydroxyapatite?

a.   Abnormal cellular structures seen in osteoporosis
b.   The calcium-rich crystalline structure of teeth and bones
c.   A calcium regulatory hormone secreted from the trabeculae region of bone
d.   A compound in plant foods that binds to calcium and phosphorus and inhibits absorption

c   404;409;(A) 53.   All of the following characteristics are shared by calcium and
     411;414   magnesium EXCEPT

          a.   both are involved in blood clotting.
          b.   both are involved in bone formation.
          c.   both are found in abundance in dairy products.
          d.   both may result in tetany when blood levels become
                abnormally low.

c   404(K)   54.   Which of the following regulates the level of calcium in the
                        blood?

          a.   Dietary intake of calcium
          b.   Glucagon and epinephrine
          c.   Parathormone and calcitonin
          d.   Dietary intake of phosphorus

c   404-409(A)   55.   Which of the following represents the LEAST likely cause for
                        an abnormal blood calcium level?

          a.   Diseases of the liver
          b.   Diseases of the kidney
          c.   Insufficient dietary intake
          d.   Altered secretion of parathormone

b   404-405(K)   56.   Calcium absorption is facilitated by the presence of

          a.   fiber.
          b.   lactose.
          c.   phytic acid.
          d.   oxalic acid.

b   404(A)   57.   How much calcium would be typically absorbed by a normal
                        adult with a calcium intake of 1,000 mg?

          a.   100 mg
          b.   300 mg
          c.   600 mg
          d.   950 mg

c   404-405(K)   58.   All of the following are known to enhance calcium absorption
                        from the GI tract EXCEPT

          a.   lactose.
          b.   pregnancy.
          c.   oxalic acid.
          d.   stomach acid.

b   404(K)   59.   What is calmodulin?

   a.   A drug that treats osteoporoses
   b.   A messenger molecule activated by calcium
   c.   A calcium supplement with high bioavailability
   d.   A form of calcium used in fortifying soy products

b   404(A)   60.   Calcium-binding protein acts on the

   a.   kidneys.
   b.   intestines.
   c.   cortical bone.
   d.   trabecular bone.

b   404-405;(K)   61.   All of the following dietary substances are known to adversely
       411   affect calcium balance <u>EXCEPT</u>

   a.   high fiber diet.
   b.   lactose in the diet.
   c.   phytic acid in the diet.
   d.   phosphorus in the diet at a level 3 times that of calcium.

d   406(K)   62.   Which of the following are good sources of dietary calcium?

   a.   Fruits
   b.   Breads
   c.   Enriched grains
   d.   Certain green vegetables

b   406(K)   63.   Which of the following vegetable greens shows the <u>lowest</u>
                           bioavailability of calcium?

   a.   Kale
   b.   Spinach
   c.   Broccoli
   d.   Mustard greens

c   406(K)   64.   Which of the following shows the highest bioavailability for
                           calcium?

   a.   Milk
   b.   Spinach
   c.   Broccoli
   d.   Pinto beans

d   407(A)   65.   On a per kcalorie basis, which of the following are the best sources of magnesium?

a.   Meats
b.   Fruits
c.   Breads
d.   Vegetables

c   409(A)   66.   What is the calcium Adequate Intake for college-age students?

a.   500 mg
b.   800 mg
c.   1000 mg
d.   1200 mg

b   409(K)   67.   Which of the following is a feature of osteoporosis?

a.   It is most common in men over 45 years of age
b.   It has virtually no effect on blood calcium levels
c.   It results from short-term deprivation of dietary calcium
d.   It causes significant alterations in the blood levels of parathormone and calcitonin

a   409(K)   68.   Which of the following is a feature of phosphorus?

a.   Involved in energy exchange
b.   Activates fat-soluble vitamins
c.   Ranks lowest among the minerals in amount present in the body
d.   Ranks highest among the minerals in amount present in the body

d   409(K)   69.   Which of the following minerals is involved in the transportation of lipids through the body's lymph and blood systems?

a.   Iron
b.   Sodium
c.   Calcium
d.   Phosphorus

d   409(A)   70.   Which of the following minerals is LEAST likely to be deficient in anyone's diet?

a.   Iron
b.   Calcium
c.   Chromium
d.   Phosphorus

d   409-410(K)   71.   Which of the following is a feature of phosphorus in nutrition?

    a.   Dietary sources include fresh vegetables
    b.   Absorption is known to be reduced by soft drink consumption
    c.   It's participation in bone synthesis requires equivalent intake of dietary calcium
    d.   Dietary deficiencies are virtually unknown in major dietary sources include fresh vegetables

c   411(K)   72.   Which of the following is a major function of magnesium?

    a.   Transport of oxygen
    b.   Prevention of anemia
    c.   Catalyst in energy metabolism
    d.   Production of thyroid hormone

a   411(K)   73.   Where is the majority of the body's magnesium found?

    a.   Bones
    b.   Teeth
    c.   Fatty tissue
    d.   Cells of soft tissue

d   411(K)   74.   Which of the following is a feature of magnesium in nutrition?

    a.   Toxicity is common in people taking diuretics
    b.   High intakes interfere with stability of tooth enamel
    c.   The amounts present in hard water are poorly utilized
    d.   Average intakes from food are below recommendations

b   413(K)   75.   Sulfur is present in practically all

    a.   vitamins.
    b.   proteins.
    c.   fatty acids.
    d.   carbohydrates.

a   413(K)   76.   Some amino acids can link to each other by bridges made of

    a.   sulfur.
    b.   calcium.
    c.   chloride.
    d.   magnesium.

c   413;388(A)   77.   All of the following are known to have a high sulfur content EXCEPT

     a. skin.
     b. hair.
     c. teeth.
     d. nails.

b   413(K)   78.   What is the major source of dietary sulfur?

     a. Fats
     b. Protein
     c. Mineral salts
     d. Carbohydrates

b   420-421(K)   79.   Which of the following is a feature of Type I osteoporosis?

     a. It shows onset after 70 years of age
     b. It can be prevented by taking estrogen
     c. It leads to formation of the "dowager's hump"
     d. Its prevalence is similar between males and females

c   420(K)   80.   Which of the following is a function of trabecular bone?

     a. Synthesis of vitamin D
     b. Synthesis of calcitonin
     c. Storage site for calcium
     d. Storage site for vitamin D

b   421(A)   81.   The strongest predictor for loss of bone density is a person's

     a. sex.
     b. age.
     c. calcium intake.
     d. blood estrogen level.

d   422-423(K)   82.   All of the following are known to have a high correlation with risk for osteoporosis EXCEPT

     a. being thin.
     b. being female.
     c. having anorexia nervosa.
     d. consuming a high-protein diet.

b   422(A)   83.   A person's bone density is highest at around age

a.   18 years.
b.   30 years.
c.   55 years.
d.   70 years.

c   423(K)   84.   Among the following ethnic groups, which has the highest bone density?

a.   Japanese
b.   Caucasian
c.   African-American
d.   South America Hispanic

c   425(K)   85.   To minimize the risk of calcium toxicity, total daily intakes should be limited to under

a.   500 mg
b.   1,000 mg
c.   2,500 mg
d.   5,000 mg

d   425(K)   86.   Calcium supplements most likely to be contaminated with toxic minerals are those made from

a.   oyster shells.
b.   calcium citrate.
c.   calcium carbonate.
d.   powdered animal bones.

Matching (Answers can be used only once)

D	389	87.	Typical amount (in ml) of water lost from lungs every day
M	409	88.	Soft drinks are usually high in this substance
G	289	89.	Recommended water intake (in ml) for infant expending 1,000 kcal
H	389	90.	Enzyme released by kidneys
O	389	91.	Stimulates retention of sodium by kidneys
R	389	92.	Stimulates retention of water by kidneys
S	392	93.	A cation
T	392	94.	An anion
C	395	95.	Number of times more acidic a substance with pH of 4 is versus a substance with pH of 2
J	396	96.	Most prevalent major mineral in the body
L	396	97.	Least prevalent major mineral in the body
N	405	98.	Substance that inhibits absorption of calcium
Q	403	99.	Crystalline structure of bone
P	404	100.	Hormone that helps regulate calcium balance
A	404	101.	Percentage of dietary calcium absorbed by average adult
F	409	102.	Calcium Adequate Intake for college-age students
B	405	103.	Percentage of dietary calcium absorbed by growing children
K	405	104.	Substance that enhances absorption of calcium
E	409	105.	Amount of calcium, in mg, in 2 cups of milk
I	414	106.	Mineral that accounts for the structure of many proteins

A.	30	K.	Lactose
B.	60	L.	Magnesium
C.	100	M.	Phosphorous
D.	350	N.	Oxalic acid
E.	600	O.	Aldosterone
F.	1000	P.	Parathormone
G.	1500	Q.	Hydroxyapatite
H.	Renin	R.	Antidiuretic hormone
I.	Sulfur	S.	Potassium in solution
J.	Calcium	T.	Phosphate in solution

Essay Questions

387   107.   List 8 different functions for water in the body.

387-309   108.   Discuss the advantages of a liberal daily intake of water.

389-391   109.   Explain the roles of hormones in helping to regulate the body's water balance.

391-396   110.   In what ways do the GI tract and the kidney function to help maintain fluid and electrolyte balance? How does the body defend itself when faced with conditions that induce excessive water and mineral losses (e.g. sweating; diarrhea)?

394-396   111.   Describe the role of the kidneys in regulating acid-base balance.

396-397   112.   Compare and contrast the major functions of minerals and vitamins.

397;405   113. Identify some of the common substances found in foods that combine with minerals to form complexes the body cannot absorb. In what foods are they found and what minerals are affected?

388-389;401;   114. Explain the relationship between dietary sodium and
409-414   hypertension. What are the roles of calcium, magnesium, and potassium in regulating blood pressure?

404   115. What are the major sources of sodium in the diet of the U.S. population? Describe ways in which consumers can lower intakes of salt in their diets.

404   116. Define calcium rigor and calcium tetany. What role does dietary intake of calcium play in these disorders?

404-405   117. Explain the functions of parathormone, calcitonin, and vitamin D in the regulation of calcium metabolism.

406-408   118.   List 5 nonmilk sources of calcium.

407-408   119.   Explain the cooking techniques that improve calcium extraction from ethnic foods.

420-425   120.   Discuss major risk factors in the development of osteoporosis. What population groups are most at risk? What dietary measures are advocated for high risk groups?

420-421   121.   Compare and contrast trabecular bone and cortical bone formation and function.

420-422   122.   Discuss the contributions of cortical bone and trabecular bone development of osteoporoses.

421-422   123.   Explain the difference between type I and type II osteoporoses.

422-424   124. What dietary and metabolic factors are associated with poor calcium balance in older adults?

422-423   125. Discuss the role of male and female hormones in calcium balance and bone loss.

424   126. Discuss the roles of alcohol and smoking in development of osteoporosis.

425   127. Discuss bioavailability of the various calcium supplements.

425   128. Explain the risks associated with taking calcium supplements.

CHAPTER 13
THE TRACE MINERALS

a   429(K)   01. Which of the following is a characteristic of the trace minerals?

   a. The amounts found in foods are not predictable
   b. A deficiency sign common to many trace minerals is dermatitis
   c. Deficiencies are more difficult to recognize in children than in adults
   d. The amount of all trace minerals in the average person totals approximately 100 grams

b   430(K)   02. Which of the following is a feature of iron nutrition?

   a. Most people absorb about 50-60% of dietary iron
   b. Many people do not eat enough iron-containing foods
   c. Iron plays an important role in the synthesis of thyroxine
   d. Iron deficiency represents the second most common mineral deficiency in the United States.

d   430(K)   03. What iron-containing compound carries oxygen in the bloodstream?

   a. Ferritin
   b. Myoglobin
   c. Transferrin
   d. Hemoglobin

1

b   430(K)   04.   What is the oxygen carrying protein of muscle cells?

          a.   Transferrin
          b.   Myoglobin
          c.   Hemoglobin
          d.   Cytochrome

b   430(K)   05.   Which of the following is a characteristic of iron transport?

          a.   Albumin is the major iron transport protein in the blood
          b.   Transferrin in the blood carries iron to the bone marrow
          c.   Hemochromatosis results from inability to absorb and transport iron
          d.   Ferritin functions by transporting iron from the spleen to the bone marrow

b   430(K)   06.   Which of the following is a protein that carries iron through the circulation to the tissues?

          a.   Albumin
          b.   Transferrin
          c.   Hemosiderin
          d.   Metallothionein

a   431K)   07.   What is the function of MFP factor?

          a.   Enhances iron absorption
          b.   Acts as iron enrichment nutrient
          c.   Simulates metallothionein synthesis
          d.   Acts as chelating agent for iron toxicity treatment

a   432(K)   08.   Which of the following compounds provides major a storage reservoir for iron?

          a.   Ferritin
          b.   Myoglobin
          c.   Transferrin
          e.   Hemoglobin

a   430-432;(K) 8.   When calculating the amount of iron that can be absorbed
      436-438   from a meal, all of the following factors are considered EXCEPT

          a.   fiber content.
          b.   heme iron content.
          c.   vitamin C content.
          d.   nonheme iron content.

d   431-432(K)   09.   All of the following factors are known to <u>enhance</u> the absorption of iron <u>EXCEPT</u>

    a.   MFP factor.
    b.   stomach acid.
    c.   ascorbic acid.
    d.   calcium from milk.

c   431(K)   10.   All of the following are known to <u>reduce</u> the absorption of iron <u>EXCEPT</u>

    a.   tea.
    b.   coffee.
    c.   sugars.
    d.   phytates.

b   431;(A)
    437-438   11.   Absorption of iron from supplements is improved by taking them with

    a.   tea.
    b.   meat.
    c.   milk.
    d.   whole grain bread.

c   431-432(K)   12.   All of the following characteristics are shared by iron and zinc <u>EXCEPT</u>

    a.   absorption is inhibited by fiber.
    b.   absorption is inhibited by cow's milk.
    c.   transport in the blood is primarily by albumin.
    d.   absorption rises with increased needs of the body.

a   432(A)   13.   Iron bioavailability from complete meals is known to be affected significantly by each of the following substances <u>EXCEPT</u>

    a.   caffeine.
    b.   phytates.
    c.   Vitamin C.
    d.   MFP factor.

b   432(K)   14.   All of the following are known to reduce the absorption of iron <u>EXCEPT</u>

    a.   phytates.
    b.   MFP factor.
    c.   tannic acid in tea.
    d.   EDTA in food additives.

c   432(K)   15.   What is the average lifespan of red blood cells?

                         a.   Two weeks
                         b.   One month
                         c.   Four months
                         d.   Six months

b   432(K)   16.   Under normal circumstances, what is the average percentage of dietary iron that is absorbed?

                         a.   2 to 5
                         b.   10 to 15
                         c.   50 to 60
                         d.   90 to 95

a   432-433(K)   17.   Which of the following is a characteristic of iron utilization?

                         a.   Most of the body's iron is recycled
                         b.   The chief storage site for iron is the intestinal epithelium
                         c.   Iron is absorbed better from supplements than from foods
                         d.   Iron from nonheme food sources is absorbed better than from heme food sources

a   432(A)   18.   How would the body respond typically to loss of blood from hemorrhage?

                         a.   More transferrin is produced to allow absorption and transport of more iron
                         b.   The average life of the red blood cell is increased in order to allow better tissue oxygenation
                         c.   Less iron storage proteins are produced which increases the amount of iron available for synthesis of new red blood cells
                         d.   The liver and muscles release their supply of stored red blood cells which compensates, in part, for the decrease in red blood cell concentration of the circulation

b   432-433(K)   19.   Which of the following is a feature of iron absorption?

                         a.   It is lower in people with iron toxicity
                         b.   It is higher in people with severe iron deficiency
                         c.   It is lower when iron is in the form of heme rather than non-heme
                         d.   It is higher in adults than children due to more mature intestinal function

b   432;440(A)   20. Which of the following characteristics is shared by zinc and iron?

    a.   Good food sources include dairy products
    b.   Proteins in the blood are needed for their transport
    c.   Severe deficiencies lead to delay in the onset of puberty
    d.   Doses of 10 times the RDA are known to cause death in children

b   428-434(A)   21. Low levels of blood hemoglobin indicate a possible deficiency of

    a.   zinc.
    b.   iron.
    c.   copper.
    d.   manganese.

c   433-434(A)   22. The most common tests to diagnose iron deficiency include all of the following measures EXCEPT

    a.   size of red blood cells.
    b.   number of red blood cells.
    c.   DNA content of red blood cells.
    d.   hemoglobin content of red blood cells.

d   433;435(A)   23. Which of the following population groups is LEAST susceptible to iron deficiency anemia?

    a.   Older infants
    b.   Children 2-10 years of age
    c.   Women of childbearing age
    d.   Men 20-45 years of age

a   434(A)   24. Iron deficiency in children is likely to result from a diet that overemphasizes

    a.   milk.
    b.   cereals.
    c.   vegetables.
    d.   dried beans.

b   433(A)   25.   Taking into account the intestinal absorption efficiency of iron, approximately how much dietary iron must be consumed to account for the iron lost by donating a pint of blood?

      a.   5 mg
      b.   25 mg
      c.   50 mg
      d.   100 mg

a   433(A)   26.   Which of the following is found in the first stage of iron deficiency?

      a.   Iron stores decline as assessed by serum ferritin
      b.   Hemoglobin levels fall, as assessed by complete blood count
      c.   Red blood cell count falls, as assessed by hematocrit count
      d.   Hemoglobin synthesis declines, as assessed by erythrocyte protoporphyrin

c   433(K)   27.   Approximately how many of the world's population are thought to be affected by iron-deficiency anemia?

      a.   One million
      b.   100 million
      c.   One billion
      d.   Two billion

b   433(K)   28.   What is erythrocyte protoporphyrin?

      a.   Iron chelating drug
      b.   Hemoglobin precursor
      c.   Indicator of iron toxicity
      d.   Inherited iron deficiency disease

c   433(K)   29.   The erythrocyte protoporphyrin level is used as an indicator of

      a.   late iron toxicity.
      b.   early iron toxicity.
      c.   late iron deficiency.
      d.   early iron deficiency.

b   433-434(A)   30.   What is the major cause of iron deficiency?

      a.   Blood loss
      b.   Poor nutrition
      c.   Hereditary defect
      d.   Parasitic infections of the GI tract

c   433(K)   31. Why are hemoglobin and hematocrit tests of limited usefulness in the assessment of iron status?

　　a. They are expensive to perform
　　b. They are notoriously inaccurate
　　c. They are late indicators of iron deficiency
　　d. The range of normal value is usually wide

c   433(A)   32. Which of the following individuals would most likely need an iron supplement?

　　a. One-year old
　　b. Elderly female
　　c. Pregnant female
　　d. Adolescent female

c   434-436;(K)   33. Signs of iron <u>toxicity</u> include all of the following <u>EXCEPT</u>
　　439

　　a. apathy.
　　b. fatigue.
　　c. hypochromic anemia
　　d. increases in infections.

a   434(K)   34. What is the name given to the ingestion of nonnutritive substances?

　　a. Pica
　　b. Goiter
　　c. Tetany
　　d. Hemosiderosis

d   434(A)   35. Which of the following symptoms would ordinarily <u>NOT</u> be found in individuals with iron-deficiency anemia?

　　a. Fatigue
　　b. Headaches
　　c. Concave nails
　　d. Diminished sense of smell

c   434(K)   36. What type of anemia results from iron deficiency?

　　a. Hemolytic
　　b. Megaloblastic
　　c. Hypochromic microcytic
　　d. Hyperchromic macrocytic

a   435(K)   37.   Which of the following describes one aspect of iron toxicity?

      a.   Among men in the United States, it is twice as common as iron-deficiency anemia
      b.   In adults, the consumption of alcohol is somewhat protective against absorption of excess iron
      c.   In most people with this disorder, infections are rare because bacteria are killed by excess iron in the blood
      d.   It is usually caused by a virus that attacks the intestinal mucosal cells leading to unregulated and excessive iron absorption

c   435-436(A)   38.   Which of the following foods should be especially limited in the diet of individuals with hemochromatosis?

      a.   Dairy products
      b.   Fluoridated water
      c.   Iron-fortified cereals
      d.   Carbonated beverages

c   435(A)   39.   Which of the following disorders is positively correlated with the presence of high blood iron?

      a.   Dermatitis
      b.   Diverticulosis
      c.   Heart disease
      d.   Neural tube defects

b   435(K)   40.   The most common cause of iron overload is

      a.   an injury to the GI tract.
      b.   a genetic predisposition.
      c.   excessive use of iron cookware.
      d.   excessive use of iron supplements.

d   436-437(A)   41.   Which of the following is the most effective and least costly strategy for preventing an iron deficiency?

      a.   Consume iron supplements at a level 2-3 times the RDA
      b.   Switch to iron cooking utensils and eat 4 servings of red meat daily
      c.   Eat small amounts of citrus products and increase intake of low fat milk
      d.   Eat small quantities of meat, fish, and poultry frequently together with liberal amounts of vegetables and legumes

c   436(A)   42. Approximately how much iron would be provided by a balanced diet supplying 2000 kcalories?

    a.   3 mg
    b.   6 mg
    c.   12 mg
    d.   30 mg

b   436(K)   43. In the United States, iron is currently added to which of the following foods?

    a.   Milk and cheese
    b.   Breads and cereals
    c.   Peanut butter and jellies
    d.   Orange juice and tomato juice

b   436(A)   44. A child diagnosed with iron-deficiency anemia would most likely benefit from increasing the consumption of

    a.   milk.
    b.   red meat.
    c.   fresh fruits.
    d.   yellow vegetables.

c   436-438(A)   45. Which of the following foods provides iron in the most absorbable form?

    a.   Rice
    b.   Spinach
    c.   Hamburger
    d.   Orange juice

d   436;438(K)   46. Which of the following nutrients enhances iron absorption from the intestinal tract?

    a.   Biotin
    b.   Calcium
    c.   Vitamin D
    d.   Vitamin C

c   436;438(K)   47. Which of the following is known to enhance iron absorption?

    a.   Tea
    b.   Coffee
    c.   Foods containing vitamin C
    d.   Foods containing vitamin E

c   436;439(K)   48.   What is the RDA for iron for females 11-50 years old?

    a.   8 mg
    b.   10 mg
    c.   15 mg
    d.   22 mg

d   436(A)   49.   If a normal, healthy young adult woman loses an average of 2 mg/day of iron from the body, approximately what minimum amount (mg/day) should she consume from the diet to prevent negative iron balance?

    a.   2
    b.   4
    c.   10
    d.   20

c   438(A)   50.   When eaten in the same meal, which of the following foods enhances the absorption of iron in legumes?

    a.   Nuts
    b.   Fiber
    c.   Oranges
    d.   Whole-grain breads

a   438(A)   51.   Which of the following is a common example of iron contamination in the diet?

    a.   Using an iron skillet to scramble eggs can triple their iron content
    b.   Cooking acidic foods in a copper pot can extract chelate iron from the pot
    c.   Simmering acidic foods in glass dishes leads to leaching of iron salts from the glass
    d.   Cooking leafy vegetables in a galvanized pot leads to a six-fold increase in iron content

b   438(A)   52.   Why is taking vitamin C ineffective at enhancing iron-absorption from standard iron supplements?

    a.   The iron in the supplement is in a chelated form
    b.   The iron in the supplement is already in the ferrous form
    c.   The iron in the supplement binds irreversibly with vitamin C
    d.   The iron supplement already contains MFP to enhance absorption

c   438(A)   53. Which of the following is a common side effect from taking iron supplements?

a. Itching
b. Diarrhea
c. Constipation
d. Black tongue

c   438(A)   54. Which of the following has been shown to improve absorption of iron from iron supplements?

a. Taking then with milk
b. Taking them with orange juice
c. Taking them on an empty stomach rather than with meals
d. Taking them in the form of the ferric salt rather than the ferrous salt

d   440(K)   55. Which of the following is a major binding protein for zinc?

a. Ligand
b. Ferritin
c. Hemosiderin
d. Metallothionein

d   439;443(A)   56. Zinc is known to play an important role in all of the following functions EXCEPT

a. wound healing.
b. synthesis of retinal.
c. production of sperm.
d. oxidation of polyunsaturated fatty acids.

b   439(K)   57. Among the following, which contains the highest concentration of the body's zinc?

a. Liver
b. Muscle
c. Blood cells
d. Prostate gland

d   440(A)   58.   Which of the following characteristics are shared by iron and zinc?

    a.   Neither functions in the maintenance of blood glucose
    b.   Neither is circulated from the pancreas to the intestines and back to the pancreas
    c.   Both are absorbed into intestinal mucosal cells and bound to metallothionein for transport first to the liver
    d.   Both are absorbed into intestinal epithelial cells but may then be lost by normal villus cell renewal processes

a   440(K)   59.   Which of the following is thought to regulate the absorption of zinc?

    a.   Metallothionein in the intestinal cells
    b.   Zinc releasing enzymes in the intestinal mucosa
    c.   Pancreatic juice containing zinc-absorption enhancers
    d.   Bile acids which form a complex with zinc to promote its absorption

a   440(K)   60.   What is the chief transport substance for zinc in the circulation?

    a.   Albumin
    b.   Metallothionein
    c.   Carbonic anhydrase
    d.   High-density lipoproteins

b   440(K)   61.   Which of the following minerals undergoes enteropancreatic circulation during normal metabolism?

    a.   Iron
    b.   Zinc
    c.   Copper
    d.   Fluoride

d   440(K)   62.   What dietary ratio of iron to zinc inhibits zinc absorption?

    a.   0.5 to 1
    b.   1 to 1
    c.   Less than 2 to 1
    d.   Greater than 2 to 1

c   440(A)   63. Which of the following would be the minimum amount of dietary iron known to impair zinc absorption in an individual with a zinc intake of 15 mg?

    a.   5 mg
    b.   15 mg
    c.   30 mg
    d.   60 mg

c   440(K)   64. What is the bioavailability of dietary zinc?

    a.   2-5%
    b.   5-10%
    c.   15-40%
    d.   50-60%

a   440(K)   65. Which of the following conditions is known to lead to copper deficiency?

    a.   Excess zinc
    b.   Excess protein
    c.   Insufficient iodine
    d.   Insufficient calcium

b   441;443(K)   66. Deficiency of which of the following minerals is associated with retarded growth and sexual development in children?

    a.   Iron
    b.   Zinc
    c.   Iodine
    d.   Chromium

b   442-443(K)   67. All of the following are known to result from excessive zinc intake EXCEPT

    a.   inhibition of iron absorption.
    b.   galvanized liver and kidneys.
    c.   inhibition of copper absorption.
    d.   decreases in high-density lipoproteins.

b   442-443(K)   68. Conditions associated with zinc deficiency include all of the following EXCEPT

    a.   altered taste.
    b.   kidney failure.
    c.   abnormal night vision.
    d.   poor healing of wounds.

a   442-443(K)   69.   All of the following are recognized symptoms of zinc deficiency EXCEPT

    a.   anemia.
    b.   altered taste acuity.
    c.   impaired dark vision.
    d.   increased susceptibility to infection.

c   442(A)   70.   Which of the following is a known side effect of prolonged ingestion of excessive amounts of zinc supplements?

    a.   Iron toxicity due to increased ferritin synthesis
    b.   Zinc salt deposits in soft tissues such as the heart and kidneys
    c.   Copper deficiency due to interference with copper absorption
    d.   Mineral binding protein deficiency due to a decrease in metallothionein production

d   442(K)   71.   Which of the following represents the most reliable dietary source of zinc?

    a.   Milk
    b.   Fiber
    c.   Fruits
    d.   Meat and whole-grain cereals

c   442;443(A)   72.   Zinc is highest in foods that also contain a high amount of

    a.   fat.
    b.   fiber.
    c.   protein.
    d.   carbohydrate.

c   442(K)   73.   Commercially available zinc-containing lozenges are advertised to be effective against

    a.   fatigue.
    b.   vitamin A toxicity.
    c.   the common cold.
    d.   slowing of the BMR.

c   442(A)   74. Under which of the following conditions are certain supplements of zinc known to be beneficial?

     a. In the treatment of colds
     b. In the treatment of Menkes' syndrome
     c. In the treatment of toxicity from certain other metals
     d. In the treatment of slow growth syndrome in U.S. children

d   442(K)   75. What formulation of zinc has been found effective in treating the symptoms of the common cold?

     a. Zinc chelator
     b. Zinc plus ferrous iron
     c. Zinc plus copper salt
     d. Unbound zinc gluconate

a   440-442(K)   76. Which of the following is a feature of zinc in nutrition?

     a. Pancreatic enzymes are rich in zinc
     b. The body's primary excretory route is urine
     c. Good food sources are whole grain products
     d. Toxicity symptoms include constipation and low body temperature

c   443(K)   77. What mineral is critical to the synthesis of thyroxin?

     a. Iron
     b. Copper
     c. Iodine
     d. Magnesium

d   445(A)   78. If cow's milk is found to contain unusually high levels of iodine, what is the most likely explanation?

     a. Storage of milk in galvanized tanks
     b. Grazing of cows on high iodine soils
     c. Addition of fortified salt at the milk processing plant
     d. Exposure of cows to iodide-containing medications and disinfectants

b   445(K)   79. Which of the following may result from iodine deficiency?

     a. Gout
     b. Goiter
     c. Anemia
     d. Hypertension

c   445(A)   80. A woman with a severe iodine deficiency during pregnancy may have a child who develops

    a.   anemia.
    b.   rickets.
    c.   cretinism.
    d.   allergies.

c   445(A)   81. What is the response of the pituitary gland of a person who is deficient in iodine?

    a.   Increase in its size to trap more iodine
    b.   Increase in its size to trap more thyroxine
    c.   Increased release of thyroid-stimulating hormone
    d.   Decreased release of thyroid-stimulating hormone

a   445(A)   82. What nutrient deficiency during pregnancy may give rise to a child with cretinism?

    a.   Iodine
    b.   Copper
    c.   Chromium
    d.   Molybdenum

c   445(K)   83. Which of the following is a feature of iodide utilization?

    a.   Ingestion of plants of the cabbage family stimulates iodide uptake
    b.   It is an integral part of pituitary thyroid stimulating hormone
    c.   A deficiency or a toxicity leads to enlargement of the thyroid gland
    d.   The amount in foods is unrelated to the amount of iodine present in the soil

b   445(A)   84. A person ingesting large amounts of thyroid antagonist substances is at high risk of developing

    a.   cretinsm.
    b.   simple goiter.
    c.   high blood T_3 levels.
    d.   high blood thyroxin levels.

c   445(A)   85. Which of the following foods are known to contain goitrogens?

    a.   Shellfish
    b.   Whole grains
    c.   Cauliflower and broccoli
    d.   Strawberries and raspberries

b   445(A)   86.   Which of the following is the richest source of iodine?

     a.   Corn
     b.   Seafood
     c.   Orange juice
     d.   Cruciferous vegetables

d   445(A)   87.   Which of the following would most likely result from an excessive intake of iodine?

     a.   Diarrhea
     b.   Skin rashes
     c.   Dehydration
     d.   Thyroid gland enlargement

b   445(A)   88.   Which of the following would be the most appropriate food source of iodide for a person who lives inland?

     a.   Fresh water fish
     b.   Iodized table salt
     c.   Locally grown produce
     d.   Plants of the cabbage family

b   445-436(K)   89.   Which of the following is a prominent feature of iodine deficiency?

     a.   Gout
     b.   Weight gain
     c.   Demineralization
     d.   Discoloration of teeth

c   445(K)   90.   What is a goitrogen?

     a.   One of the hormones produced by the thyroid gland
     b.   A substance that enhances absorption of dietary iodide
     c.   A substance that interferes with the functioning of the thyroid gland
     d.   A compound used to supplement salt as a way to increase iodide intake

a   445(K)   91.   The most common cause of iodine deficiency is

     a.   insufficient intake of iodine from foods.
     b.   overconsumption of other trace elements.
     c.   overconsumption of anti-thyroid substances.
     d.   pituitary deficiencies of thyroid-stimulating hormone.

b   446(A)   92. Which of the following nutrients has functions similar to those of vitamin E?

   a. Iron
   b. Selenium
   c. Chromium
   d. Molybdenum

b   446(K)   93. Which of the following is a property of selenium in nutrition?

   a. It participates in the functioning of insulin
   b. Severe deficiency is associated with heart disease in China
   c. Significant food sources include dairy and unprocessed vegetables
   d. It has no RDA but the estimated safe and adequate dietary intake is only 2-3 µg/day

c   447(K)   94. The rare genetic disorders Menkes disease and Wilson's disease result from abnormal utilization of

   a. iron.
   b. zinc.
   c. copper.
   d. manganese.

c   446(K)   95. What trace element is part of the enzyme glutathione peroxidose?

   a. Iron
   b. Zinc
   c. Selenium
   d. Chromium

b   446(K)   96. Which of the following is an important function of selenium?

   a. Helps blood to clot
   b. Inhibits the formation of free radicals
   c. Stabilizes the alcohol content of beer
   d. Acts as a cross-linking agent in collagen

b   446(A)   97. Approximately how much iodized salt must be consumed to meet but not exceed the RDA for iodine?

   a. 1 mg
   b. ½ teaspoon
   c. 1 teaspoon
   d. 1 tablespoon

b   447(A)   98. Which of the following minerals is a cofactor in the formation of hemoglobin?

    a. Iodine
    b. Copper
    c. Sodium
    d. Calcium

b   447(K)   99. Which of the following minerals functions primarily in reactions that consume oxygen?

    a. Zinc
    b. Copper
    c. Chromium
    d. Molybdenum

a   447;449(A)   100. Which of the following characteristics are shared by copper and fluoride?

    a. Both may be obtained from drinking tap water
    b. Both serve as cofactors for a number of enzymes
    c. Neither is involved in the integrity of bones and teeth
    d. Neither is known to be toxic at intakes of 10 times the estimated safe and adequate dietary intake

d   447(K)   101. Which of the following does NOT have an RDA?

    a. Iron
    b. Zinc
    c. Iodine
    d. Copper

b   447(A)   102. Which of the following meats would be the best source of copper?

    a. Ham
    b. Liver
    c. Beefsteak
    d. Hamburger

b   447(K)   103. Which of the following is a feature of copper nutrition?

    a. Absorption efficiency is similar to that of iron
    b. It is involved in collagen synthesis and wound healing
    c. Soft water may provide significant amounts in the diet
    d. Deficiency is common in children of Middle East countries

b   448(K)   104. Characteristics of manganese in nutrition include all of the following EXCEPT

   a.   good sources are plant foods.
   b.   deficiencies are seen primarily in the elderly.
   c.   absorption is inhibited by calcium supplements.
   d.   toxicity is more common from environmental contamination than from the diet.

c   448(A)   105. Which of the following represents the most likely cause of manganese toxicity?

   a.   Consumption of supplements
   b.   Increased absorption due to genetic defect
   c.   Inhalation of dust contaminated with manganese
   d.   Consumption of foods grown on manganese-rich soils

b   449(A)   106. Which of the following mechanisms explains why fluoride is effective in controlling tooth decay?

   a.   It helps regulate calcium levels in saliva
   b.   It helps form decay-resistant fluorapatite
   c.   It inhibits growth of decay-producing bacteria
   d.   It changes the pH of the mouth, inhibiting bacterial growth

a   449(K)   107. What is the most reliable source of dietary fluoride?

   a.   Public water
   b.   Dark green vegetables
   c.   Milk and milk products
   d.   Meats and whole-grain cereals

a   449(A)   108. What is the optimal fluoride concentrated in community water supplies?

   a.   1 ppm
   b.   2 ppm
   c.   2.5 ppm
   d.   4 ppm

d   449(K)   109. What is the primary mechanism associated with the role of fluoride in prevention of dental caries?

    a. Fluoride increases calcium absorption which increases crystal formation of teeth
    b. Decay is inhibited due to neutralization of organic acids produced by bacteria on the teeth
    c. Decay is reduced due to the inhibitory effects of fluoride on growth of bacteria on the teeth
    d. Fluoride becomes incorporated into the crystalline structure of teeth making them less susceptible to decay

a   449(K)   110. Which of the following is known to cause discolored enamel of the teeth?

    a. Excessive fluoride in the water
    b. Insufficient fluoride in the water
    c. Excessive intake of simple sugars
    d. Inability of the body to absorb fluoride

a   449(K)   111. Fluoride deficiency is best known to lead to

    a. dental decay.
    b. osteoporosis.
    c. discoloration of teeth.
    d. nutritional muscular dystrophy.

c   449-450(K)   112. One of the chief functions of chromium is participation in the metabolism of

    a. iron.
    b. proteins.
    c. carbohydrates.
    d. metallothionein.

b   450(K)   113. Chromium deficiency is characterized by

    a. hypertension.
    b. hyperglycemia.
    c. enlargement of the liver.
    d. enlargement of the thyroid gland.

c   450(A)   114.   Which of the following has been found to result from excessive intakes of molybdenum?

    a.   Goiter
    b.   Diabetes
    c.   Gout-like symptoms
    d.   Atherosclerotic lesions

b   450(K)   115.   Which of the following is a characteristic of the mineral molybdenum?

    a.   Enhances the activity of insulin
    b.   Deficiency symptoms in animals and people are unknown
    c.   Unusually poor food sources are milk and leafy green vegetables
    d.   Toxicity symptoms in human beings include damage to red blood cells

c   450(K)   116.   As far as is known, what hormone is dependent upon chromium for optimal activity?

    a.   Renin
    b.   Gastrin
    c.   Insulin
    d.   Antidiurectic hormone

b   451(K)   117.   What mineral is part of vitamin B_{12}?

    a.   Copper
    b.   Cobalt
    c.   Nickel
    d.   Vanadium

c   451(K)   118.   Which of the following trace minerals is known to be essential in bone development?

    a.   Tin
    b.   Cobalt
    c.   Silicon
    d.   Barium

b   451(A)   119. Evidence to date in animals and/or human beings suggests that normal bone metabolism requires all of the following trace minerals <u>EXCEPT</u>

    a.   boron.
    b.   silver.
    c.   silicon.
    d.   nickel.

c   451(A)   120. Which of the following elements has proved useful in the treatment of certain leukemias?

    a.   Tin
    b.   Arsenic
    c.   Selenium
    d.   Molybdenum

c   458(K)   121. What term designates foods that contain nonnutrient substances which may provide health benefits beyond basic nutrition?

    a.   Health foods
    b.   Organic foods
    c.   Functional foods
    d.   Disease preventative foods

a   459(K)   122. Which of the following is most descriptive of the term probiotics?

    a.   Living microbes in foods
    b.   Concentrated phytonutrients
    c.   Vitamins and essential trace elements
    d.   Vitamin supplements that include biotin

Matching (Answers can be used only once)

H	432	123.	Iron storage protein
N	431	124.	Enhances absorption of nonheme iron
E	430	125.	Form of iron found only in animal flesh
I	431	126.	Form of iron found in both plant and animal foods
M	430	127.	Oxygen-carrying protein in muscle
P	432	128.	Substance in coffee and tea that reduces iron absorption
C	434	129.	Craving for non-food substances
B	435	130.	Mineral showing highest prevalence of toxicity in Americans
S	439	131.	Condition characterized by large deposits of iron protein in body tissues
T	440	132.	Zinc binding protein of intestine
D	440	133.	A deficiency of this element retards growth and arrests sexual maturation
O	430	134.	Iron-containing protein in erythrocytes
F	445	135.	Iodine deficiency disease
R	445	136.	Major dietary source of iodine
I	446	137.	Disease associated with severe selenium deficiency
Q	449	138.	Stabilized form of tooth crystal
K	450	139.	Deficiency leads to hyperglycemia
L	450	140.	Condition associated with discoloration of tooth enamel
A	450	141.	Significant dietary source of fluoride
G	451	142.	Mineral that forms integral part of vitamin B_{12}

A.	Tea	K.	Chromium
B.	Iron	L.	Fluorosis
C.	Pica	M.	Myoglobin
D.	Zinc	N.	MFP Factor
E.	Heme	O.	Hemoglobin
F.	Goiter	P.	Tannic acid
G.	Cobalt	Q.	Fluorapatite
H.	Ferritin	R.	Fortified salt
I.	Keshan	S.	Hemosiderosis
J.	Nonheme	T.	Metallothionein

Essay Questions

429   143.   Make several general statements about trace elements in nutrition, including common food sources, deficiencies, toxicities, and interactions.

430-450   144.   Choose any 3 trace elements and discuss their major functions, deficiency symptoms, toxicity symptoms, and food sources.

430-432   145.   What factors are known to reduce or enhance iron absorption?

430-432; 146.   Discuss factors that influence the bioavailability of dietary iron. What are good sources of bioavailable iron? What factors interfere with iron absorption?
436-438

430-431   147.   Explain the difference between heme and nonheme iron. How can the efficiency of absorption be increased for both types of iron?

433-434   148.   In the proper sequence, describe the three stages in the development of iron deficiency.

435-436   149.   Discuss the pros and cons of increasing the iron level of enriched bread in the United States.

440-442   150.   What are the signs and symptoms of zinc deficiency? Which ones have similarities to other nutrient deficiencies?

445-446   151.   `What factors account for the above average intake of iodine by many people in the U.S. population?

445   152.   What are the effects of iodine deficiency and iodine excess? What population groups show iodine abnormalities?

446   153.   Discuss iodine availability and sources of iodine in the U.S. diet.

460-461   160.   Briefly explain the laws governing the marketing of functional foods.

461   161.   Explain the meaning and significance of structure-function claims on food labels. Support your discussion with examples.

461   162.   Cite examples of advertising claims permitted by the Federal Trade commission but not by the FDA.

CHAPTER 14
FITNESS: PHYSICAL ACTIVITY, NUTRIENTS, AND BODY ADAPTATIONS

Ans   Page

d   468(K)   01. According to the American College of Sports Medicine, which of the following would meet the exercise schedule to maintain an appropriate level of fitness?

   a. 2 hours of aerobic exercise daily
   b. 1 hour of strength training 4 times a week
   c. 5 minutes of aerobic exercise 2 times a week
   d. 20 minutes of any continuous activity using large muscle groups 3 times a week

c   469(K)   02. All of the following are acceptable definitions of the term fitness EXCEPT

   a. the ability of the body to resist stress.
   b. the ability of the body to perform physical activity without undue stress.
   c. the ability to maintain a normal body composition and remain free of injury while performing strenuous physical tasks.
   d. the ability to meet normal physical demands while maintaining an energy reserve sufficient to overcome an immediate challenge.

b   470(A)   03. Three hours per week of brisk walking by adults is known to lower the risk of heart attach by at least

    a.   10%
    b.   30%
    c.   75%
    d.   90%

a   470-471(K) 04. Which of the following is generally NOT associated with a regular program of physical fitness?

    a.   Lowering of bone density
    b.   Lowering of blood pressure
    c.   Lowering of blood cholesterol
    d.   Lowering of resting pulse rate

c   471(K)   05. The components of fitness include all of the following EXCEPT

    a.   strength.
    b.   flexibility.
    c.   bone fragility.
    d.   cardiovascular endurance.

b   472(A)   06. A muscle that increases size in response to use is an example of

    a.   atrophy.
    b.   hypertrophy.
    c.   muscular endurance.
    d.   muscle engorgement.

c   472(A)   07. Athletes can safely add muscle tissue by

    a.   tripling protein intake.
    b.   taking hormones duplicating those of puberty.
    c.   putting a demand on muscles by making them work harder.
    d.   relying on protein for muscle fuel and decreasing intake of carbohydrates.

a 472(K) 08. What is muscle atrophy?

  a. Loss of muscle size and strength
  b. Muscle cramps arising from insufficient warm-up
  c. Muscle spasms resulting from too rapid progressive overloading
  d. Alterations in heart muscle contractions when first initiating a fitness program

c 472(K) 09. Two definitive indicators of the physical fitness of older adults are strength and

  a. VO$_2$ max.
  b. jumping ability.
  c. walking endurance.
  d. resting heart rate below 70,

a 472-473(A) 10. In weight training, muscle strength can best be emphasized by combining a

  a. low number of repetitions with heavy weight.
  b. low number of repetitions with lighter weight.
  c. high number of repetitions with heavy weight.
  d. high number of repetitions with lighter weight.

a 473(K) 11. Which of the following is <u>NOT</u> derived directly from cardiorespiratory conditioning?

  a. Increased flexibility
  b. Slowed resting pulse
  c. Increased breathing efficiency
  d. Increased blood volume and oxygen delivery

d 473(K) 12. The effect of regular exercise on heart and lung function is known as

  a. muscle fitness.
  b. muscle endurance.
  c. cardiopulmonary adaptation.
  d. cardiorespiratory conditioning.

b   473-474(K)   13. What is VO_2 max?

    a.   An individual's maximum velocity on a test treadmill
    b.   An individual's maximum rate of oxygen consumption
    c.   An individual's maximum intake of oxygen while at rest
    d.   An individual's maximum intake of air at 70% physical exhaustion

d   473-474(A)   14. With cardiorespiratory conditioning muscle cells show all of the following changes <u>EXCEPT</u>

    a.   they hold more myoglobin.
    b.   they become stronger in the lungs.
    c.   they hold more fat oxidizing enzymes.
    d.   they draw less oxygen due to increased efficiency of aerobic metabolism.

a   425(K)   15. What substance contains the chemical energy that drives immediate muscle contraction?

    a.   ATP
    b.   NAD
    c.   Glucose
    d.   Fatty acids

d   475(K)   16. What high-energy compound acts as a reservoir of energy for the maintenance of a steady supply of ATP?

    a.   Glycerol
    b.   Glycogen
    c.   Fatty acids
    d.   Phosphocreatine

b   475(K)   17. During physical performance, what is the role of creatine phosphate?

    a.   Removal of lactic acid
    b.   Transfer of energy to make ATP
    c.   Removal of nitrogen waste products
    d.   Transfer of phosphate to muscle fiber

b   475(A)   18. A person who suddenly begins sprinting will exhaust the muscle's supply of creatine phosphate in about

        a.   1 second.
        b.   10 seconds.
        c.   1 minute.
        d.   10 minutes.

a   475-476(A) 19. If muscle work is anaerobic, which of the following can <u>NOT</u> serve as fuel?

        a.   Fat
        b.   Protein
        c.   Carbohydrate

a   476(A)   20. What is the usual fate of muscle glycogen during exercise?

        a.   Utilized as a fuel within the muscle cell only
        b.   Released into the bloodstream to provide fuel for brain cells
        c.   Released into the bloodstream to replenish liver glycogen as needed
        d.   Utilized to support lung and heart function under conditions of intense physical performance

c   476(A)   21. What dietary nutrients are most effective at raising muscle glycogen concentrations?

        a.   Fats
        b.   Proteins
        c.   Carbohydrates
        d.   Chromium and iron

a   476(K)   22. What is the predominant fuel used by muscle cells during low or moderate intensity activity?

        a.   Fat
        b.   Protein
        c.   Glycogen
        d.   Blood glucose

d   445-447(A)   23. Which of the following activities depletes glycogen most quickly?

                         a.   Hiking
                         b.   Jogging
                         c.   Walking
                         d.   Quarter-mile run

b   476-477(A)   24. A tissue deprived of an oxygen supply during exercise would
                         have an accumulation of

                         a.   ATP.
                         b.   lactic acid.
                         c.   glucose-1-phosphate.
                         d.   TCA cycle intermediates.

a   476-477(A)   25. Which of the following is a common product of anaerobic
                         metabolism?

                         a.   Lactic acid
                         b.   Phytic acid
                         c.   Phosphoric acid
                         d.   Hydrochloric acid

c   476-477(A)   26. Which of the following substances increases in muscles during
                         increasing exercise intensity?

                         a.   ATP
                         b.   Glycogen
                         c.   Lactic acid
                         d.   Phosphocreatine

b   478(K)   27. How much time is usually needed in vigorous activity to cause
                         depletion of glycogen reserves?

                         a.   1 hour
                         b.   2 hours
                         c.   3 hours
                         d.   4 hours

b   477(K)   28. What is the Cori cycle?

    a.   The coordinated muscle contraction sequence of slow-twitch and fast-twitch fibers
    b.   A process in the liver that regenerates glucose from lactic acid released by muscles
    c.   An exercise machine that allows development of both aerobic and anaerobic capacities
    d.   A group of enzymatic reactions to accelerate muscle glycogen repletion in the trained athlete

d   477(K)   29. During the first 20 minutes of moderate exercise, the body uses about

    a.   50% of the available fat.
    b.   10% of the available water.
    c.   90% of the available protein.
    d.   20% of the available glycogen.

c   478(A)   30. When a marathon runner experiences the phenomenon known as "hitting the wall," what nutrient is most likely depleted?

    a.   Water
    b.   Protein
    c.   Glucose
    d.   Fatty acids

c   478-479(A)   31. Which of the following is LEAST likely to affect the size of the body's glycogen stores?

    a.   Exercise regimen
    b.   Fat content of the diet
    c.   Type of supplements taken
    d.   Carbohydrate content of the diet

c   478-479(A)   32. Which of the following diets promotes superior physical performance in athletes?

    a.   High fat diet
    b.   High protein diet
    c.   High carbohydrate diet
    d.   Normal mixed diet with vitamin supplements

b   478-479(K)   33. Which of the following is a property of conditioned muscles?

    a.   They can store more glycogen
    b.   They are more efficient at converting fat to glucose
    c.   They contain less mitochondria due to increased glucose utilization
    d.   They rely less on fat breakdown and more on glucose oxidation for energy

d   479(A)   34. What type of meal and time of its ingestion promote the most rapid repletion of glycogen stores after physical activity?

    a.   Mixed meal taken within 4 hours
    b.   Mixed meal taken within 30 minutes
    c.   High-carbohydrate meal taken within 2½ hours
    d.   High-carbohydrate meal taken within 15 minutes

c   479(A)   35. During a physical activity, what hormone blunts the response of insulin to consumption of a surgery drink?

    a.   Leptin
    b.   Glucagon
    c.   Epinephrine
    d.   Neuropeptide-y

c   480(K)   36. What cellular organelles are responsible for producing ATP aerobically?

    a.   Ribosomes
    b.   Golgi bodies
    c: Mitochondria
    d.   Cell membranes

c   480(A)   37. Which of the following describes fat utilization during physical activity?

    a.   Fat that is stored closest to the exercising muscle is oxidized first
    b.   Fat oxidization makes more of a contribution as the intensity of the exercise increases
    c.   Fat oxidation may continue at an above normal rate for some time after cessation of physical activity
    d.   Fat is burned in higher quantities during short high-intensity exercises than prolonged low-intensity exercises

c   481(A)   38. Which of the following is an effect of physical fitness on fat
                       metabolism?

                       a. Fatty acid release from adipose cells into muscle cells
                           becomes more efficient
                       b. Fat oxidation by the whole body is higher throughout the
                           day rather than only during exercise
                       c. Fatty acid energy release requires less oxygen on a per-
                           kcal basis than does the use of glucose
                       d. Fat utilization slows down and liver glucose release rises in
                           response to adaptation of the body's hormonal profile

b   482(A)   39. Which of the following is an effect of exercise on protein
                       metabolism?

                       a. Protein use as a fuel is lowest in endurance athletes
                       b. Protein synthesis is inhibited during exercise and for some
                           time thereafter
                       c. Protein use during physical performance is generally not
                           related to carbohydrate content of the diet
                       d. Protein synthesis is increased slightly during exercise but
                           diminishes by a like amount to remain in balance

c   . 482(K)   40. Which of the following is a feature of protein nutrition in physical
                       activity?

                       a. Protein contributes 30% more to total fuel used versus that
                           in the resting state
                       b. Body protein synthesis rates are increased about 10%
                           during the physical activity
                       c. Protein contributes about the same percentage of total fuel
                           used versus that in the resting state
                       d. Body protein synthesis rates are increased about 30% for
                           several hours after the physical activity

d   482-484(A) 41. Which of the following is NOT known to modify the body's use of
                       protein?

                       a. Diet
                       b. The degree of training
                       c. Exercise intensity and duration
                       d. Vitamin supplements above the RDA

b   482-483(A)   42. Which of the following is a role for diet in physical activity?

    a. Diets high in fat lead to a fall in amino acid utilization for fuel
    b. Diets lacking in carbohydrates lead to increased amino acid utilization for fuel
    c. Deficiencies of vitamins have no effect on performance provided that all other nutrients are adequate
    d. Deficiencies of minerals have no effect on performance provided that all other nutrients are adequate

b   483(A)   43. According to several recognized health organizations, about how many grams of protein per day are recommended for a 70 kg strength athlete?

    a. 56
    b. 112
    c. 140
    d. 168

c   483(A)   44. Which of the following describes the role of protein in the diet of competitive athletes?

    a. The need for protein per kg body weight is higher in females than male athletes
    b. The need for protein is best met by increasing the level to 20-25% of total energy content of the diet
    c. The need for protein in weight lifters and marathon runners may be up to 75-100% higher than the RDA
    d. The need for protein in most athletes generally could <u>NOT</u> be obtained from diets meeting energy requirements but containing only 10% of the energy as protein

c   487(A)   45. According to several recognized health organizations, about how many grams of protein per day are recommended for a 50 kg marathon runner?

        a.   45-52
        b.   55-70
        c.   72-96
        d.   120-154

d   484(K)   46. Which of the following represents current knowledge of the role of vitamin and mineral supplements in physical performance?

        a.   When taken right before an event, they have been shown to benefit performance
        b.   Moderate amounts have been shown to improve the performance of most elite athletes
        c.   Except perhaps for iron, they are needed in high amounts to meet the needs of athletes exposed to hot and humid weather conditions
        d.   Except perhaps for iron and vitamin E, supplements are not recommended since there is no difference in the RDA of physically active people compared with sedentary people

a   484(A)   47. What nutrient is important in transport of oxygen in blood and in muscle tissue and energy transformation reactions?

        a.   Iron
        b.   Calcium
        c.   Thiamin
        d.   Vitamin C

d   484-485(K)   48. Which of the following is a known feature of iron nutrition in athletes?

        a.   Iron in sweat represents the major route of iron loss from the body
        b.   Iron deficiency affects a higher percentage of male athletes than female athletes
        c.   Sports anemia is successfully treated by increasing dietary iron to levels 2-3 times the RDA
        d.   Iron losses in runners occur when blood cells are squashed by the impact of the foot on a hard surface

a   485(A)   49. What would be the minimum amount of body water loss
                       necessary to bring about a reduction in work capacity of an
                       average 165 pound individual?

                       a.   1½ liters
                       b.   3½ liters
                       c.   6 liters
                       d.   10 liters

b   485(K)   50. Which of the following is a characteristic of sports anemia?

                       a.   It requires a prolonged treatment period
                       b.   It is a temporary condition requiring no treatment
                       c.   It responds to treatment only with high doses of iron
                       d.   It is due primarily to increased iron loss via perspiration

a   485(K)   51. The first sign of dehydration is typically

                       a.   fatigue.
                       b.   dizziness.
                       c.   intense thirst.
                       d.   intense sweating.

a   485(K)   52. Physical performance is noticeably affected when body water
                       loss first reaches

                       a.   1-2%.
                       b.   5-10%.
                       c.   15-20%.
                       d.   25-30%.

a   485(K)   53. Which of the following is a feature of sports anemia?

                       a.   It is not a true iron deficiency anemia
                       b.   It is usually corrected by iron supplementation
                       c.   It is found primarily in over-conditioned athletes
                       d.   It is associated with reduced cardiorespiratory fitness

d   485(A)   54. A person engaged in an endurance event has lost two liters of body water by sweating. What would be the approximate energy loss from the evaporation of the sweat?

     a.   100 kcal
     b.   500 kcal
     c.   850 kcal
     d.   1200 kcal

a   485(K)   55. All of the following are characteristics of heat stroke EXCEPT

     a.   it is rarely fatal.
     b.   it is due, in part, to dehydration.
     c.   it is caused by heat buildup in the body.
     d.   its symptoms include headache, nausea, and mental changes.

b   485(A)   56. A person engaged in physically active work in hot humid weather and who wears a rubber suit to promote weight loss is at high risk of experiencing

     a.   ketosis.
     b.   heat stroke.
     c.   hypothermia.
     d.   overhydration.

b   485(K)   57. What nutrient becomes depleted most rapidly during physical exercise?

     a.   Iron
     b.   Water
     c.   Glucose
     d.   Glycogen

a   486(A)   58. In the endurance athlete, the first priority of nutrient repletion should be

     a.   fluids.
     b.   protein.
     c.   glycogen.
     d.   electrolytes.

b   486(K)   59. Which of the following are common early symptoms of
                          hypothermia in athletes?

                          a.   Headache and nausea
                          b.   Euphoria and shivering
                          c.   Confusion and delirium
                          d.   Dizziness and clumsiness

c   486(K)   60. Which of the following is a feature of water metabolism during
                          exercise?

                          a.   The maximum loss of fluid per hour of exercise is about 0.5
                               liters
                          b.   In cold weather, the need for water falls dramatically
                               because the body does not sweat
                          c.   Sweat losses can exceed the capacity of the GI tract to
                               absorb water resulting in some degree of dehydration
                          d.   Heavy sweating leads to a marked rise in the thirst
                               sensation to stimulate water intake which delays the onset
                               of dehydration

b   486-487(K)   61. All of the following are valid reasons for consuming sports drinks
                          by most physically active people EXCEPT

                          a.   they may provide a psychological advantage.
                          b.   they are better than water at preventing sodium depletion.
                          c.   they contain a source of fuel which may enhance
                               performance in endurance events.
                          d.   they have a good taste which encourages their
                               consumption and ensures adequate hydration.

c   486-487(A)   62. Which of the following would be the best choice for physically
                          active people who need to rehydrate?

                          a.   "Sweat" replacers
                          b.   Salt tablets and tap water
                          c.   Diluted juice or cool water
                          d.   Water warmed to body temperature

a   486(K)   63. What is the recommended amount of water to meet the needs of athletes?

    a.   1-1½ ml per kcal expended
    b.   5-7 ml per kcal expended
    c.   1,000 ml per hour of activity
    d.   1,500 ml per hour of activity

c   486-487(K)   64. All of the following are characteristics of electrolyte metabolism in sports EXCEPT

    a.   the trained athlete actually loses fewer electrolytes than the untrained person.
    b.   replenishment of lost electrolytes in most athletes can be accomplished by ingesting a regular diet.
    c.   sweating leads to significant losses of calcium, sulfur, and chromium which can be replaced by including milk and whole grains in the diet.
    d.   salt tablet supplements to replace electrolyte losses of sweat are known to cause fluid retention in the GI tract, irritation of the stomach, and vomiting.

c   487(K)   65. Which of the following is a benefit of glucose polymer sports drinks as compared with sugar containing drinks?

    a.   They supply more energy per gram of carbohydrate
    b.   They require less digestion and therefore are absorbed faster into the circulation
    c.   They attract less water in the GI tract and thus allow more water to remain in the circulation
    d.   They are absorbed much more slowly and therefore provide a more even carbohydrate load to the body

a   487(A)   66. Which of the following describes an effect of caffeine use in the athlete?

    a.   It induces fluid losses
    b.   It enhances performance for almost all athletes
    c.   It raises blood pH to counteract the buildup of lactic acid
    d.   It promotes absorption of electrolytes from the intestinal tract

c   487(A)   67. The optimal carbohydrate concentration of sports drinks for the
                      endurance athlete is

                      a.   1-2%.
                      b.   5%.
                      c.   6-10%.
                      d.   15-20%.

b   488(A)   68. What is the minimum amount of fluid that an athlete should
                      drink for each pound of body weight lost during an activity?

                      a.   ¼ liter
                      b.   ½ liter
                      c.   1 liter
                      d.   2 liters

c   488(A)   69. Which of the following should be a component of a healthy diet
                      for athletes?

                      a.   Salt tablets
                      b.   Protein powders
                      c.   Nutrient dense foods
                      d.   Vitamin and mineral supplements

c   488(A)   70. The recommended amount of dietary carbohydrate for an
                      athlete training for a marathon is

                      a.   2 g/kg body weight.
                      b.   4 g/kg body weight.
                      c.   8 g/kg body weight.
                      d.   12 g/kg body weight.

c   490(A)   71. What should be the composition of the last (pregame) meal
                      before an athletic event?

                      a.   High-protein, providing 30 kcal per kg body weight
                      b.   Vegetable and fruit juices, providing 100 to 200 kcal
                      c.   High-carbohydrate, low-fiber, providing 300 to 800 kcal
                      d.   High-fiber, providing 200 to 300 kcal and liberal amounts of
                           fluid which is beneficially retained by the fiber in the GI tract

d   490(A)   72. What is the recommended composition of the postgame meal of
                             the athlete?

                             a.   Low-protein
                             b.   High-protein
                             c.   Low-carbohydrate
                             d.   High-carbohydrate

d   490(K)   73. Why should fiber-rich foods be avoided in an athlete's pregame
                             meal?

                             a.   The fiber delays absorption of fat
                             b.   The fiber interferes with glycolysis
                             c.   The meal crowds out more energy-dense foods
                             d.   The fiber retains water in the GI tract that would otherwise
                                  be absorbed

d   490(A)   74. Why should high proteins or high fat foods be avoided during
                             the first few hours after physical activity?

                             a.   They induce GI cramping
                             b.   They suppress protein synthesis
                             c.   They promote continued water loss and this increase the
                                  risk for dehydration
                             d.   They are known to suppress hunger and thereby reduce
                                  carbohydrate intake

c   496(K)   75. What is the source of whey protein sold as supplements to body
                             builders?

                             a.   An alkaline extract of brewer's yeast
                             b.   An acid extract of soybean processing
                             c.   A waste product of cheese manufacturing
                             d.   A complementary protein composed of animal and legume
                                  extracts

a   497(A)   76. Research results of carnitine supplementation as an ergogenic
                             aid showed that it

                             a.   produced diarrhea in half of the subjects.
                             b.   enhanced carbohydrate oxidation rate but not fat oxidation.
                             c.   raised muscle carnitine concentration but did not improve
                                  performance.
                             d.   promoted retention of amino acids but did not lead to
                                  increased muscle mass.

a 497(K) 77. Which of the following is a feature of specific ergogenic acids?

  a. Vitamin E in high doses seems to protect against exercise-induced oxidative stress
  b. Branched-chain amino acid supplementation appears to lower blood ammonia levels
  c. Carnitine supplementation appears to increase the concentration of muscle carnitine
  d. Chromium supplementation (as chromium picolinate) appears to enhance fat oxidation in most athletes

b 498(A) 78. An athlete who believes in soda loading as a means of improving performance would, right before the event, consume

  a. caffeine tablets.
  b. sodium bicarbonate.
  c. a carbonated beverage.
  d. a lactose containing beverage.

d 498-501(K) 79. Which of the following ergogenic aids increases the risk for acromegaly?

  a. HMB
  b. Creatine
  c. Octacosanol
  d. Growth hormone

a 501(K) 80. What type of chemicals are DHEA and androstendione?

  a. Hormones
  b. Estrogens
  c. Phytonutrients
  d. Herbal extracts

a 501(K) 81. Which of the following is a characteristic of human growth hormone use in athletes?

  a. Excessive use shortens life span
  b. Low cost accounts for some of its popularity
  c. Excessive use leads to shrinking of internal organs
  d. Laboratory tests can differentiate between the naturally occurring form and the drug form of growth hormone

Matching (Answers can be used only once)

H	469	82	The body's ability to deal with stress
O	471	83.	The capacity of the joints to move with less chance of injury
Q	472	84.	Increase in muscle size and strength
G	473	85.	Required for aerobic metabolism
L	475	86.	Used as precursor to form a high-energy compound in muscle cells
P	477	87.	A chief substance of the Cori cycle
M	478	88.	Depletion of this substance leads runners to experience "hitting the wall"
D	478	89.	Recommended amount of carbohydrate as percentage of total energy intake of endurance athletes
K	479	90.	Substance in muscle that serves as a source of energy and water
C	480	91.	Number of minutes after starting a physical activity for blood fatty acid concentrations to rise
E	483	92.	Recommended protein intake (g per day) for a 70 kg competitive body builder
T	485	93.	Transient condition of low blood hemoglobin in athletes
S	485	94.	Early symptoms of this disorder include nausea and stumbling
F	485	95.	Number of kcalories expended from evaporation of one liter of sweat
R	486	96.	Early symptoms of this disorder are shivering and euphoria
N	486	97.	The replacement of fluids during physical activities
A	486	98.	Water intake recommendation for physically active people, in ml/kcal expended
J	487	99.	Stimulant that promotes urine losses during exercise
I	487	100.	Depressant that promotes urine losses
B	488	101.	Recommended carbohydrate intake, in g/kg body weight, of athletes in heavy training

A.	1	K.	Glycogen
B.	8	L.	Creatine
C.	20	M.	Glucose
D.	70	N.	Hydration
E.	112	O.	Flexibility
F.	600	P.	Lactic acid
G	Oxygen	Q	Hypertrophy
H.	Fitness	R.	Hypothermia
I.	Alcohol	S.	Hyperthermia
J.	Caffeine	T.	Sports anemia

Essay Questions

468-471   102. Discuss the physiological and psychological benefits of being
                    physically fit.

471-472   103. Explain the recommended training procedure (i.e., overload
                    principle) for mastering the components of fitness.

473-474   104. Explain the meaning and significance of cardiorespiratory
                    endurance.

476-483   105. Discuss the use of protein, fat, and carbohydrate as fuels
                    during low, moderate, and intense exercise.

478-480   106. Explain the training technique of glycogen loading. What are
                    its advantages and disadvantages?

480-482   107. Describe three factors that influence fat use during physical activity.

480-482   108. Discuss the pros and cons of high-fat diets for athletic performance.

484-485   109. Discuss the effects of athletic training on iron nutrition.

485   110. Compare and contrast the characteristics of sports anemia with the anemia that would be found in marathon runners.

485-487   111. Discuss the need for water in maintaining physical performance. What are the symptoms of dehydration? What are the recommendations for ensuring that the body is well-hydrated prior to an athletic event?

488-490   112. Describe an appropriate diet for physically active people.

497   113.   Under what circumstances might supplemental vitamin E be of benefit for physically active people?

496-499   114.   Discuss the use of 6 substances promoted as aids to enhance athletic performance.

497-499   115.   Discuss the use and abuse of caffeine, carnitine, and creatine as ergogenic substances.

499-501   116.   Describe the hazards of using anabolic steroids and human growth hormone as ways of improving physical performance.

CHAPTER 15
LIFE CYCLE NUTRITION: PREGNANCY AND LACTATION

Ans   Page

a   500(K)   01.   What is the placenta?

     a.   An organ from which the infant receives nourishment
     b.   A muscular organ within which the infant develops before birth
     c.   The developing infant from the eighth week after conception until birth
     d.   The developing infant during its second through eighth week after conception

c   500(K)   02.   What organ of the pregnant woman is central to the exchange of nutrients for waste products with the fetus?

     a.   Uterus
     b.   Vagina
     c.   Placenta
     d.   Amniotic sac

b   500(K)   03.   What is the name given to the human organism two to eight weeks after fertilization and the stage at which the digestive system is formed?

     a.   Fetus
     b.   Embryo
     c.   Ectoderm
     d.   Mesoderm

a   500(K)   04.   At what stage of pregnancy does an embryo show a beating heart and a complete central nervous system?

      a.   8 weeks
      b.   12 weeks
      c.   20 weeks
      d.   29 weeks

c   500-501(K)   05.   What organ functions to prepare the mother's breasts for lactation?

      a.   Uterus
      b.   Ovaries
      c.   Placenta
      d.   Amniotic sac

d   500-501(K)   06.   During development of the fetus, what organ(s) are the first to reach maturity?

      a.   Heart and lungs
      b.   Liver and kidneys
      c.   Gastrointestinal tract
      d.   Central nervous system and brain

a   500-501(K)   07.   What is the term given to the developing infant from the eighth week after conception until birth?

      a.   Fetus
      b.   Ovum
      c.   Zygote
      d.   Embryo

d   502(K)   08.   Gestation is generally divided into equal periods of

      a.   4 weeks, called quarters.
      b.   9 weeks, called quartiles.
      c.   4 months, called semesters.
      d.   3 months, called trimesters.

c   502(A)   09.   All of the following statements are specific to the critical periods of cell division <u>EXCEPT</u>

a.   malnutrition during pregnancy can affect fetal cell division.
b.   malnutrition during critical periods can have irreversible effects.
c.   high-nutrient-density food fed after the critical period can remedy a growth deficit.
d.   whatever nutrients are needed during a critical period must be supplied at that time.

b   502(K)   10.   What term is given to the time period during which irreversible damage to the fetus may occur from specific events such as malnutrition or exposure to toxins?

a.   First trimester
b.   Critical period
c.   Fertility period
d.   Conceptual period

b   502(K)   11.   The most common forms of neural tube defects are spina bifida and

a.   macrosomia.
b.   anencephaly.
c.   preeclampsia.
d.   cesarean section.

c   502(A)   12.   What organ is most affected in anencephaly?

a.   Liver
b.   Heart
c.   Brain
d.   Pancreas

d   502-503(K)   13.   The neural tube forms the early parts of the

a.   umbilical cord.
b.   liver and pancreas.
c.   gastrointestinal tract.
d.   brain and spinal cord.

a   502-503(K)   14.   Which of the following is a characteristic of neural tube defects?

    a.   They affect about 0.1% of newborns in the United States
    b.   They include common disorders such as liver and kidney disease
    c.   They can be prevented by supplementation of the pregnant woman's diet with vitamin B_{12}
    d.   They can be prevented by supplementation of the pregnant woman's diet with vitamins A and E

d   503(K)   15.   Studies report that folate supplements for women may lower the incidence of neural tube defects of infants when the vitamin is taken during the

    a.   last trimester of pregnancy.
    b.   second trimester of pregnancy.
    c.   second and third trimesters of pregnancy.
    d.   month before conception through the first trimester of pregnancy.

b   503-504(K)   16.   Which of the following nutrients taken as a prenatal supplement has been found to be associated with a lower incidence of neural tube defects?

    a.   Iron
    b.   Folate
    c.   Calcium
    d.   Cobalamin

a   504(K)   17.   Which of the following is the most potent single indicator of an infant's future health status?

    a.   Infant's birthweight
    b.   Mother's weight before pregnancy
    c.   Mother's weight gain during pregnancy
    d.   Mother's nutrition status prior to pregnancy

b   505(K)   18.   What is the minimum recommended weight gain for the obese pregnant woman?

    a.   10 lbs
    b.   15 lbs
    c.   25 lbs
    d.   35 lbs

c   505-506(K)   19.   What is the recommended range of weight gain during pregnancy for a normal-weight woman?

     a.   10-18 lbs
     b.   19-24 lbs
     c.   25-30 lbs
     d.   35-40 lbs

b   505(A)   20.   Which of the following increases the risk of macrosomia?

     a.   Folate deficiency
     b.   Prepregnancy obesity
     c.   Postpregnancy infection
     d.   Gestational oxygen deprivation

b   506(K)   21.   In pregnancy, a large weight gain over a short time is usually an indication of

     a.   excessive fat deposition.
     b.   excessive fluid retention.
     c.   abnormal fetal development.
     d.   normal pregnancy only if it occurs during the second trimester.

c   506-507;   22.   Adaptational responses in the woman who becomes pregnant
     511(K)   include all of the following <u>EXCEPT</u>

     a.   a 50% increase in blood volume.
     b.   an increase in calcium absorption.
     c.   an increase in serum albumin concentration.
     d.   a decline in blood hemoglobin concentration.

c   507(A)   23.   The component of weight gain during pregnancy that is similar to the average weight of the infant at birth is the

     a.   placenta.
     b.   amniotic sac fluid.
     c.   maternal fat stores.
     d.   uterus and supporting muscles.

b   507(K)   24.   Which of the following is a characteristic of body weight changes associated with pregnancy?

    a.   Weight gain is generally steady throughout pregnancy for normal-weight women
    b.   Most women are unable to lose all of the weight that was gained during pregnancy
    c.   Sudden, large, weight gain in pregnancy may signal the development of hypotension
    d.   Overweight pregnant women should gain as much weight as underweight pregnant women

a   507-508(K)   25.   To maintain physical fitness during pregnancy, all of the following activities are considered acceptable <u>EXCEPT</u>

    a.   saunas.
    b.   swimming.
    c.   playing singles tennis.
    d.   45-minute balanced exercise sessions 3 times/week.

a   508(A)   26.   Edema in a pregnant woman who does not have high blood pressure or protein in the urine is   .

    a.   expected and normal.
    b.   a sign of dietary deficiencies.
    c.   very rare and life threatening.
    d.   a warning signal of a difficult labor.

c   508(K)   27.   All of the following are normal body responses to pregnancy <u>EXCEPT</u>

    a.   breast size increases.
    b.   blood volume increases.
    c.   body water level decreases.
    d.   joints become more flexible.

b   509;511(A)   28.   Which of the following nutrients are required in higher amounts during pregnancy due to their roles in the synthesis of red blood cells?

    a.   Protein and chromium
    b.   Folate and vitamin B_{12}
    c.   Calcium and vitamin A
    d.   Vitamin E and vitamin C

c   509;   29.   For women 25 years and older who are pregnant, an
     511-512(K)   increased intake of at least 50% is recommended for all of the
                           following EXCEPT

                           a.   calcium.
                           b.   vitamin D.
                           c.   potassium.
                           d.   phosphorus.

b   510(K)   30.   What is the recommended increase in energy intake for the
                          second and third trimester of pregnancy?

                          a.   200 kcal/day
                          b.   300 kcal/day
                          c.   450 kcal/day
                          d.   440 kcal/day

d   510(A)   31.   Over the course of the entire pregnancy, approximately how
                          much extra energy does the average pregnant woman need to
                          consume?

                          a.   10,500 kcal
                          b.   26,000 kcal
                          c.   39,000 kcal
                          d.   55,000 kcal

d   510(K)   32.   Which of the following statements characterizes energy needs
                          during pregnancy?

                          a.   The need is proportionally greater than for most other
                               nutrients
                          b.   The increased needs are similar at the beginning and end
                               of pregnancy
                          c.   The needs increase by similar amounts in teenagers and
                               30 year-old women
                          d.   The increased need is equivalent to the amount supplied
                               by about 4 to 5 extra slices of bread per day

b   510-512(A)   33.   According to the recommended food intake for pregnancy,
                          which of the following food groups is the only one that is
                          provided in sufficient amounts by this menu?

                          a.   Milk
                          b.   Meats
                          c.   Vegetables
                          d.   Bread/cereal

b   511(A)   34.   In the United States, what is the minimum daily amount of protein that should be consumed by a 135-pound woman during pregnancy?

            a.   49 g
            b.   59 g
            c.   108 g
            d.   135 g

Examine the following menu for a pregnant woman.

BREAKFAST LUNCH		SUPPER
2 scrambled eggs	2 pieces (4 oz) fried	3 oz pork chop
1 crushed wheat	chicken	1 ear corn on the cob
English muffin	2 wheat rolls w/butter	Lettuce and tomato salad
1 cup orange juice	1/2 cup mashed potatoes	with 2 tbsp dressing
	and gravy	1 slice bread
	Iced tea	

a   511-512(K)   35.   Of the following nutrient needs, which is considered the most difficult to meet during pregnancy?

            a.   Iron
            b.   Protein
            c.   Vitamin D
            d.   Vitamin B_6

c   511-512(K)   36.   During pregnancy, which of the following nutrients shows a dramatic increase in absorption?

            a.   Salt and sugar
            b.   Protein and fat
            c.   Calcium and iron
            d.   Thiamin and ascorbic acid

d   511(K)   37.   All of the following reflect a state of iron nutrition in pregnancy EXCEPT

            a.   absorption of the mineral increases three-fold.
            b.   the mineral is well-conserved during this period.
            c.   stores of the mineral diminish slowly during this period.
            d.   most women enter pregnancy with adequate stores of the mineral.

b   512(A)   38.   Why is routine vitamin D supplementation during pregnancy NOT recommended?

    a.   The RDA does not change
    b.   It may be toxic to the fetus
    c.   Self-synthesis rate of vitamin D increases markedly in pregnancy
    d.   Pregnancy leads to increased absorption efficiency of calcium and therefore extra vitamin D is not needed

b   512(K)   39.   All of the following are features of zinc nutrition in pregnancy EXCEPT

    a.   typical intakes are lower than the recommended amount.
    b.   supplements are effective in preventing neural tube defects.
    c.   the mineral is needed for nucleic acid synthesis and thus cell development.
    d.   a secondary deficiency may develop when iron supplements are taken.

b   512(K)   40.   Which of the following is a feature of calcium nutrition in pregnancy?

    a.   The RDA increases by over 100%
    b.   Intestinal absorption increases by over 100%
    c.   Supplements are recommended for most women due to the increased needs
    d.   Transfer of calcium from maternal stores to the fetus increases rapidly at the beginning of the second trimester

c   512(K)   41.   Since repeated pregnancies occurring within short time frames lead to depletion of the mother's nutrient reserves, what is the optimal interval between pregnancies?

    a.   ½ year
    b.   1 year
    c.   1 ½-2 years
    d.   3-4 years

a   513(K)   42.   What is the most likely reason for a pregnant woman to crave pickles?

    a.   A change in hormones
    b.   A hypoglycemic episode
    c.   A physiologic need for fluid
    d.   A physiologic need for sodium

d   513(A)   43.   To help alleviate pregnancy-related nausea, all of the following actions are recommended <u>EXCEPT</u>

        a.   eat dry toast or dry crackers.
        b.   avoid milk when feeling nauseated.
        c.   avoid orange juice when feeling nauseated.
        d.   eat large, infrequent meals so as to limit contact time with food.

d   513(K)   44.   The common problems of pregnancy include all of the following <u>EXCEPT</u>

        a.   nausea.
        b.   heartburn.
        c.   constipation.
        d.   low blood pressure.

a   513(K)   45.   Which of the following is one of the recommendations to treat pregnancy-associated heartburn?

        a.   Eat many small meals
        b.   Drink fluids only with meals
        c.   Exercise within 30 minutes after eating
        d.   Lie down within 15 minutes after eating

d   513-514(K)   46.   Which of the following statements reflects current knowledge of food choices in pregnancy?

        a.   A craving for pickles is a strong indicator that the body needs salt
        b.   A craving for milk is a strong indicator that the body needs calcium and/or phosphorus
        c.   Careful and appropriate selection of foods can meet all nutrient needs for most women
        d.   Cravings and aversions to certain foods are probably the result of altered taste and smell sensitivities induced by hormones

a   513(K)   47.   A craving for non-food substances is known as

        a.   pica.
        b.   bulimia.
        c.   toxemia.
        d.   hyperemesis.

d   515(K)   48. What is WIC?

   a. A serious neural tube defect
   b. The World Intervention and Conception program of the United Nations
   c. An environmental contaminant that may interfere with breast milk production
   d. A food and nutrition education program for pregnant women, children, and infants

c   515(K)   49. Which of the following is the standard classification for a low birthweight infant?

   a. 3½ lbs or less
   b. 4 lbs or less
   c. 5½ lbs or less
   d. 6½ lbs or less

b   515(K)   50. Risks from malnutrition in women or men before conception include all of the following EXCEPT

   a. it may lead to cessation of menstruation.
   b. it affects ovulation but not sperm quality.
   c. it may result in a poorly developed placenta.
   d. it results in more complications during pregnancy in both overweight and underweight women.

c   516(K)   51. Which of the following is a characteristic of gestational diabetes?

   a. It predicts risk of diabetes for the infant
   b. It occurs in over one-half of normal weight women
   c. It leads to adult-onset diabetes in about a third of the women
   d. It occurs more often in women with a history of having premature births

b   516(K)   52. All of the following are features of gestational diabetes EXCEPT

   a. Asian ancestry is a risk factor.
   b. infant birthweights are typically low.
   c. it usually develops during the second half of pregnancy.
   d. the most common consequences include labor and delivery complications.

b 516-517(K) 53. Preeclampsia typically develops during the

  a. first half of pregnancy.
  b. second half of pregnancy.
  c. first month after delivery.
  d. first trimester of pregnancy.

b 517(K) 54. All of the following are features of preeclampsia <u>EXCEPT</u>

  a. edema.
  b. diabetes.
  c. proteinuria.
  d. high blood pressure.

a 517(K) 55. What is the name of the condition characterized by high blood pressure, edema, and protein in the urine of a pregnant woman?

  a. Preeclampsia
  b. Gestational diabetes
  c. Teratogenic hypertension
  d. Pregnancy-induced blood pressure crisis

c 517(K) 56. What is the approximate percentage of babies born to teenagers in the United States?

  a. 2
  b. 6
  c. 12
  d. 25

a 517-518(K) 57. Which of the following is a characteristic associated with adolescent pregnancy?

  a. The recommended weight gain is approximately 35 lbs
  b. The incidence of stillbirths and preterm births is 5-10% lower compared with adult women
  c. The incidence of pregnancy-induced hypertension is 5-10% lower compared with older women
  d. The time in labor is usually shorter than for older women because there are fewer overweight teenagers

a   518(K)   58.   All of the following are features of older pregnant women in comparison with younger pregnant women <u>EXCEPT</u>

    a.   maternal mortality rates are lower.
    b.   fetal mortality rates are twice as high.
    c.   cesarean delivery is twice as common.
    d.   complications that arise typically reflect chronic conditions such as diabetes and hypertension.

d   518(K)   59.   What term best describes a factor that causes abnormal fetal development and birth defects?

    a.   Toxigenic
    b.   Mutagenic
    c.   Neonagenic
    d.   Teratogenic

a   518-519(K)   60.   Which of the following recommendations for pregnant women and alcohol intake that has been issued by the U.S. Surgeon General?

    a.   They should drink absolutely no alcohol
    b.   They should refrain from drinking hard liquor only
    c.   They are permitted to ingest no more than 2 drinks per day
    d.   They are permitted to ingest small amounts of alcohol during the first 3 months but none thereafter

c   519-520(A)   61.   With few exceptions, all of the following substances or practices should be totally eliminated during pregnancy <u>EXCEPT</u>

    a.   cigarette smoking.
    b.   weight-loss dieting.
    c.   artificial sweeteners.
    d.   alcohol consumption.

d   519(K)   62.   Relationships between the use of tobacco products and complications of pregnancy include all of the following EXCEPT

    a.   smoking during pregnancy increases the risk of vaginal bleeding.
    b.   chewing tobacco during pregnancy leads to lower birthweight infants.
    c.   smoking during pregnancy increases the risk of sudden infant death syndrome.
    d.   taking zinc supplements prevents the development of pregnancy-induced hypertension in smokers.

b   519(K)   63.   All of the following are effects of tobacco use in pregnancy EXCEPT

    a.   an increased risk for fetal death
    b.   an increased risk for macrosomia.
    c.   an increased risk for vaginal bleeding.
    d.   an association with SIDS and cigarette smoking during pregnancy.

d   520(K)   64.   What are the known effects of heavy caffeine use on human pregnancy?

    a.   It may worsen edema
    b.   It may increase the risk of birth defects
    c.   It may increase the risk of stillborn infants
    d.   It may increase the risk of spontaneous abortion

d   521(K)   65.   Which of the following is a function of probating?

    a.   Acts to reverse the effects of certain mutagens
    b.   Acts to reverse the effects of certain teratogens
    c.   Acts on mammary glands to stimulate milk release
    d.   Acts on mammary glands to promote milk production

c   521(k)   66.   Which of the following is a function of prolactin?

    a.   Acts to reverse the effects of certain mutagens
    b.   Acts to reverse the effects of certain teratogens
    c.   Acts on mammary glands to stimulate milk release
    d.   Acts on mammary glands to promote milk production

b   521(K)   67.   What causes the "let-down reflex?

    a.   Oxytocin
    b.   Estrongen
    c.   Prepartum amenorhea
    d.   Postpartum amenorrhea

c   522-523(K) 68.   In general, what are the chief consequences of nutritional deprivation in the lactating mother?

    a.   Cessation of lactation
    b.   Reduced quality of milk
    c.   Reduced quantity of milk
    d.   Reduced quality and quantity of milk

b   522-523(K) 69.   Which of the following statements describes an association between nutrient intake and lactation?

    a.   Milk production is increased by higher fluid intake
    b.   Ingestion of garlic may lead to an off-flavor of the milk
    c.   Inadequate protein intake lowers the protein concentration of the milk
    d.   The energy RDA for milk production calls for an additional 1,000 kcal/day

d   523(K)   70.   Which of the following describes the findings from studies of lactating women who exercised intensely compared with sedentary lactating women?

    a.   They had similar energy intakes
    b.   Their milk was more nutrient-dense
    c.   They had a slightly greater amount of body fat
    d.   Their milk contained more lactic acid which alters taste

c   524(K)   71.   Which of the following reflects one of the effects of alcohol intake on lactation?

    a.   It does not pass into the milk
    b.   It mildly stimulates milk production
    c.   It hinders the infant's ability to breastfeed
    d.   It passes into the milk but is degraded by enzymes in breast tissue

b   524(K)   72.   Which of the following is an effect of alcohol intake in the mother who breastfeeds?

a. It stimulates lactation
b. It hinders breastfeeding
c. It first appears in the milk approximately 12 hours after ingestion
d. It passes into the milk and stimulates the infant's acceptance

c   524-525(A)   73.   Under which of the following circumstances would it still be acceptable for a mother to breastfeed?

a. She has alcohol abuse
b. She has a drug addiction
c. She has an ordinary cold
d. She has a communicable disease

a   531(K)   74.   A less severe form of fetal alcohol syndrome is known as

a. fetal alcohol effects.
b. fetal toxigenic disorder.
c. fetal development disorder.
d. infant development sydrome.

a   531-532(K)   75.   According to many experts, what <u>MINIMUM</u> level of alcohol intake increases the risk of giving birth to an infant with fetal alcohol syndrome?

a. 1 drink/day
b. 2 drinks/day
c. 4 drinks/day
d. 7 drinks/week

a   532-533(K)   76.   Which of the following statements describes a relationship between alcohol intake and fetal development?

a. Birth defects are most severe when the woman drinks around the time of conception
b. Infants born with fetal alcohol syndrome typically show immediate signs of brain impairment
c. Eating well and maintaining adequate nutrient stores will prevent alcohol-induced placenta damage
d. Toxicity to the fetus begins to occur when fetal blood alcohol levels rise above maternal blood alcohol levels

b   532-533(K)   77.   In what period of pregnancy would most damage occur from alcohol consumption?

　　　　　　　　　　a.　Before conception
　　　　　　　　　　b.　First trimester
　　　　　　　　　　c.　Second trimester
　　　　　　　　　　d.　Third trimester

Matching (Answers can be used only once)

K	500	78.	A newly fertilized ovum
L	500	79.	Developing infant from 2 to 8 weeks after conception
O	500	80.	Fluid in which the fetus floats
E	502	81.	Number of days after conception during which the neural tube is highly vulnerable to nutrient deficiency
J	503	82.	Adequate intakes of this nutrient within the first 30 days of conception are especially important to lower risk of birth defects
A	502	83.	Percentage of U.S. newborns with a neural tube defect
P	504	84.	Most reliable indicator of an infant's health
G	505	85.	An infant born prior to this number of weeks of pregnancy is classified as preterm
F	505	86.	Upper limit for the recommended number of pounds that a pregnant woman of normal weight should gain
B	506	87.	Approximate weight, in pounds, of average newborn baby
C	511	88.	Number of grams of extra protein per day recommended for the pregnant woman
H	511	89.	Dietary supplements of this nutrient are recommended for the last 6 months of pregnancy
S	513	90.	A recommended practice to prevent or relieve heartburn
T	513	91.	A recommended practice to prevent or alleviate constipation
I	513	92.	A craving for non-food substances
Q	517	93.	A condition characterized by high blood pressure and protein in the urine
N	517	94.	A condition characterized by convulsions
D	517	95.	Percentage of U.S. babies born to teenagers
M	518	96.	Excess intake of this substance in pregnancy is known to result in mental retardation of the child
R	521	97.	A practice that may reduce risk of breast cancer

A.	0.1	K.	Zygote
B.	7	L.	Embryo
C.	10	M.	Alcohol
D.	13	N.	Eclampsia
E.	17-30	O.	Amniotic
F.	35	P.	Birthweight
G.	38	Q.	Preeclampsia
H.	Iron	R.	Breastfeeding
I.	Pica	S.	Eat small, frequent meals
J.	Folate	T.	Drink at least 8 glasses of liquid a day

Essay Questions

500-501   98. Describe the three major stages of fetal growth and development.

505-506   99. Compare the recommended weight gains for pregnancy in women who, at conception, are normal weight, underweight, overweight, or obese.

507-508   100. What are several benefits of exercise specifically for the pregnant woman? What types of exercise should be avoided and why?

508-512   101. What nutrients are needed in larger amounts during pregnancy and what physical changes account for the increased needs?

513   102. What steps can be taken to minimize the development and discomfort of nausea, heartburn, and constipation during pregnancy?

514-515   103.   Discuss 6 factors and conditions that lead to high-risk pregnancies

515   104.   Describe the consequences of malnutrition on conception and early pregnancy.

516-517   105.   Describe the condition known as preeclampsia. What are its risk factors and what is known about its prevention?

516   106.   Define gestational diabetes and list risk factors. How is it managed?

517   107.   Explain the development of pregnancy-induced hypertension and the consequences if not properly managed.

517-518   108.   Describe the risks associated with adolescent pregnancy.

518   109.   Describe the risks associated with pregnancy of older women.

518-520   110.   What practices should be avoided during pregnancy and why?

519   111.   Discuss the effects of tobacco use in the pregnant woman and its effects on health of the newborn.

521-522   112.   List the benefits of breastfeeding for the infant and for the mother

523-524   113.   Explain the energy needs for breastfeeding in light of the mother's desire to lose the extra weight from pregnancy.

523   114.   Give examples of associations between maternal food choices and breastmilk flavor.

524   115.   Discuss the effects of maternal alcohol intake and tobacco use on breastfeeding.

531-533   116.   Discuss the consequences of maternal alcohol intake on fetal development?

531-533   117.   Describe the physical and mental abnormalities associated with fetal alcohol syndrome.

531-532   118.   Describe distinguishing facial characteristics associated with fetal alcohol syndrome.

CHAPTER 16
LIFE CYCLE NUTRITION: INFANCY, CHILDHOOD, AND ADOLESCENCE

Ans   Page

c   535(A)   01.   What would be a normal body weight after 1 year for a healthy infant with a birthweight of 8 lbs?

a.   12 lbs
b.   16 lbs
c.   24 lbs
d.   35 lbs

a   525(A)   02.   Infants showing symptoms of acidosis, dehydration, diarrhea, elevated blood ammonia and urea, and fever may be reacting to the nutritional problem of

a.   protein overload.
b.   milk protein intolerance.
c.   carbohydrate intolerance.
d.   insufficient protein and energy.

d   535(A)   03.   The recommended amounts of vitamins and minerals for infants are based on

     a.   The average amounts present in body tissues of thriving infants
     b.   The adult RDA scaled down to infants on a per kg body weight basis
     c.   The older child's RDA scaled down to the infant on a per kg body weight basis
     d.   The average amounts ingested by thriving infants breastfed by well-nourished mothers

a   535(K)   04.   What is the approximate energy requirements of infants, in kcal/kg body weight?

     a.   25
     b.   35
     c.   75
     d.   100

d   536-537(K)   05.   According to the American Academy of Pediatrics and the Canadian Pediatric Society, breastfeeding of full-term infants is

     a.   optional.
     b.   mildly recommended.
     c.   moderately recommended.
     d.   strongly recommended.

b   537(A)   06.   When expressed per kilogram body weight, the nutrient needs of infants are markedly higher than those of adults for all of the following nutrients EXCEPT

     a.   iron.
     b.   folate.
     c.   calcium.
     d.   vitamin D.

d   537-538(K)   07.   Breast milk as the sole source of nutrition, up to the first 6 months in healthy infants is satisfactory for all nutrients with the possible EXCEPTION(S) OF

     a.   fluoride.
     b.   vitamin D.
     c.   iron and folate.
     d.   zinc and vitamin A.

d   538(K)   08.   What is the chief protein in human breast milk?

     a.   Casein
     b.   Lactose
     c.   Albumin
     d.   alpha-Lactalbumin

d   538-539(K)   09.   Nutrient characteristics of human breast milk include all of the following EXCEPT

     a.   the sodium content is low.
     b.   the zinc is highly bioavailable.
     c.   the iron is highly bioavailable.
     d.   the vitamin D content meets optimal growth requirements.

b   538(K)   10.   What is the chief difference in the fatty acid content of breast milk and infant formula?

     a.   Linoleic acid and linolenic acid are found in infant formula but not breast milk
     b.   Arachidonic acid and docosahexaenoic acid are found in breast milk but not infant formula
     c.   Medium-chain fatty acids are present in higher concentrations in infant formula than in breast milk
     d.   Short-chain fatty acids are present in higher concentrations in infant formula than in breast milk

d   538(K)   11.   Which of the following vitamin-mineral supplements need NOT be prescribed for an infant breastfed beyond 6 months of age?

     a.   Iron
     b.   Fluoride
     c.   Vitamin D
     d.   Vitamin E

d   539(K)   12.   What is colostrum?

     a.   Clot in the bloodstream
     b.   Major protein in breast milk
     c.   Hormone that promotes milk production
     d.   Milk-like substance secreted right after delivery

b   539(K)   13.   Which of the following is an advantage of breastfeeding compared with formula feeding?

         a.   There is no limit to the supply
         b.   It provides immunological protection
         c.   The mother can be sure the baby is getting enough milk
         d.   It is the only way to develop a true loving relationship with the baby

b   539(K)   14.   Which of the following is associated with bifidus factors?

         a.   Increased iron absorption
         b.   Increased bacterial growth
         c.   Decreased allergy protection
         d.   Decreased hormone production

b   539(K)   15.   What is the factor in breast milk that binds iron and prevents it from supporting the growth of the infant's intestinal bacteria?

         a.   Colostrum
         b.   Lactoferrin
         c.   Lactalbumin
         d.   Bifidus factor

b   539(K)   16.   To gradually replace breast milk with infant formula or other foods appropriate to an infant's diet is to

         a.   feed.
         b.   wean.
         c.   nurse.
         d.   breastfeed.

c   539(K)   17.   What is lactadherin?

         a.   An iron-binding protein in breast milk
         b.   A vitamin D-binding protein in breast milk
         c.   A breast milk protein that inactivates a GI virus that causes diarrhea
         d.   A protein supplement to infant formulas that simulates the digestibility properties of alpha-lactalbumin

a   539-540(K)   18.   Features of infant formulas include all of the following <u>EXCEPT</u>

    a.   they contain antibodies.
    b.   they breed bacteria in bottles left at room temperature.
    c.   they typically contain over twice the amount of iron compared with breast milk.
    d.   they contain fat and carbohydrate at concentrations resembling those in breast milk.

a   539(A)   19.   In comparison with cow's milk, breast milk contains

    a.   less protein and minerals.
    b.   less lactose and vitamin C.
    c.   more fat and less carbohydrate.
    d.   more energy and less vitamin E.

b   540(A)   20.   Which of the following sources of nutrition for infants is LEAST likely to become contaminated with microorganisms?

    a.   Soy formula
    b.   Breast milk
    c.   Iron-fortified formula
    d.   Liquid concentrate formula

b   540(A)   21.   What type of formula is available for infants with milk allergy?

    a.   Egg
    b.   Soy
    c.   Meat
    d.   Peanut

c   539(K)   22.   Which of the following is a common source of lead poisoning in infants?

    a.   Maternal passage of lead to fetus
    b.   Baby bottles made from lead crystal
    c.   Contaminated water used to make infant formula
    d.   Preparation of infant formula in galvanized containers

c   539;550(A)   23.   What is the most realistic advice for reducing lead exposure content of tap water used to prepare infant formula?

    a.   Whenever possible boil the water to vaporize the lead and thus decrease the amount remaining in the water
    b.   Since upon sitting overnight the lead in hot water pipes settles out, draw the drinking water from this source first
    c.   Since the first water drawn from the tap each day is highest in lead, let the water run a few minutes before using it
    d.   Add a small amount of citrus juice to the water to provide citric acid to complex with the lead and inhibit its absorption

c   540(K)   24.   Which of the following defines nursing bottle tooth decay?

    a.   Caries development resulting from frequent use of non-sterile bottles and nipples
    b.   Bacterial attack of teeth due to severe tooth misalignment from sucking on oversized bottle nipples
    c.   Marked tooth decay of an infant due to prolonged exposure to carbohydrate-rich fluids from a bottle
    d.   Tooth decay resulting from constant exposure to food due to inability of the infant to swallow in normal fashion

d   540(K)   25.   What term defines the condition of infant tooth deterioration resulting from chronic exposure to carbohydrate-rich fluids from a bottle?

    a.   Juice bottle erosion
    b.   Suckling enamelosis
    c.   Formula-induced gingivitis
    d.   Nursing bottle tooth decay

b   540(A)   26.   Goat's milk is inappropriate for infants due to its low content of

    a.   iron.
    b.   folate.
    c.   protein.
    d.   calcium.

a   541(K)   27.   Which of the following should <u>NOT</u> be used to feed an infant?

    a.   Whole milk
    b.   Ready-to-feed formula
    c.   Liquid concentrate formula appropriately diluted
    d.   Powdered formula or evaporated milk formula appropriately reconstituted

a   541(K)   28.   The metabolic bone disease osteopenia is common in

    a.   preterm infants.
    b.   overweight infants.
    c.   overweight mothers.
    d.   late-for-gestational age infants.

c   541(K)   29.   Which of the following feeding practices is recommended for preterm infants?

    a.   They should be fed exclusively on breast milk
    b.   They should be fed on breast milk enriched in a 1 to 1 ratio with cow's milk
    c.   They should be fed preterm breast milk occasionally fortified with specific nutrients
    d.   They should be fed only on special formula because breast milk nutrient content is too low

b   541(K)   30.   During the first year of life, cow's milk is considered an inappropriate food due to all of the following <u>EXCEPT</u>

    a.   it is too low in iron.
    b.   it is too low in sodium.
    c.   it is too high in protein.
    d.   it is too low in vitamin C.

c   541(A)   31.   Which of the following represents a good age to introduce solid foods to infants?

    a.   Two weeks
    b.   Two months
    c.   Five months
    d.   One year

a 541(K) 32. What adverse side effect is most likely to develop in infants who are deprived of solid foods for the entire first year of life?

   a. Delayed growth
   b. Impaired speech
   c. Mental dysfunction
   d. Impaired eye coordination

c 541(K) 33. What is beikost?

   a. An oral rehydration solution
   b. A term that describes a type of malnutrition in infants
   c. A term that describes any nonmilk food offered to an infant
   d. A fermented milk product used as a substitute for breastmilk

c 542(K) 34. At what age does the normal infant first develop the ability to swallow solid food?

   a. 3-5 weeks
   b. 26-32 weeks
   c. 4-6 months
   d. 9-12 months

c 542(K) 35. What should be the first cereal introduced to the infant?

   a. Oat
   b. Corn
   c. Rice
   d. Wheat

b 542(K) 36. Why should new foods be introduced to an infant one at a time?

   a. It prevents overfeeding
   b. Any allergic reactions can be detected
   c. Immunological protection hasn't been developed
   d. The swallowing reflex is not under voluntary control

d 542(A) 37. Of the following cereals, which is <u>MOST</u> likely to result in an allergic reaction upon first feeding?

    a. Oat
    b. Rice
    c. Corn
    d. Wheat

a 543(K) 38. Which of the following nutrients need to be supplied first by solid foods in a baby's diet?

    a. Vitamin C and iron
    b. Vitamin A and zinc
    c. Vitamin B_{12} and fluoride
    d. Vitamin E and magnesium

c 543(K) 39. Low-fat or nonfat milk should not be given routinely to a child until after the age of

    a. two weeks.
    b. three months.
    c. two years.
    d. six years.

c 543(K) 40. Infants should not be given canned vegetables due to excessive amounts of

    a. tin.
    b. fiber.
    c. sodium.
    d. botulinum spores.

b 543(K) 41. Which of the following is the primary factor in the development of milk anemia?

    a. Impaired absorption of iron
    b. Excessive intake of cow's milk
    c. Low iron content of breast milk
    d. Insufficient intake of whole cow's milk

a 543(A) 42. A child who drinks a lot of milk at the expense of other foods is at high risk of showing signs of

    a. anemia.
    b. rickets.
    c. hyperkeratosis.
    d. ariboflavinosis.

b   543(A)   43.   The consumption of milk by children should not exceed 4 cups per day in order to lower the risk for

       a.   solute overload.
       b.   iron deficiency.
       c.   vitamin A toxicity.
       d.   vitamin D toxicity.

a   543(K)   44.   Young children who drink more than 2 to 31/2 cups of milk a day are most likely at increased risk for deficiency of

       a.   iron.
       b.   folate.
       c.   vitamin A.
       d.   vitamin C.

c   544(A)   45.   What should be the parent's response when a one-year-old child wants to clumsily spoon-feed himself?

       a.   Punish the child
       b.   Let the child eat with his fingers instead
       c.   Let the child try to feed himself so that he will learn
       d.   Gently take the spoon back and feed the child with it

d   545(K)   46.   Which of the following is associated with energy metabolism of the preschool child?

       a.   Food intake is remarkably similar from meal to meal
       b.   Overweight individuals have appetites similar to normal weight individuals
       c.   Energy needs per kg body weight increase from 1 year of age to 5 years of age
       d.   A 1-year old who needs 1000 kcal/day would require only about 1300 kcal at 3 years of age

c   545(K)   47.   Approximately how many kcal per day does an average 3-year old need to obtain?

       a.   500
       b.   800
       c.   1300
       d.   2400

c   545(A)   48.   How much more total energy does a normal 10 year old
                             need vs. a 1-year old?

                             a.   25%
                             b.   50%
                             c.   100%
                             d.   200%

b   545(A)   49.   A reasonable fiber intake for a 5-year old would be

                             a.   2 grams.
                             b.   5 grams.
                             c.   Age plus 5 grams.
                             d.   Age plus 10 grams.

a   546(K)   50.   Which of the following is characteristic of children who
                             regularly eat breakfast or skip breakfast?

                             a.   Breakfast-skippers actually show lower scores on IQ
                                   tests than those who eat breakfast
                             b.   Attention spans are similar but a significant number of
                                   breakfast-skippers show hyperglycemia
                             c.   Breakfast-skippers initially show decreased mental
                                   performance but with time they adapt and show almost
                                   identical achievements
                             d.   Breakfast-skippers who change to eating breakfast
                                   show a temporary improvement in mental concentration
                                   but also a moderate degree of hypoglycemia

c   547(A)   51.   Which of the following is the most likely reason that teachers
                             promote the consumption of midmorning snacks for
                             children?

                             a.   It provides an opportunity to learn about nutrition
                             b.   It meets federally mandated school nutrition guidelines
                             c.   It provides carbohydrate for maintenance of blood
                                   glucose and brain function
                             d.   It helps decrease the symptoms of attention-deficit-
                                   hyperactivity disorder in 5% of school-age children

c   548(K)   52.   Which of the following is a feature of iron nutrition in the very young?

     a.   Iron deficiency is most prevalent in children aged 2 to 3 years old
     b.   The supply of stored iron becomes depleted after the birthweight triples
     c.   Infants with iron-deficiency anemia demonstrate abnormal motor development
     d.   Serum ferritin concentrations fall in infants who start drinking whole milk at 3 months of age but not at 6 months of age

a   548(K)   53.   Which of the following is a characteristic of iron deficiency in children?

     a.   It affects brain function before anemia sets in
     b.   It rarely develops in those with high intakes of milk
     c.   It is the primary factor in tension-fatigue syndrome
     d.   Mild deficiency enhances mental performance by lowering physical activity level thereby leading to increased attention span

d   549-550(K)   54.   All of the following are characteristics of hyperactivity in children EXCEPT

     a.   it impairs learning ability.
     b.   it occurs in approximately 5% of young, school-age individuals.
     c.   it is managed, in part, by prescribing stimulant drugs when necessary.
     d.   it responds favorably to dietary manipulations such as limiting sugar intake.

d   549(K)   55.   What is the term given to the child who is hyperactive with severe and impulsive behavior?

     a.   Food hypersensitivity
     b.   Fetal alcohol syndrome
     c.   Caffeine hypersensitivity
     d.   Attention-deficit/hyperactivity disorder

c   549(A)   56.   All of the following are common signs of mild lead toxicity
                      EXCEPT

                      a.   diarrhea.
                      b.   lethargy.
                      c.   dermatitis.
                      d.   irritability.

a   549(K)   57.   Which of the following is a characteristic of lead exposure
                      and health?

                      a.   Absorption of lead is higher on an empty stomach
                      b.   Lead toxicity is most prevalent in children around the
                            time of puberty
                      c.   Lead-induced anemia is similar to the anemia of vitamin
                            B12 deficiency
                      d.   The symptoms of lead toxicity can be reversed by
                            adding iron to the diet

b   551(K)   58.   An adverse reaction to food that does NOT signal the body
                      to form antibodies is termed a

                      a.   food allergy.
                      b.   food intolerance.
                      c.   mild food challenge.
                      d.   transient food episode.

a   551(A)   59.   A child who develops antibodies to a certain food is said to
                      have a

                      a.   food allergy.
                      b.   food intolerance.
                      c.   specific inducible episode.
                      d.   transient immune suppression.

b   551-552(K)   60.   Which of the following is a characteristic of a food allergy?

                      a.   It always elicits symptoms in the person
                      b.   It always involves the production of antibodies
                      c.   It usually shows up immediately after exposure to the
                            allergic food
                      d.   It is usually elicited from very small, simple molecules as
                            well as large, complex molecules

a   551(A)   61.   Which of the following foods are most often the cause of allergies?

     a.   Eggs, peanuts, and milk
     b.   Bananas, juice, and cola
     c.   Apples, noodles, and rice
     d.   Pears, oatmeal, and chocolate

b   552-553(A)   62.   Which of the following is a feature of nutrition and behavior in children?

     a.   Hyperactivity responds favorably to a low sugar diet
     b.   Television commercials featuring snack foods have been found to affect children's food preferences
     c.   The adverse effects from caffeine intake typically first appear only after drinking 6 cans of cola in one day
     d.   Most children are able to control their intake of cola beverages since they are more sensitive to the stimulating effects of caffeine

b   552(K)   63.   Which of the following two conditions are associated with television's influence?

     a.   Anorexia and nutrient deficiencies
     b.   Obesity and high blood cholesterol
     c.   Drug abuse and teenage pregnancy
     d.   Hyperactivity and lower body weight

d   552(K)   64.   What is the most likely explanation for the increased prevalence of obesity in children over the past 30 years?

     a.   Genetics
     b.   They sleep more hours
     c.   They consume more kcalories
     d.   They are less active physically

a   553(K)   65.   What is the leading cause of high blood pressure in children?

     a.   Obesity
     b.   High sodium intake
     c.   Insufficient calcium intake
     d.   Insufficient potassium intake

a   554-556(K)   66.   Even in preschoolers whose habits are being established, existing dietary attitudes are relatively resistant to change. How should wise parents react?

    a.   Be patient and persistent
    b.   Impose their own eating habits on the children
    c.   Wait until the children start school to initiate changes
    d.   Exert continuous pressure to initiate good food habits

c   554(K)   67.   To lower the risk of obesity in children, which of the following practices should parents institute for their children?

    a.   Serve them smaller portions
    b.   Serve them 3 meals a day without dessert
    c.   Teach them to take appropriate food portions
    d.   Serve them more beverages and less solid food

b   554(A)   68.   Which of the following is an effective strategy for dealing with obesity in a child?

    a.   Encourage the individual to eat quickly and then leave the table
    b.   Teach the individual to take small portions first and then second helpings if desired
    c.   Institute new eating habits such as teaching the individual to clean the food plate
    d.   Take control and strongly encourage the individual to lose weight by dieting and regular exercise

a   555-536(K)   69.   Which of the following steps should be undertaken by the parent or guardian to ensure that young people eat well?

    a.   Control the availability of food
    b.   Control the consumption of food
    c.   Prohibit eating except at mealtime
    d.   Provide an emotional climate that discourages snacking

d   555-537(K)   70.   Which of the following practices is NOT among the recommendations to help children develop an interest in vegetables?

    a.   Serve vegetables warm, not hot
    b.   Serve vegetables separately on the plate
    c.   Serve vegetables undercooked and crunchy
    d.   Serve vegetables with the promise that after they are eaten, dessert will follow

d   555-556(K)   71.   Which of the following is <u>NOT</u> among the recommended methods for introducing new foods to children?

    a.   Offer foods one at a time
    b.   Offer foods in small amounts
    c.   Create a pleasant eating atmosphere
    d.   Present new foods at the end of the meal

c   556(K)   72.   If a child is reluctant to try a new food, it is best to

    a.   send the child to his/her room.
    b.   withhold dessert until all food on the plate is eaten.
    c.   quietly remove it and present it again at another time.
    d.   encourage other family members to coax the child to eat it.

c   556-557(K)   73.   When children are allowed to eat freely from a variety of foods, they usually select foods that are high in

    a.   iron.
    b.   fiber.
    c.   sugar.
    d.   protein.

a   557(A)   74.   The single most effective way to teach nutrition to children is by

    a.   example.
    b.   punishment.
    c.   singling out only hazardous nutrition practices for attention.
    d.   explaining the importance of eating new foods as a prerequisite for dessert.

c   559(K)   75.   What minimum fraction of the RDA for children 10-12 years of age should be provided by public school lunches?

    a.   1/8
    b.   1/4
    c.   1/3
    e.   ½

a   559(K)   76. Which of the following is a feature of public school food programs?

    a. They must meet the Dietary Guidelines over a week's menus
    b. They allow for low fat menus while still meeting the needs for iron
    c. They ensure a lunch period is long enough to consume the entire meal
    d. They are overwhelmingly preferred over the foods obtained by students through on-site vending machines and snack bars

c   560(K)   77. What is the approximate time period of the adolescent growth spurt?

    a. 6 months
    b. 1 year
    c. 2 ½ years
    d. 6 years

d   560(K)   78. The adolescent growth spurt

    a. affects the brain primarily.
    b. decreases total nutrient needs.
    c. affects every organ except the brain.
    d. begins and ends earlier in girls than in boys.

a   561(K)   79. Which of the following is a characteristic of the adolescent period?

    a. Obesity occurs more often in African-American females
    b. Appetite for red meat increases in females to meet iron needs
    c. More nutrient-dense foods are needed by males because of their faster development
    d. The risk for calcium insufficiency is greatest in males due to their high intake of soft drinks

a   562(A)   80. Approximately what fraction of an average teenager's daily energy intake is derived from snacks?

    a. 1/4
    b. 1/3
    c. 1/2
    d. 2/3

d   562(K)   81.   What is considered to be the minimum pharmacologically active dose of caffeine?

       a.   5 mg
       b.   100 mg
       c.   200 mg
       d.   500 mg

b   562(K)   82.   Approximately how much caffeine is delivered by a typical cola beverage?

       a.   5 mg
       b.   50 mg
       c.   100 mg
       d.   500 mg

b   562(A)   83.   About how many meals each week are eaten outside the home in adolescents?

       a.   3
       b.   7
       c.   12
       d.   15

d   562(K)   84.   Which of the following is a feature of beverage intake in adolescents?

       a.   Juice intake is spread throughout the day
       b.   Milk intake occurs primarily between meals
       c.   Males are more likely to drink less milk than are females
       d.   Four standard colas a day provides enough caffeine to alter behavior

a   563(A)   85.   Users of hard drugs or narcotics face all of the following problems EXCEPT

       a.   they tend to overeat during "high" periods.
       b.   they spend money for drugs rather than food.
       c.   they often have hepatitis, which causes taste changes.
       d.   they often develop infectious diseases which increase needs for nutrients.

b   563(K)   86.   Approximately what percentage of high school seniors admit
                             having used cocaine at least once?

                             a.   2
                             b.   8
                             c.   15
                             d.   22

a   563(K)   87.   Which of the following is a characteristic of marijuana use?

                             a.   Appetite for sweet foods is increased
                             b.   Regular use leads to excessive weight gain
                             c.   Smoking it dulls the sense of taste and smell
                             d.   The active ingredient is cleared from the body within 24
                                   hours

b   563-564(K)   88.   Associations between cigarette smoking and nutrition
                             include all of the following EXCEPT

                             a.   smokers have blunted hunger sensations.
                             b.   smokers have higher intakes of carotene-rich foods.
                             c.   smokers have lower body weights than nonsmokers.
                             d.   smokers degrade vitamin C faster than nonsmokers.

c   563(K)   89.   Which of the following is a characteristic of use of the drug
                             ectasy?

                             a.   Its primary action is on the liver
                             b.   It leads to low body temperature
                             c.   Using it regularly leads to weight loss
                             d.   Its potency is increased when taken with caffeinated
                                   beverages

a   564(K)   90.   Which of the following is a characteristic of tobacco use and
                             adolescents?

                             a.   Smokers require about two times as much vitamin C to
                                   maintain body stores
                             b.   The prevalence of smokeless tobacco use in high
                                   school is one in 100 students
                             c.   Supplements of beta-carotene are recommended for
                                   tobacco users in this population group
                             d.   The risk of mouth cancer is slightly lower for users of
                                   smokeless tobacco compared with smokers

c   571-572(K)   91.   The association of cholesterol to the health of children is described by all of the following <u>EXCEPT</u>

    a.   cholesterol intake should be limited beginning at 2 years of age.
    b.   blood cholesterol levels in children are good predictors of their adult levels.
    c.   there appears to be only a very weak correlation between obesity in children and their blood cholesterol levels.
    d.   serum cholesterol is higher in children viewing television for 2 hours per day compared with more active individuals.

a   572-573(K)   92.   Which of the following is a characteristic of blood cholesterol in childhood and health?

    a.   Acceptable total cholesterol leads are up to 240 mg/d
    b.   Cholesterol levels at birth are similar in all populations
    c.   Childhood obesity and high cholesterol levels show a strong association
    d.   Children with high cholesterol levels usually have parents with high cholesterol levels

Matching (Answers can be used only once)

B	535	93.	Expected weight, in pounds, of an infant with a birthweight of seven pounds who reaches one year of age
E	535	94.	Typical daily energy need, in kcalories per kg body weight, of an infant
O	538	95.	Nutrient that is low in human milk but adequate in infant formulas
L	538	96.	Essential fatty acid in breast milk
T	538	97.	Chief protein in human breast milk
F	538	98.	Chief protein in cow's milk
P	538	99.	Substance in breast milk that deprives intestinal bacteria of iron
K	538	100.	Process whereby breast milk is gradually replaced by formula or semi-solid foods
Q	539	101.	A breast milk protein that fights virus-induced diarrhea
N	539	102.	Pre-milk substance from the breast, containing antibodies
S	539	103.	Substance in breast milk that promotes growth of beneficial bacteria in the intestines
G	540	104.	Low content of this nutrient makes goat's milk inappropriate for infants
R	541	105.	Metabolic bone disease in pre-term infants
I	541	106.	Another term for supplemental or weaning foods
H	543	107.	Possible source of infant botulism
A	552	108.	Approximate percentage of young children with food allergies
D	551	109.	Percentage of all adverse reactions to foods that are caused by eggs, peanuts, or milk
J	560	110.	Period in life when an individual becomes physically capable of reproduction
C	563	111.	Percentage of teenagers who drink alcohol regularly
M	564	112.	Substance known to suppress appetite and increase rate of energy expenditure

A.	5		K.	Weaning
B.	21		L.	Linoleic
C.	50		M.	Nicotine
D.	75		N.	Colostrum
E.	100		O.	Vitamin D
F.	Casein		P.	Lactoferrin
G.	Folate		Q.	Lactadherin
H.	Honey		R.	Osteopenia
I.	Beikost		S.	Bifidus factors
J.	Puberty		T.	Alpha-lactalbumin

Essay Questions

539   113. Describe substances present in breast milk that affect immunologic function of the infant.

540-541   114. Discuss the special nutritional needs of the preterm infant and ways to meet these needs.

541   115. Why is preterm breast milk suitable to meet the special needs of the preterm infant?

541-543   116. Discuss guidelines for introducing first foods to an infant.

541-544   117. Explain the appropriate procedure for introducing new foods to children.

546-549   118. Give examples of how hunger and nutrient deficiencies affect behavior in children.

551-552   119. Discuss the effects of food allergies and food intolerances on nutritional status.

552-555   120. Discuss the effects of obesity in childhood. What steps can be taken to prevent and to treat this condition in the child?

562   121. Describe common eating patterns of teenagers and suggest appropriate changes to foster better eating habits.

562-564   122. List 6 nutrition problems associated with drug abuse and tobacco use in adolescents.

572-573   123. Describe relationships among obesity, hypertension, and blood cholesterol in children and adolescents.

INTRODUCTION TO TEST BANK

A Note on Test Bank Style and Use
For the Clinical Nutrition Chapters
(17-29)

The test bank for the Clinical Nutrition section includes both multiple-choice and essay questions. For each chapter, the multiple-choice questions are provided first followed by the essay questions.

MULTIPLE-CHOICE QUESTIONS

Some of the multiple-choice questions are descriptive or knowledge based and are designated with the symbol (k). Others are more analytical and require analysis, application, or computation before a solution can be identified. These questions are designated with the symbol (a). In addition, the page number reference and the correct answer for each question is provided.

These multiple-choice questions can be utilized in two ways. First, they may be used to test the students' ability on a day-to-day basis in the form of short quizzes. Second, they may be combined with the essay questions to form the foundation of longer tests such as mid-terms or final examinations.

ESSAY QUESTIONS

These questions are designed to test the students' understanding of chapter objectives. Not only do the essay questions require fundamental knowledge, but they demand that the students communicate this knowledge in an organized and comprehensive manner. If the instructor is able to return the essay questions to the students with comments, the students will be given the opportunity to check their thinking against the standards of someone with more experience in the field.

Melaney A. Jones

Chapter 17
Illness and Nutrition Status

a   567 (k)

1. The provision of a client's nutrient and nutrition education needs based on a complete nutrition assessment is
   a. medical nutrition therapy.
   b. nutrition care process.
   c. nutrition screening.
   d. medical history.

d   567 (k)

2. Clients can be put at risk for malnutrition by situations
   a. interfering with digestion and absorption.
   b. impairing a person's ability to eat.
   c. altering metabolism and excretion.
   d. all of the above

c   568 (k)

3. Which of the following affects nutrition status by reducing nutrient and food intake?
   a. loss of bile salts
   b. elevated metabolic rate
   c. nausea and Vomiting
   d. infection

b   568 (a)

4. Kidney failure, and hyperglycemia affect nutrition status by
   a. reducing nutrient and food intake.
   b. altering metabolism and excretion.
   c. impairing digestion and absorption.
   d. all of the above

1

d   568 (k)   5. The breakdown of skin and underlying tissues due to constant pressure and lack of oxygen to the affected area is
a. pressure sores.
b. bedsores.
c. decubitus ulcers.
d. all of the above

b   569 (k)   6. A nutrition care plan is
a. the client's diet prescription ordered by the physician.
b. the dietitian's goals for determining and meeting the client's nutrition and nutritional education needs.
c. the nurse's documentation of how well the client is eating.
d. nutritional formulas showing minimum daily requirements.

b   569 (k)   7. In a health care facility, who holds the ultimate responsibility for ensuring that all the patient's nutritional needs are met?
a. clinical dietitians
b. physicians
c. nurses
d. pharmacists

c   569 (k)   8. A client's diet prescription that the physician writes in the medical record is called
a. diet menu.
b. food list.
c. diet order.
d. food order.

d   570 (k)   9. The purposes of a nutritional assessment is to
a. detect malnutrition.
b. detect people at risk for malnutrition.
c. identify areas for dietary improvement.
d. all of the above

a   570 (a)   10. Is Mrs. Albert a candidate for nutritional screening?
a. Yes, because she is underweight.
b. Yes, because she is going to have a bunionectomy.
c. No, because her weight reveals adequate nutrition.
d. No, because a bunionectomy is a minor surgical procedure.

a   570 (k)   11. Basic nutritional screening would include all of the
following *except*
a. weighing the client.
b. observing the client.
c. obtaining a food record.
d. checking blood glucose levels.

d   570 (k)   12. A tool for quickly identifying clients at risk for malnutrition
so that they can receive complete nutrition assessments
is called
a. nutrition questionnaire.
b. health history.
c. health screening.
d. nutrition screening.

b   570 (a)   13. Which of the observations by the nurse would indicate
the need for a complete nutrition assessment?
a. refusal to eat breakfast
b. weight loss of 10% in two weeks
c. weight gain of 2 lbs in seven days
d. increased consumption of dairy products

c   571 (k)   14. According to the Joint Commission on Accreditation of
Healthcare Organizations, nutrition screenings should be
completed on each clients within _____ after
admission.
a. 12 hours
b. 18 hours
c. 24 hours
d. 48 hours

d   571 (k)   15. The purpose of obtaining historical information is to
assess for
a. low socioeconomic status
b. food and drug interactions
c. nutrient deficiencies
d. health factors that affect nutrition status

d   571 (k)   16. Historical data used in the development of a nutrition
care plan are health history, socioeconomic history, and
a. diet history.
b. medication history.
c. physical activity history.
d. a and b
e. a, b, and c

d   572 (k)   17. Which of the following data is the least important component of a client's nutritional assessment?
                                   a. weight
                                   b. medication
                                   c. eating habits
                                   d. current address

a   572 (k)   18. Which of the following is *not* considered a personal factor included in the personal history of a client?
                                   a. current health problems
                                   b. role in family
                                   c. economic status
                                   d. gender

d   572 (k)   19. Which of the following is a socioeconomic factor that can affect food choices?
                                   a. education
                                   b. age
                                   c. income
                                   d. all of the above

c   573 (k)   20. All of the following are examples of diet history *except*
                                   a. usual intake.
                                   b. 24-hour recall.
                                   c. physical examination.
                                   d. food record.

d   573 (a)   21. By analyzing the data collected from the diet history, dietitians can address which of the following?
                                   a. "Does the diet meet the dietary guidelines?"
                                   b. "Is the percent of total kcalories from fat and saturated fat appropriate?"
                                   c. "Are all of the food groups adequately represented in the diet?"
                                   d. all of the above

b   574 (k)   22. The easiest method used by nurses to collect food intake data is a
                                   a. food diary.
                                   b. 24-hour recall or usual intake.
                                   c. diet history.
                                   d. food frequency questionnaire.

c 574 (k) 23. If a client is asked to recount everything eaten or drunk in a typical day, the assessor is using the _____ to collect the data.
a. food record
b. kcalorie count
c. usual intake method
d. 24-hour recall

a 574 (a) 24. A 24-hour recall was used to collect a diet history. The client states she didn't eat breakfast. She had a soft drink and an apple for lunch, and for dinner, she had a slice of pizza. What is the best question the health care professional could ask next regarding this finding?
a. "Is this a usual day's food intake?"
b. "What was on the slice of pizza?"
c. "Do you normally skip breakfast?"
d. "Are you on a busy schedule?"

d 574 (a) 25. Which of the following statements is the *best* way to begin the interview for a 24-hour dietary history?
a. "What did you have for breakfast today?"
b. "You do eat breakfast everyday, don't you?"
c. "Do you begin the day with juice or coffee?"
d. "What is the first thing you ate or drank when you woke up?"

b 575 (k) 26. Assuming that each method is performed reliably, valuable food intake data can be obtained from the
a. usual intake.
b. food record.
c. 24-hour recall.
d. food frequency checklist.

d 574 (a) 27. Which of the following is a limitation to the value of 24-hour recall?
a. The process is time consuming.
b. Clients often keep poor records.
c. The method excludes recording of beverages.
d. A 24-hour period may not be typical.

d   575 (k)   28. The method for collecting diet history that is best for pinpointing nutrients that may be excessive or deficient in a diet is
a. 24-hour recall.
b. usual diet.
c. observing food intake.
d. food frequency checklist.

b   575 (k)   29. An extensive, accurate log of foods eaten over a period of several days or weeks is called a(n)
a. food-frequency checklist.
b. food record.
c. usual intake.
d. 24-hour recall.

d   575 (k)   30. Which of the following statements describe advantages of food records?
a. Food intake is recorded promptly after eating.
b. The individual assumes an active role in record keeping.
c. The individual becomes aware of personal food choices.
d. all of the above

d   568 (k)   31. Illness can affect nutrition status by affecting all of the following *except*
a. digestion and absorption.
b. metabolism.
c. emotional health.
d. all of the above

d   575 (k)   32. A food frequency questionnaire is typically used to compare a client's usually food intake with the Daily Food Guide to help identify
a. energy intakes.
b. nutrient imbalances.
c. amount of fat in the diet.
d. all of the above

a   576 (k)   33. All of the following are purposes of anthropometric measurements *except*
a. to diagnose medical conditions.
b. to evaluate growth.
c. to detect undernutrition and overnutrition.
d. to measure changes in body composition.

d   577 (k)   34. Anthropometric measurements compare an individual with
a. another individual.
b. population standards specific for age.
c. population standards specific for gender.
d. population standards specific for gender and age.

a   577 (k)   35. Head circumference in an infant can help predict all of the following *except*
a. age.
b. brain size.
c. growth rate.
d. protein-energy malnutrition.

d   577 (k)   36. Head circumference is used to
a. monitor infant growth.
b. help detect PEM.
c. evaluate brain size.
d. all of the above

b   577 (k)   37. In infants and children, length or height and weight below the ____ percentile suggests growth retardation, a sign of malnutrition.
a. 15th
b. 25th
c. 50th
d. 75th

a   577 (k)   38. A BMI-for age below the ____ percentile indicates that the child is underweight.
a. 5th
b. 15th
c. 25th
d. 50th

d   578 (k)   39. Which of the following measurements are used to detect undernutrition and overnutrition?
a. height-weight
b. % IBW
c. fatfold
d. a and b
e. a, b, and c

For question 40: Mrs. Falwell is 5'4" and weighs 110 lbs. During the interview, she mentions she has lost "a lot of weight" over the last five years. She reports her highest weight at 135 lbs

c   580 (a)

40. What is her *ideal* body weight?
    a. 100 lbs
    b. 110 lbs
    c. 120 lbs
    d. 135 lbs

b   580 (a)

41. The ideal weights for a female 5'5" tall and a male 5'10" are
    a. 120 lbs, 160 lbs
    b. 125 lbs, 166 lbs
    c. 130 lbs, 160 lbs
    d. 135 lbs, 165 lbs

b   577 (k)

42. The equation for body mass index is
    a. weight (lbs) / height (ft)^2.
    b. weight (kg) / height (m)^2.
    c. height (ft)^2 / weight (lbs).
    d. height (m)^2 / weight (kg).

c   579 (a)

43. Henry is 28 years old and is 5'9". What is his estimated desirable body weight?
    a. 151 lbs
    b. 157 lbs
    c. 160 lbs
    d. 169 lbs

b   579 (a)

44. Kathy is 21 years old and is 5'4". What is her estimated desirable body weight?
    a. 115 lbs
    b. 120 lbs
    c. 126 lbs
    d. 131 lbs

b   580 (a)

45. Danny is 37 years old, weighs 179 lbs, and is 5'8". Regarding his % IBW, Danny is considered
    a. obese.
    b. overweight.
    c. adequate.
    d. mildly underweight.

c   580 (a)   46. Cindy is a 28-year-old female who is 5'7". Her usual weight is 130 lbs, but her current weight is 110 lbs. Regarding her % UBW, Cindy is considered
        a. adequate.
        b. mildly underweight.
        c. moderately underweight.
        d. severely underweight.

        For question 47: Mrs. Sealy is an 85-year-old woman who states she has a poor appetite. She is 5'2" and weighs 80 lbs.

c   580 (a)   47. The correct nursing diagnosis is altered nutrition: less than body requirements because
        a. she states she has a poor appetite.
        b. she is elderly.
        c. her percent IBW is 73%.
        d. her percent IBW is 82%.

a   579 (k)   48. After unclotted blood is centrifuged, the fluid that remains is called
        a. plasma.
        b. serum.
        c. electrolytes.
        d. platelets.

d   581 (k)   49. Laboratory tests used in assessing fluid balance include
        a. blood urea nitrogen.
        b. hemoglobin.
        c. hematocrit.
        d. all of the above

d   580 (k)   50. Protein can be found in
        a. serum.
        b. skeletal muscle.
        c. internal organs.
        d. all of the above

c   581 (k)   51. All of the following biochemical tests are used to detect PEM *except*
        a. phosphorus.
        b. albumin.
        c. serum creatinine.
        d. transferring.

b   581 (k)   52. Hematocrit, hemoglobin, and mean corpuscular volume are all hematology tests used to detect
a. PEM.
b. anemia.
c. dehydration.
d. all of the above

a   581 (k)   53. All of the following enzymes are used to monitor heart function *except*
a. alkaline phosphatase.
b. creatinine phosphokinase.
c. lactic dehydrogenase.
d. alanine transaminase.

a   580 (k)   54. Which of the following nutrition assessment techniques is a measure of protein status?
a. serum albumin
b. body mass index
c. tricep skinfold thickness
d. visual assessment of the oral cavity

d   582 (a)   55. A serum albumin of 2.5 g/100 ml in a stable adult male with malnutrition suggests
a. iron deficiency.
b. a normal finding.
c. short-term protein malnutrition.
d. long-term protein malnutrition.

c   582 (a)   56. Donna Davis is an 18-year-old girl who is 5'4" and weighs 90 lbs. Her serum albumin level is 2.0 g/100 ml. From this information, what can you conclude about Donna's nutrition status?
a. She is undergoing short-term exposure to stress.
b. Her nutrition status is adequate for her age.
c. Her biochemical data reflects long-term protein depletion.
d. Not enough information is provided to speculate.

b   580 (k)   57. Which of the following proteins is the most abundant serum protein?
a. transferrin
b. albumin
c. transthyretin
d. retinol-binding protein

b   580 (k)   58. Which of the following proteins reflect both protein and iron status?
   a. albumin
   b. transferrin
   c. transthyretin
   d. retinol-binding protein

b   580 (k)   59. During iron deficiency, transferrin concentrations ___ and during severe PEM, transferrin concentrations ___.
   a. increase, increase.
   b. increase, decrease.
   c. decrease, increase.
   d. decrease, decrease.

d   580 (k)   60. Which of the following proteins is best for monitoring quick changes in protein status?
   a. transthyretin
   b. transferrin
   c. retinol-binding protein
   d. a and c
   e. a, b, and c

d   580 (k)   61. Another name for Transthyretin is
   a. prealbumin.
   b. thyroxin-binding protein.
   c. both a and b
   d. none of the above

c   582 (a)   62. The classification of PEM is made through all of the following *except*
   a. biochemical analysis.
   b. physical examination.
   c. docioeconomic status.
   d. anthropometric measures.

c   578 (a)   63. Which of the following clients is at *greatest* risk of malnutrition?
   a. A body builder 5'8" and 190 lbs taking amino acid supplements
   b. An 85-year-old woman 5'4" and a body weight of 122 lbs
   c. A 30-year-old woman, 5'6", 192 lbs with a recent unexplained weight loss of 25 lbs
   d. A 15-year-old boy 5'8", 132 lbs, with a good appetite going through a growth spurt

d   580 (k)   64. Which of the following proteins provide the most sensitive test for protein status?
         a. albumin
         b. transthyretin
         c. retinol-Binding Protein
         d. b and c

         For questions 65 and 66: Nancy has a WBC count of 6750 mm^3 with 17% lymphocytes. Use this data to answer the following questions.

b   581 (a)   65. Nancy's total lymphocyte count equals
         a. 397 mm^3.
         b. 1,148 mm^3.
         c. 10,750 mm^3.
         d. 39,706 mm^3.

b   582 (a)   66. What does Nancy's total lymphocyte count suggest regarding her immune system?
         a. mildly depleted
         b. moderately depleted
         c. severely depleted
         d. adequate

a   582 (k)   67. Chronic PEM, liver disease and pregnancy are factors that affect
         a. tranferrin.
         b. transthyretin.
         c. total lymphocyte count.
         d. all of the above

c   582 (k)   68. Which of the following factors affect retinal-binding protein levels?
         a. eclampsia
         b. iron deficiency
         c. vitamin A deficiency
         d. infection

d   583 (k)   69. A physical symptom of dehydration is
         a. hollow cheekbones
         b. weight loss
         c. thirst
         d. all of the above

d   583 (k)   70. All of the following are signs of fluid retention *except*
    a. ascites.
    b. weight gain.
    c. elevated blood pressure.
    d. sunken eyes.

b   582 (a)   71. Physical findings are most appropriately used to
    a. pinpoint vitamin deficiencies.
    b. reveal problems for other assessment techniques to confirm.
    c. verify hydration state.
    d. diagnose patients.

a   583 (k)   72. Which of the following physical findings reflect PEM?
    a. dull, brittle, dry, loose hair
    b. spoon-shaped, brittle, ridged nails
    c. sore, smooth, purplish, swollen tongue
    d. discolored, decayed teeth

c   583 (k)   73. What do the symptoms of the eyes that include pale membranes, spots, redness and slow adjustment to darkness reflects?
    a. PEM
    b. vitamin C and vitamin D status
    c. vitamin A, B vitamins and iron status
    d. essential fatty acid deficiency

a   583 (k)   74. A young adult with spoon-shaped ridged, brittle nails might be deficient in
    a. iron.
    b. calcium.
    c. vitamin A.
    d. vitamin B.

ESSAY QUESTIONS

1. Illustrate the steps in the nutrition care process and explain its applications.

2. In what ways are the needs of a client addressed in both an individualized and holistic manner through the nutrition care process?

3. Describe the roles of health care professionals in meeting client's nutritional needs.

4. Describe the interrelationships among health, medications, nutrition status, and personal factors.

5. Compare and contrast the methods for collecting diet history and provide advantages and disadvantages for each.

6. Give examples of anthropometric measurements and tell how they are used in nutrition assessment.

7. Describe how laboratory tests are used to determine nutritional status and how are they affected.

Chapter 18
Nutrition, Medications, and Complementary Therapies

b   591 (k)

1. Most health care professionals have not received formal training in
   a. conventional therapies.
   b. complementary therapies.
   c. over-the-counter medicines.
   d. prescription medicines.

c   591 (k)

2. With enough research and experience to support its use, _____ may become _____.
   a. conventional therapy, complementary therapy
   b. conventional therapy, alternative therapy
   c. complementary therapy, conventional therapy
   d. complementary therapy, alternative therapy

a   591 (k)

3. Chemicals that alter one or more body functions that are marketed only with approval of the Food and Drug Administration are
   a. medications.
   b. dietary supplements.
   c. over-the-counter medicines.
   d. all of the above

d   591 (k)

4. Which of the following are examples of dietary supplements?
   a. herbs
   b. vitamin and minerals
   c. coenzyme Q
   d. all of the above

b   592 (k)   5. An example of alternative medicine for mind-body
                            interventions is
                            a. ayurveda.
                            b. faith healing.
                            c. ozone therapy.
                            d. all of the above

c   592 (k)   6. Homeopathic medicine and naturopathic medicine are
                            examples of
                            a. mind-body interventions.
                            b. manual healing methods.
                            c. alternative systems of medical practice.
                            d. pharmacological treatments.

d   592 (k)   7. Conventional medical therapies include
                            a. over-the-counter medications.
                            b. prescription medications.
                            c. herbal products.
                            d. a and b
                            e. all of the above

b   592 (k)   8. Which of the following statements is true?
                            a. Over-the-counter medications are stronger than
                               prescription medications.
                            b. Prescription medications are often used for longer
                               periods of time than over-the-counter medications.
                            c. Clients who use over-the-counter medications are at
                               greater risk of serious side effects.
                            d. Using prescription medications is far more difficult
                               compared to over-the-counter medications.

d   593 (k)   9. Which of the following statements is true?
                            a. Aspirin is an over-the-counter medication used for
                               treating headaches or pain.
                            b. Over-the-counter medications are less potent than
                               prescription medications.
                            c. People are more likely to self-medicate with
                               prescription medications rather than over-the-counter
                               medications.
                            d. a and b
                            e. all of the above

c   593 (k)   10. The FDA is responsible for
- a. studying the effectiveness and safety of dietary supplements.
- b. proving dietary supplements are safe.
- c. documenting the effectiveness and safety of medications.
- d. all of the above

c   593 (a)   11. Which of the following statements would you expect to see on a label of the herb ginseng?
- a. Enhances energy level.
- b. Alleviates insomnia.
- c. Has not been evaluated by the FDA.
- d. all of the above

b   594 (k)   12. What percentage of the US population is taking prescription medications?
- a. 33
- b. 44
- c. 55
- d. 66

a   595 (k)   13. St. John's wort claims to
- a. relieve depression and anxiety.
- b. protect liver tissue.
- c. lower blood lipids.
- d. enhance memory.

d   595 (k)   14. Which of the following herb has claims associated with promoting sleep and reducing stress and anxiety?
- a. ginseng
- b. saw palmetto
- c. valerian
- d. kava

c   595 (k)   15. Risks associated with taking the herbal supplement _____ include hypertension, insomnia and edema.
- a. St. John's wort
- b. ginkgo
- c. ginseng
- d. valerian

d   595 (k)   16. Drug guides can provide information about
- a. prescription and over-the-counter medications.
- b. interactions between medications and herbs and dietary supplements.
- c. self-medicating.
- d. a and b
- e. all of the above

d   595 (a)   17. Which of the following increases a client's risk for adverse nutrition-related side effects from medications, herbs, and dietary supplements?
- a. failure to use medications as directed
- b. take medications over long periods of time
- c. drink alcohol regularly
- d. all of the above

a   596 (a)   18. Mr. Williams, 88 yrs. old, has just been discharged from the hospital after suffering from a MI. The physician wrote three prescriptions for him to get filled. Which of the following statements needs consideration?
- a. Mr. Williams needs assistance obtaining the prescriptions due to financial difficulties.
- b. Mr. Williams has already had a previous MI.
- c. Mr. Williams' regular physician is out of town.
- d. all of the above

b   596 (k)   19. In order to limit the risks of drug-related side effects, the most important step health care professionals can take is to know
- a. how diet and drugs interaction.
- b. what and how much medications and supplements a client is taking.
- c. when the client is taking the medications and supplements.
- d. why the client is taking the medications and supplements.

a   596 (a)   20. Susan, a 30-year-old teacher, started taking calcium
supplements after her mother was diagnosed with
osteoporosis. Her physician should
a. examine Susan's eating habits to see if diet
modification is needed to ensure the adequate
amount of calcium and vitamin D is in her diet.
b. encourage Susan to continue her calcium supplement.
c. order Susan to undergo a bone density test.
d. instruct Susan to increase the amount of her calcium
supplement.

b   597 (k)   21. A medication prescribed for obesity is
a. ephedra.
b. amphetamines.
c. dronabinol.
d. antidepressants.

d   597 (k)   22. Medications can reduce food intake by
a. suppressing the appetite.
b. heightening the appetite.
c. causing complications that make it difficult to eat.
d. a and c
e. all of the above

a   597 (k)   23. Which of the following medications is not intended for
weight gain?
a. antianxiety agents
b. growth hormone
c. testosterone
d. megestrol acetate

d   597 (k)   24. Amphetamines are used to
a. suppress the appetite.
b. improve concentration.
c. reduce depression.
d. a and b
e. all of the above

For questions 25 and 26: Ms. Brown has experienced
unwanted weight loss and has been complaining of nausea.

c   598 (a)

25. After reviewing her chart, the physician discovered Ms. Brown was prescribed _____ at her last appointment.
    a. calcium supplements
    b. vitamin c supplements
    c. iron supplements
    d. antiemetics

a   598 (a)

26. In order to reduce her nausea, the physician should prescribe
    a. antiemetics.
    b. chamomile.
    c. ginkgo.
    d. megestrol acetate.

b   598 (a)

27. Mr. Jerkins has been prescribed captopril to control is hypertension. When he picks up his prescription, the pharmacist instructs Mr. Jerkins to
    a. take the medicine with food.
    b. take the medicine on an empty stomach.
    c. take the medicine with grapefruit juice.
    d. take the medicine with water only.

b   598 (k)

28. Which of the following statements is true about aspirin.
    a. It works faster on a full stomach.
    b. It works faster on an empty stomach.
    c. It can irritate the GI tract when taken with certain foods.
    d. a and c
    e. b and c

c   598 (k)

29. Oxalates are nonnutrients found in all of the following except
    a. chocolate.
    b. tea.
    c. legumes.
    d. wheat bran.

d   598 (k)

30. Phytates are nonnutrients found in
    a. grain husks.
    b. seeds.
    c. wheat bran.
    d. a and b
    e. all of the above

e   598 (k)   31. Which of the following can affect medication absorption?
    a. fiber
    b. phytates
    c. minerals
    d. a and b
    e. all of the above

b   599 (a)   32. A possible side effect of antibiotic use that can affect
nutrition status is
    a. GI distress.
    b. vomiting.
    c. constipation.
    d. all of the above

a   599 (a)   33. Betty has been prescribed an antiulcer agent. Her
physician will monitor _____ for side effects.
    a. iron absorption
    b. GI distress
    c. renal function
    d. sodium excretion

c   599 (a)   34. Altered excretion of potassium, magnesium, and calcium
are side effects associated with the use of
    a. narcotics.
    b. antihypertensives.
    c. diuretics.
    d. laxatives.

c   599 (k)   35. Which of the following statements is true?
    a. Laxatives can interfere with nutrient excretion.
    b. Some laxatives move foods rapidly through the
intestine, increasing the time available for nutrient
absorption.
    c. Some laxatives can reduce calcium absorption.
    d. all of the above

d   600 (k)   36. Amphetamines can alter food intake by
    a. suppressing the appetite.
    b. changing taste perception.
    c. producing mouth ulcers.
    d. a and b
    e all of the above

d   600 (k)   37. Which of the following medications alter food intake by
                            causing dry mouth?
                            a. amphetamines
                            b. digitalis
                            c. methotrexate
                            d. Phenobarbital

b   600 (k)   38. Chemotherapy alters nutrient absorption by
                            a. binding to nutrients.
                            b. damaging mucosal cells.
                            c. displacing nutrients from their plasma protein carriers.
                            d. all of the above

a   600 (k)   39. Vitamin __ can alter urinary pH and limit excretion of __.
                            a. C, aspirin
                            b. C, sodium
                            c. K, aspirin
                            d. K, sodium

d   600 (k)   40. In what way can foods alter medication absorption?
                            a. binding to drugs
                            b. competing for absorption sites in the intestine
                            c. stimulating secretion of digestive juices
                            d. all of the above

c   600 (a)   41. All of the following statements are true *except*
                            a. Warfarin is an anticlotting agent that resembles
                               vitamin K.
                            b. The prescribed warfarin dose is dependant on the
                               amount of vitamin K in the diet.
                            c. Dietary supplements of vitamin A can interact with
                               warfarin.
                            d. Garlic is an herb that can interact with warfarin.

d   600 (k)   42. Dietary and herbal supplements that can interact with
                            warfarin include
                            a. omega-3 fatty acids and ginger.
                            b. vitamin E and ginkgo.
                            c. vitamin D and ginseng.
                            d. a and b
                            e. all of the above

d   600 (a)   43. In order to maximize the effectiveness of aldendronate
sodium, Adequate supply of ____ must be present.
a. calcium
b. vitamin D
c. iron
d. a and b
e. all of the above

a   601 (a)   44. Mr. Brown has been given a new prescription from his
physician. He was instructed not to consume grapefruit
juice. What was Mr. Brown prescription for?
a. hypertension
b. diabetes
c. weight-loss
d. all of the above

c   601 (k)   45. Caffeine can accentuate the actions of ____ and limit the
effectiveness of ___.
a. methotrexate, barbituates
b. amphetamines, corticosteroids
c. ephedra, barbituates
d. ephedra, corticosteroids

b   601 (a)   46. When physicians prescribe the use of corticosteroids,
they raise the risk of
a. osteomalacia.
b. osteoporosis.
c. iron deficiency.
d. folate deficiency.

d   601 (k)   47. Methotrexate resembles the structure of
a. niacin.
b. calcium.
c. iron.
d. folate.

a   601 (a)   48. Prolonged use of aspirin can affect
a. folate metabolism.
b. calcium metabolism.
c. iron metabolism.
d. vitamin D metabolism.

For questions 49 and 50: Mrs. Appleton has been diagnosed with depression and her physician has prescribed a monoamine oxidase inhibitor. He instructs her to avoid consuming large amounts of tyramine.

d   602 (a)

49. The interaction of MAO and tyramine can alter metabolism by
   a. stimulating the release of norepinephrine.
   b. stimulating the release of epinephrine.
   c. blocking the action of the enzyme responsible for inactivating tyramine.
   d. a and c
   e. b and c

b   602 (a)

50. All of the following foods should be restricted on Mrs. Appleton's diet *except*
   a. aged cheese.
   b. baker's yeast.
   c. snow peas.
   d. sausage.

d   603 (k)

51. Medications include both active and inactive ingredients. An example of an inactive ingredient is
   a. caffeine.
   b. lactose.
   c. sorbitol.
   d. all of the above

c   603 (a)

52. Mr. Barton has just been diagnosed with diabetes. He is instructed to monitor his carbohydrate intake. What inactive ingredient found in some medications does Mr. Barton need to be aware of?
   a. caffeine
   b. cellulose
   c. sugar
   d. sodium

a   603 (k)

53. Lactose is composed of glucose and
   a. galactose.
   b. glucose.
   c. fructose.
   d. sucrose.

ESSAY QUESTIONS

1. Differentiate between conventional and complementary therapies.

2. In what ways are over-the-counter and prescription medications different?

3. What are the problems associated with dietary supplements?

4. Explain the risks of drug-related side effects and discuss how health care professionals can work together to limit them.

5. Why is it important to recognize the need to research diet-drug interactions?

6. How can absorption be affected in relation to diet-drug interactions? Give examples.

7. How can metabolism be affected in relation to diet-drug interactions? Give examples.

8. How can excretion be affected in relation to diet-drug interactions? Give examples.

Chapter 19
Nutrition Intervention

c   613 (k)   1. For a dietitian, the basis of the nutrition care plan is the
                           a. critical pathway.
                           b. medical nutrition therapy.
                           c. nutrition problem list.
                           d. nutrition education needs.

d   613 (k)   2. The nutrition care plan sets goals and identifies
                           interventions that aim to
                           a. resolve the client's long-term nutrition problems.
                           b. resolve the client's short-term nutrition problems.
                           c. resolve the client's needs for nutrition education.
                           d. all of the above

b   613 (k)   3. Charts or tables that outline a coordinated plan of care
                           for a specific medical diagnosis, treatment, or procedure
                           are
                           a. diet manuals.
                           b. clinical pathways.
                           c. nutrition care plans.
                           d. none of the above

e   613 (k)   4. Which of the following is an example of a nursing
                           diagnosis with nutrition implications?
                           a. feeding self-care deficit
                           b. body image disturbance
                           c. chronic pain
                           d. a and b
                           e. a, b, and c

1

b   613 (a)   5. What part of the nursing process corresponds to nutritional problems in the nutrition care process?
   a. goals
   b. nursing diagnosis
   c. objective data
   d. diet prescriptions

For questions 6 and 7: Jane Collins has just delivered her first infant and plans to breastfeed. She expresses self-doubt about her abilities, and her infant is fretful. Jane is being cared for by a nurse and a dietitian.

a   613 (a)   6. Jane's care should include
   a. nursing and nutrition plans complementary to one another.
   b. nursing plan only, since this is really an emotional problem.
   c. nutrition plan only, since breast milk reflects Jane's nutrition status.
   d. nursing and nutrition plans independent from one another.

d   613 (a)   7. What would be the appropriate nursing diagnosis for the infant?
   a. Altered nutrition: more than body requirements.
   b. Altered nutrition: less than body requirements.
   c. Altered nutrition: high risk for more than body requirements.
   d. Altered nutrition: high risk for less than body requirements.

c   613 (k)   8. Which of the following *best* describes a nutrition care plan?
   a. documentation of a client's dietary intake
   b. diet prescription ordered by the physician
   c. goals developed by a dietitian for meeting a client's nutritional needs
   d. analysis of nutrition assessment data

b   613 (a)   9. Dietitians can use analyzed assessment data for all of the following *except*
   a. generating a nutrition problem list.
   b. predicting client responses to the nutrition care plan.
   c. determining nutrition education strategies.
   d. estimating nutrient needs.

a   613 (a)   10. In a hospital setting, implementation of a nutrition care plan includes all of the following *except*
   a. assessing the client's progress.
   b. supplying the appropriate diet.
   c. providing nutrition education.
   d. monitoring the client's compliance with the treatment.

   For questions 11 and 12: Mr. Whitaker is 5'8", 145 lbs. and has been diagnosed with esophageal cancer. His hematocrit is 28 and albumin level is 3.1 g/dl.

c   613 (a)   11. Which of the following would be noted in his nutritional care plan?
   a. need for a low-kcalorie diet
   b. need to reduce protein intake
   c. need to improve energy-protein status
   d. need to limit milk

a   613 (a)   12. Which of the following additional findings is *most* detrimental to Mr. Whitaker's nutritional status?
   a. weight loss of 25 lbs in the last month
   b. preference of high-sodium foods
   c. need to eat with a family member
   d. transferrin level of 275 mg/dl

a   615 (k)   13. Diet modifications usually work *best* if
   a. clients understand the needed modifications.
   b. they are independent of medical therapies.
   c. they represent real change from the normal diet.
   d. all of the above

c   615 (k)   14. When a regular diet fails to meet the nutrient needs of a client, a ___ is used.
   a. standard diet
   b. nutrition care plan
   c. modified diet
   d. nursing diagnosis

For question 15: You met with Susan Gray eight weeks ago to plan a weight-loss plan. At that time, Susan was 5'4" and weighed 185 lbs. She was instructed to eat a 1000 kcalorie diet. Today, Susan weighs 180 lbs.

c   615 (a)

15. At this phase in the nutrition care process you would
   a. assess her nutrition status.
   b. redefine the nutrition-related problem.
   c. evaluate the nutrition plan previously developed.
   d. refer Susan to a weight-loss clinic.

b   615 (k)

16. Is it important to monitor the progress of clients on a nutrition care plan on a regular basis?
   a. Yes, because it may take time for health benefits to become apparent.
   b. Yes, because client responses to the nutrition care plan reveal the individual's needs.
   c. No, because responses to nutrition care plans are basically the same.
   d. No, because the desired response will develop eventually.

d   615 (k)

17. The characteristics of a standard diet include
   a. reduced intake of fat and saturated fat.
   b. all foods.
   c. meets the nutrient needs of a normal healthy individual.
   d. b and c

c   616 (k)

18. Delivery of nutrient solutions directly into the vein is called
   a. standard nutrition.
   b. enteral nutrition.
   c. parenteral nutrition.
   d. tube feeding.

b   616 (a)

19. Enteral nutrition is to tube feeding as
   a. parenteral nutrition is to standard diet.
   b. parenteral nutrition is to intravenous feeding.
   c. diet order is to client.
   d. diet order is to modified diet.

b   616 (k)   20. All of the following statements are true *except*
- a. Tube feedings can only be used if the client is able to digest and absorb an adequate amount of nutrients.
- b. Intravenous feedings are preferred over tube feedings.
- c. A client who is unable to use the GI tract to absorb nutrients will require intravenous feedings.
- d. Enteral nutrition includes both oral diets and tube feedings.

a   616 (k)   21. A ___ diet is changed to meet the nutritional and medical needs of a client.
- a. modified
- b. restricted
- c. progressive
- d. liquid

d   616 (k)   22. To meet the specific needs of a client, a modified diet can be adjusted by
- a. excluding certain foods.
- b. changing the number of meals.
- c. altering food consistency.
- d. all of the above

a   616 (a)   23. A diet order is to physician as a
- a. diet prescription is to dietitian.
- b. nutrition health plan is to client.
- c. nutrition health plan is to nurse.
- d. diet prescription is to nurse.

c   616 (a)   24. A low-sodium diet is prescribed by the physician. As a dietitian working with the client, you would first
- a. provide the client with a modified diet.
- b. consult the client for his/her favorite foods.
- c. clarify the diet order with the physician.
- d. send the client a diet providing 2000mg of sodium.

b 616 (k) 25. The purpose of a diet order is to
- a. provide guidelines of the foods allowed and restricted on a diet, the rationale and indications for use of the diet, and sample menus.
- b. provide a written statement in the medical record of what diet a client should receive by the physician.
- c. provide a running record of the dietary intake of the client.
- d. provide the client with a reference of food listings and their corresponding nutrient content.

d 617 (k) 26. The objective of diet manuals is to
- a. provide a description of foods allowed and restricted on a diet.
- b. provide the rationale for the diet.
- c. provide a written statement in the medical record of what diet a client should receive by the physician.
- d. a and b

c 617 (a) 27. A nurse was receiving new orders written in the patient chart. The order read, NPO, which means
- a. the patient will receive only beverages and medications.
- b. the patient will receive only medications.
- c. the patient will receive nothing by mouth.
- d. the patient will receive anything orally.

c 617 (a) 28. Your client is on a 1200 kcalorie, 2 gram sodium diet. You find each diet in the diet manual but not the combined diet. Where could you *best* find information regarding this diet?
- a. the National Formulary
- b. the client's physician
- c. the client's dietitian
- d. no resources; improvise

d 617 (k) 29. An institution may choose to have diet manuals
- a. developed by the nutrition health care team.
- b. adopt the diet manual of another hospital.
- c. adopt the diet manual of the state dietetic association.
- d. all of the above

a   617 (a)   30. A client has just been admitted to your unit at 11:30 PM on Saturday. He states he is hungry and wants something to eat. You note he is on a low-fat diet, but have questions regarding what is allowed. Your *best* resource at this time of night is the
        a. diet manual.
        b. client's physician.
        c. client's dietitian.
        d. nursing supervisor.

d   617 (a)   31. Which of the following clients would be on a progressive diet?
        a. Betty, who just had gallbladder surgery and now is out of recovery.
        b. Jim, who has been receiving nutrients by tube feeding and now is ready to start eating again.
        c. Susan, who has been experience nausea.
        d. all of the above

b   617 (k)   32. A diet that changes with the client's tolerance level is called a
        a. clear-liquid diet.
        b. progressive diet.
        c. low-fat diet.
        d. manual diet.

c   617 (a)   33. After surgery, the physician ordered Tina to put on a progressive diet. The first food Tina would receive would be
        a. bread.
        b. eggs.
        c. gelatin.
        d. milk.

b   617 (k)   34. In regards to a clear-liquid diet, which of the following statements is false?
        a. The liquids are transparent at body temperature.
        b. The liquids provide maximal stimulation o the GI tract.
        c. The liquids are almost completely absorbed.
        d. The liquids help test if the digestive system is ready for complex foods.

d   618 (a)   35. Which of the following foods is included in a full-liquid diet?
- a. fruit drinks
- b. vegetable juices
- c. plain ice cream
- d. all of the above

c   618 (a)   36. Which food is excluded from a clear-liquid diet?
- a. bouillon
- b. honey
- c. pudding
- d. sugar

d   619 (k)   37. Soft diets include foods that are
- a. high in fiber.
- b. easy to digest.
- c. easy to absorb.
- d. b and c
- e. a, b, and c

c   620 (k)   38. All of the following statements are true *except*
- a. soft diets minimize the risk of indigestion and nausea.
- b. soft diets can include fish, eggs, and milk products.
- c. soft diets can include crackers, sugar, and nuts.
- d. soft diets limit highly seasoned foods.

c   620 (a)   39. Low-fiber diets restrict all of the following *except*
- a. high-fiber foods.
- b. tough meats.
- c. milk products.
- d. certain fruits and vegetables.

d   621 (a)   40. Burt has been placed on a low-fiber diet. Which food is included in his diet?
- a. poultry
- b. nuts
- c. bananas
- d. all of the above

a   620 (k)   41. A legal document used to record a client's history, assessment, treatment, and results of therapy is a(n)
- a. medical record.
- b. informal record.
- c. diagnosis.
- d. nutrition care plan.

d   620 (k)   42. The main reason nurses, dietitians, and physicians document their plans of care in the client's chart is to
a. communicate plans with other health care professionals.
b. meet accreditation requirements.
c. protect themselves legally.
d. all of the above

d   621 (a)   43. Nutrition-related information that should be documented in a client's medical record is
a. nutrition screening.
b. medical nutrition therapy and goals.
c. diet education.
d. all of the above

ESSAY QUESTIONS

1. Discuss the steps involved in developing a nutrition care plan and strategies used in monitoring the progress of implemented plans.

2. Compare and contrast enteral and parenteral nutrition.

3. Using an example, explain how and why health care professionals use diet modification.

4. Outline a progressive diet for a patient who has just had open-heart surgery. How should the diet progress and what kinds of foods might be introduced at each stage.

5. Explain how health care professionals use medical records to communicate the needs of their clients. Why is it so important that good communication techniques are used?

Chapter 20
Nutrition and Disorders of
the Upper GI Tract

Ans	Page	
a	630 (k)	1. A client having difficulty with chewing is usually started on a(n) a. mechanical soft diet. b. enteral feeding. c. pureed diet. d. full liquid diet.
d	630 (k)	2. A diet that includes foods that are easy to chew and swallow is called a a. pureed diet. b. mechanical soft diet. c. dental soft diet. d. b and c e. a, b, and c
a	631 (k)	3. Foods that have been strained and blenderized to a thickened, near-liquid consistency are called a. pureed foods. b. mechanical soft foods. c. liquid supplements. d. mashed foods.

1

b   630 (a)   4. An example of a strategy used by dietitians to encourage clients on mechanical soft diets to eat is to
a. allow them to eat all desired foods.
b. identify foods they can tolerate and encourage them to eat foods similar to a regular diet.
c. restrict all their favorite foods.
d. allow them to eat just one meal a day.

a   631 (k)   5. A technique to help ease the task of chewing is
a. providing fluids with meals.
b. limiting fluids during the meal.
c. serving cold foods.
d. limiting sugars in the diet.

b   631 (a)   6. Which of the following foods would be best for a client with problems chewing?
a. roast beef, green salad, and an apple
b. casserole, mashed potatoes, and canned peaches
c. Swiss steak, new potatoes, and fresh fruit cup
d. baked chicken, garden salad, carrot sticks, and apple pie

d   630 (k)   7. A condition most likely to impair a person's ability to chew and swallow is
a. Alzheimer's disease.
b. broken jaw.
c. ill-fitting dentures.
d. all of the above

c   630 (a)   8. What do the following three conditions have in common: dysphagia, strokes, and Parkinson's disease?
a. They require a person to be placed on a diet containing pureed foods.
b. They affect a person's ability to communicate.
c. They affect a person's ability to chew and swallow food.
d. They require a person to avoid salty foods.

d   631 (k)   9. What problems are associated with clients' tolerance of pureed foods for extended periods of time?
a. depression
b. a psychological block may develop
c. malnutrition
d. all of the above

c   631 (a)   10. Of the following menus, which is the most appropriate for
                          a client with mouth ulcers?
                          a. orange juice, toast, and scrambled eggs
                          b. tomato juice and a chef's salad with Italian dressing
                          c. cottage cheese, sliced peaches, and banana bread
                          d. chicken broth, jello, and grapefruit juice

d   631 (a)   11. Katy has been complaining about mouth ulcers. What
                          nutritional advice could you provide to ease her
                          discomfort while she eats?
                          a. Avoid acidic foods.
                          b. Avoid foods containing nuts and seeds.
                          c. Hot foods may intensify pain.
                          d. all of the above

e   632 (k)   12. Which of the following is useful to increasing salivary
                          secretions?
                          a. sucking on sugarless candy
                          b. chewing gum
                          c. taking medication that stimulates saliva flow
                          d. b and c
                          e. a, b, and c

a   632 (k)   13. All of the following may cause dysphagia *except*
                          a. heart disease.
                          b. aging.
                          c. strokes.
                          d. head injuries.

c   633 (a)   14. What is the primary reason why dysphagia is life-
                          threatening?
                          a. causing strokes
                          b. food entering the esophagus
                          c. development of pneumonia
                          d. none of the above

c   633 (a)   15. Of the following, the best choice for enteral feeding of a
                          client with dysphagia is
                          a. nasogastric.
                          b. gastrostomy.
                          c. jejunostomy.
                          d. orogastric.

d   632 (a)   16. All of the following conditions may lead to dysphagia *except*
    a. head injury.
    b. brain tumor.
    c. HIV infection.
    d. T7 fracture.

d   633 (k)   17. A sign and symptom of dysphagia is
    a. drooling.
    b. weight loss.
    c. refusing to swallow food.
    d. all of the above

d   633 (a)   18. Which of the following beverages is most appropriate for a client with dysphagia?
    a. water
    b. chicken broth
    c. iced tea
    d. pear nectar

For question 19: The home health care nurse is visiting Paul Cantu, an 82-year-old man, recovering from a stroke. Upon assessment, the nurse observes that Mr. Cantu has lost weight, frequently clears his throat, and exhibits drooling.

b   633 (a)   19. In this situation, the nurse should suspect
    a. reduced saliva flow.
    b. dysphagia.
    c. reflux esophagitis.
    d. peptic ulcer disease.

b   633 (k)   20. The fear of eating is called
    a. hydrophobia.
    b. sitophobia.
    c. claustrophobia.
    d. arachnophobia.

c   633 (k)   21. Examples of smooth solids that can be incorporated into a diet for a client with dysphagia include all of the following *except*
    a. pudding.
    b. custard.
    c. yogurt with fresh fruit.
    d. baby cereal.

c   632 (a)   22. Which of the following clients is likely to experience
                    dysphagia?
                    a. A 38-year-old pregnant woman
                    b. A 52-year-old executive with heart burn
                    c. An 82-year-old man with Alzheimer's disease
                    d. A 28-year-old man with a hiatal hernia

                    For questions 23 and 24: Bob has been eating pureed
                    food for six months. The nurses have noticed that his
                    skin is pale, he has lost 5 lbs., and he complains
                    constantly about the food.

d   631 (a)   23. What strategies can the dietitian use to improve Bob's
                    feelings about eating a pureed diet?
                    a. order larger portions to be given
                    b. make sure the food is served at the right temperature
                    c. have the food pureed so that it is thick and smooth
                    d. b and c
                    e. a, b, and c

d   631 (a)   24. How can Bob's nutrition support be modified to ensure he
                    is getting adequate nutrients?
                    a. supplement the diet with milk or liquid formulas
                    b. try improving the taste by adding seasonings
                    c. replace his diet with baby foods
                    d. a and b
                    e. a, b, and c

b   634 (k)   25. Vague abdominal pain is called
                    a. dysphagia.
                    b. dyspepsia.
                    c. epigastric.
                    d. none of the above

d   634 (k)   26. Indigetion is also called
                    a. dysphagia.
                    b. dyspnea.
                    c. dysgeusia.
                    d. dyspepsia.

c 634 (k) 27. The backflow or regurgitation of gastric contents from the stomach into the esophagus is
 a. esophageal stricture.
 b. hearburn.
 c. reflux esophagitis.
 d. all of the above

a 634 (k) 28. Frequent reflux of highly acidic gastric fluids results in
 a. inflammation and scarring of the esophagus.
 b. stomach ulcers.
 c. tooth decay.
 d. inability to swallow.

d 634 (k) 29. Which of the following conditions increase the risk of reflux esophagitis?
 a. aging
 b. use of feeding tubes
 c. certain medications
 d. all of the above

b 634 (k) 30. Reflux esophagitis most frequently develops from
 a. aging.
 b. hiatal hernia.
 c. use of feeding tubes.
 d. medication.

c 636 (k) 31. Interventions that can help eliminate distress from reflux esophagitis include
 a. lying down for 30 minutes after meals.
 b. fluid intake with meals.
 c. small frequent feedings.
 d. pureed diet.

d 634 (k) 32. Where the esophagus joins the stomach is called the
 a. esophageal sphincter.
 b. duodenum sphincter.
 c. pharynx sphincter.
 d. lower esophageal sphincter.

d 636 (a) 33. Which of the following foods does *not* affect lower esophageal sphincter pressure?
 a. chocolate
 b. sausage
 c. peppermint candy
 d. whole wheat bread

d   634 (k)   34. Examples of substances that cause relaxation of the
                        cardiac sphincter include
                        a. garlic.
                        b. high-fat foods.
                        c. calcium channel blockers.
                        d. all of the above

d   635 (a)   35. Dietary treatment for reflux esophagitis aims to
                        a. reduce gastric acidity.
                        b. alleviate inflamed esophagus.
                        c. relax the lower esophageal sphincter.
                        d. a and b
                        e. a, b, and c

d   635 (k)   36. Management of reflux esophagitis includes all of the
                        following *except*
                        a. neutralizing gastric acid.
                        b. giving a bland diet.
                        c. performing surgery.
                        d. dilating the esophageal sphincter.

                        For question 37: Mrs. Nichols is 5'2", weighs 103 lbs.,
                        and suffers from a hiatal hernia. She smokes and
                        occasionally drinks wine. Today she is being prepared
                        for discharge.

a   636 (a)   37. Which of the following statements by Mrs. Nichols
                        indicates the need for further discharge instructions?
                        a. "I should lose weight to reduce my symptoms."
                        b. "I will avoid wine."
                        c. "I will go to the lung association classes."
                        d. "I will eat small, frequent meals."

a   638 (k)   38. Dietary interventions for nausea include all of the
                        following *except*
                        a. ice cream.
                        b. cold fluids.
                        c. dry toast.
                        d. small meals.

                        For questions 39, 40, and 41: Mr. Brown has been
                        suffering from reflux esophagitis. He is 25% above his
                        ideal body weight.

d   636 (a)   39. In order to prevent discomfort, health care professionals will instruct Mr. Brown to
a. lose weight.
b. refrain from smoking.
c. eat small meals.
d. all of the above

b   634 (a)   40. Substances that Mr. Brown should avoid are all of the following *except*
a. alcohol.
b. yogurt.
c. onions.
d. chocolate.

e   635 (a)   41. Health care professionals may prescribe medication to treat Mr. Brown's reflux esophagitis. An example includes
a. antisecretory agents.
b. cholinergics.
c. antacids.
d. a and c
e. a, b, and c

d   636 (k)   42. Which of the following can cause nausea and vomiting?
a. gallbladder disorders
b. gastritis
c. pregnancy
d. all of the above

c   638 (a)   43. A client suffering from chronic nausea should eat
a. a hot breakfast in the morning.
b. tuna salad sandwich at lunch.
c. dry toast or crackers.
d. bagels with cream cheese.

For question 44: Sam Evans has gastritis and has been experiencing nausea and vomiting for the last three days.

c   636 (a)   44. Appropriate management would include a(n)
b. liberal bland diet.
b. antacids.
c. IV therapy.
d. diet high in vitamin B_{12}.

d   636 (k)   45. Continuous nausea can lead to which of the following
                        a. weight loss.
                        b. dehydration.
                        c. malnutrition.
                        d. all of the above

d   637 (k)   46. Symptoms of gastritis include
                        a. nausea.
                        b. anorexia.
                        c. stomach pain.
                        d. all of the above

d   637 (k)   47. The dietary management of acute gastritis includes
                        a. avoiding antacids.
                        b. switching to decaffeinated coffee.
                        c. increasing aspirin for pain.
                        d. avoiding alcohol.

a   637 (k)   48. Complications that include malnutrition, dehydration, and
                        damage to the esophagus are associated with
                        a. gastritis.
                        b. nausea.
                        c. ulcers.
                        d. all of the above

                        For questions 49 and 50: Susan has been recently
                        diagnosed with Zollinger-Ellison syndrome.

d   638 (a)   49. What characteristics are associated with this condition?
                        a. tumor of the pancreas
                        b. hypersecretion of gastric acid
                        c. peptic ulcers
                        d. all of the above

a   638 (a)   50. If surgery is recommended for Susan, what is the primary
                        desired outcome?
                        a. decrease gastric acid production
                        b. increased gastric acid production
                        c. reduce inflammation
                        d. control gastric bleeding

a   638 (k)   51. In which surgical procedure does the stomach remain intact, but all or a portion of the stomach is bypassed?
a. gastric partitioning
b. vagotomy
c. pyloroplasty
d. partial gastrectomy

b   638 (k)   52. Dumping syndrome may occur when
a. the nerves of the stomach are severed.
b. the pyloric sphincter has been removed, bypassed, or disrupted.
c. a and b
d. none of the above

c   639 (k)   53. A postgastrectomy diet is a
a. protein-controlled diet to prevent hypoglycemia.
b. fat-controlled diet to prevent dumping syndrome.
c. carbohydrate-controlled diet to prevent hypoglycemia.
d. protein and fat-controlled diet to prevent dumping syndrome.

d   639 (k)   54. The postgastrectomy diet includes
a. fluid with meals.
b. refined carbohydrates.
c. high in water insoluble fiber.
d. an emphasis on fats and proteins.

b   639 (k)   55. Reductions in blood pressure caused by dumping syndrome result in all of the following *except*
a. weakness.
b. reduction in heart rate.
c. dizziness.
d. sweating.

d   638 (k)   56. Which of the following is known as a major cause of ulcers?
a. bacterial infection
b. nonsteroidal anti-inflammatory agents
c. alcohol abuse
d. a and b
e. a, b, and c

c   705 (k)   57. All of the following are used in the management of peptic ulcer disease *except*
a. antiulcer agents.
b. antibiotics.
c. low-fiber diets.
d. antisecretory agents.

For question 58: Mr. McInnis recently had a partial gastrectomy for peptic ulcer disease.

b   641 (a)   58. Which of the following statements suggest that he understands the dietary guidelines to prevent dumping syndrome?
a. "I will not eat ice cream for a snack."
b. "I will drink fluids between meals."
c. "I will avoid peanut butter."
d. "I will have raisin bran for breakfast."

d   641 (k)   59. Anemia after a gastrectomy is usually associated with all of the following *except*
a. blood loss.
b. malnutrition.
c. iron deficiencies.
d. deficiency of vitamin B_6.

For question 60: Mrs. Chang had gastric sugery six months ago. Since that time her diet has been advanced although she continues to experience dumping syndrome and frequent nausea and vomiting. Mrs. Chang's lab work reveals a hemoglobin of 14 g/dl and a hematocrit of 38%.

c   643 (a)   60. The most valid inference from these data is that Mrs. Chang has
a. bleeding from the colon.
b. steatorrhea.
c. anemia.
d. folate deficiency.

a   638 (k)   61. A sign of dumping syndrome is
a. tachycardia.
b. hyperglycemia.
c. hypervolemia.
d. edema.

a   642 (k)   62. All of the following meet the guidelines for a post-gastrectomy diet *except*
   a. liquids with meals.
   b. decrease simple sugar.
   c. small frequent meals.
   d. pectin added to meals.

b   642 (k)   63. Osteomalacia is associated with ___ of the bones.
   a. hardening
   b. softening
   c. building
   d. none of the above

c   711 (k)   64. Anemia may develop after a gastrectomy because
   a. surgery alters B_{12} absorption.
   b. folate rich foods are avoided.
   c. iron is absorbed poorly.
   d. lactose is absorbed poorly.

d   639 (k)   65. A characteristic of dumping syndrome is rapid digestion. Which of the following would be an expected outcome?
   a. increased blood glucose concentration
   b. hypoglycemia
   c. nausea
   d. all of the above

d   647 (a)   66. Which of the following is an example of a feeding skill that can be affected by disabilities?
   a. moving the tongue
   b. swallowing, sucking, and drinking
   c. hand control
   d. all of the above

a   648 (a)   67. In order to detect iron deficiency and protein status in patients with feeding disabilities, health care professionals monitor
   a. serum albumin concentrations.
   b. blood volume and body weight.
   c. plasma volume and fat folds.
   d. all of the above

   For questions 68 and 69: Mr. Henry is 58 years old and has developed severe arthritis that has affected his feeding ability.

d   648 (a)   68. What techniques can be used to assist Mr. Henry with
                             his inability to grasp feeding utensils?
                             a. allow Mr. Henry to finger food
                             b. cut food into small pieces
                             c. use plates with high, straight sides
                             d. all of the above

b   648(a)   69. What other strategies for developing feeding skill can be
                             most helpful to Mr. Henry?
                             a. strategies to improve chewing
                             b. strategies to improve hand-mouth coordination
                             c. strategies to improve swallowing
                             d. strategies to improve sucking

ESSAY QUESTIONS

1. Discuss the signs of dysphagia and explain how aging, Alzheimer's disease,
    and strokes may lead to dysphagia.

2. Illustrate the relationship of the upper GI tract to the diaphragm with reflux and
    with a hernia. Explain how these conditions develop.

3. Explain why dumping syndrome may occur in patients who have undergone
    gastric resectioning. What symptoms may be observed as a result of dumping
    syndrome?

4. Compare and contrast the symptoms and treatments of acute and chronic
    gastritis.

5. Describe strategies that can be used to contend with the inability to swallow,
    chew, and poor hand coordination associated with feeding disabilities.

Chapter 21
Nutrition and Lower GI Tract Disorders

d   652 (k)

1. Which of the following statements is true?
   a. Constipation is a condition of having difficult bowel movements.
   b. Constipation can become sever and form an obstruction.
   c. Constipation that is not treated can lead to peritonitis.
   d. all of the above

a   652 (k)

2. Which of the following is *not* a cause of constipation?
   a. excessive physical activity
   b. electrolyte imbalance
   c. chronic laxative abuse
   d. calcium supplements

d   652 (a)

3. Who would be at risk for developing constipation?
   a. Sarah, who is 30 weeks pregnant
   b. William, who is an 80-year-old man and lives in a nurslng home
   c. Joe, a CEO of a major company and is too busy to exercise
   d. all of the above

b   652 (a)

4. All of the following is included in medical nutrition therapy for constipation *except*
   a. prunes.
   b. low-fiber diet.
   c. plenty of fluids.
   d. regular physical activity.

1

c   653 (a)   5. A physician tells a client, experiencing constipation, about
                       foods that are high in fiber, like
                       a. cheddar cheese.
                       b. bananas.
                       c. legumes.
                       d. all of the above

a   653 (k)   6. Medications that help reduce intestinal gas production are
                       a. antiflatulents.
                       b. anticholinergics.
                       c. laxatives.
                       d. antidiarrheals.

d   654 (k)   7. Consequences of severe diarrhea include
                       a. weight loss.
                       b. dehydration.
                       c. multiple nutrient deficiencies.
                       d. all of the above

b   654(k)   8. Chronic diarrhea that is unresponsive to treatment is
                       known as
                       a. secretory diarrhea.
                       b. intractable diarrhea.
                       c. steatorrhea.
                       d. none of the above

d   654 (k)   9. Which of the following is known to cause chronic
                       diarrhea?
                       a. food intolerances
                       b. HIV infection
                       c. malabsorption
                       d. all of the above

b   654 (k)   10. Medication used as treatment for diarrhea is
                       a. laxatives.
                       b. antidiarrheal agents.
                       c. anti-infective agents.
                       d. a and b

a   654 (a)   11. Antidiarrheal agents are used for the treatment of diarrhea because
a. they slow GI motility, prolonging the time the toxin remains in contact with the GI cells.
b. they increase GI motility, prolonging the time the toxin remains in contact with the GI cells.
c. they decrease GI motility, decreasing the time the toxin remains in contact with the GI cells.
d. they increase GI motility, decreasing the time the toxin remains in contact with the GI cells.

For questions 12 and 13: Mrs. Thomas has been suffering from a mild case of diarrhea for the past 4 days.

d   654 (a)   12. Which of the following can Mrs. Thomas be given to replace fluid and electrolytes?
a. apple juice
b. sports drink
c. caffeine-free carbonated beverage
d. all of the above

c   654 (a)   13. Once the diarrhea stops, Mrs. Thomas should be given all of the following instructions *except*
a. gradually introduce a regular diet.
b. eat frequent, small meals.
c. high-fat foods are acceptable.
d. permanent dietary changes may be necessary.

For question 14: Mrs. Johnson is a 36-year-old female who enters the emergency room complaining of severe diarrhea of a four hour duration. Physical assessment findings reveal warm dry skin; decreased turgor; dry mucous membranes; and vital signs of T-99.6, P-104, R-24.

d   654 (a)   14. The nurse caring for Mrs. Johnson should
a. recommend over-the-counter antidiarrheal agents.
b. instruct Mrs. Johnson to remain NPO until the diarrhea subsides.
c. encourage a diet high in protein.
d. evaluate for possible fluid and electrolyte replacement.

a   654 (k)   15. If dehydration or vomiting accompanies diarrhea, then
_____ is typically used to replenish fluids and electrolytes.
a. IV solutions.
b. clear-liquid diet.
c. no fluids are permitted during this time.
d. none of the above

d   655 (k)   16. Symptoms associated with irritable bowel syndrome
include
a. indigestion, constipation, and bloating.
b. nausea, abdominal pain, and diarrhea.
c. flatulence and alternating diarrhea and constipation.
d. all of the above

d   655 (a)   17. Clients with irritable bowel syndrome should avoid foods
a. strongly seasoned.
b. containing sorbitol.
c. with caffeine.
d. all of the above

a   654 (k)   18. Oral rehydration solutions used in the treatment of
diarrhea contain
a. electrolytes.
b. minerals.
c. protein.
d. vitamins.

d   654 (k)   19. Food that may produce gas is
a. broccoli.
b. wheat.
c. fried foods.
d. all of the above

e   655 (k)   20. Medication prescribed to patients with irritable bowel
syndrome is
a. anticholinergics and antidiarrheals.
b. antidiarrheals and antimicrobials.
c. antidepressants and laxatives.
d. a and b
e. a and c

c   656 (k)

21. All of the following are symptoms of lactose intolerance *except*
    a. distention.
    b. diarrhea.
    c. constipation.
    d. cramping.

a   656 (k)

22. Among the following populations, which shows the highest prevalence of lactose intolerance?
    a. African Americans
    b. Caucasians
    c. Hispanics
    d. Scandinavians

b   656 (k)

23. The enzyme lactase splits lactose to ___ and ___.
    a. glucose, glucose
    b. glucose, galactose
    c. glucose, fructose
    d. glucose, sucrose

a   656 (a)

24. In general, most lactose-intolerant people can tolerate up to ___ cup(s) of milk a day when taken with food throughout the day.
    a. 1 to 2
    b. 2 to 3
    c. 3 to 4
    d. no milk can be tolerated

d   657 (k)

25. When milk and milk products are eliminated or restricted from the diet, what deficiencies can develop?
    a. iron
    b. vitamin D
    c. calcium
    d. b and c
    e. a, b, and c

b   657 (k)

26. Malabsorption syndromes more profoundly affect ___ absorption.
    a. carbohydrate
    b. fat
    c. protein
    d. all of the above

d   657 (a)

27. Anna has been diagnosed with steatorrhea. Regarding malabsorption what would the physician be concerned with?
    a. water-soluble vitamins
    b. fat-soluble vitamins
    c. essential fatty acids
    d. b and c
    e. a, b, and c

b   658 (k)

28. When calcium is unable to bind oxalate, it may lead to
    a. enteric hypoxaluria.
    b. kidney stones.
    c. hypercalemia.
    d. none of the above

c   659 (a)

29. A diet for a person with fat malabsorption syndrome would typically contain how many grams of fat?
    a. 15 to 25 grams
    b. 25 to 35 grams
    c. 35 to 45 grams
    d. 45 to 55 grams

d   660 (k)

30. How many servings of fat are allowed on a 35 gm fat-restricted diet?
    a. 0
    b. 1
    c. 2
    d. 3

d   660 (a)

31. Which of the following should be excluded from a fat-restricted diet?
    a. whole milk
    b. more than 3 servings of fat
    c. chocolate
    d. all of the above

a   660 (a)

32. Which of the following foods are appropriate for a fat-restricted diet?
    a. up to 6 oz. of lean meats and poultry (skinless)
    b. up to 5 oz. of lean meats and poultry (skinless)
    c. up to 6 servings of fat daily
    d. up to 5 servings of fat daily

c   659 (k)   33. MCT oil is commonly used in malabsorption syndromes
because
a. it is high in essential fatty acids.
b. the absorption occurs in the large intestine.
c. it does not require bile for absorption.
d. it can be delivered parenterally.

c   660 (a)   34. Which of the following menus *best* meets the objectives
of a fat-restricted diet for a client with steatorrhea?
a. tuna fish salad, crackers, ice cream, tea
b. baked chicken, macaroni and cheese, biscuits, milk
c. pork tenderloin, baked potato, applesauce, tea
d. sirloin steak, potato salad, broccoli augratin, milk

d   660 (a)   35. Which is the *best* dessert for a client on a fat-restricted
diet?
a. pudding
b. ice milk
c. cherry pie
d. sherbet

a   659 (k)   36. MCT contain at least how many carbon atoms?
a. 8
b. 10
c. 12
d. 14

b   659 (k)   37. What characteristics are associated with MCT?
a. Contains between 5 to 10 carbon atoms
b. Contains between 8 to 12 carbon atoms
c. Contains between 10 to 16 carbon atoms
d. None of the above

c   659 (k)   38. Pancreatic enzyme replacements is made from extracts
of ___ pancreatic enzymes to aid digestion.
a. beef
b. pork
c. a and b
d. none of the above

c   659 (k)   39. The body synthesizes oxalate through the pathway that begins with what vitamin?
a. A
b. B_{12}
c. C
d. D

b   661 (a)   40. The purpose of a tube inserted into the stomach for a client with acute pancreatitis is
a. to provide clear liquids.
b. for suction.
c. for medication delivery.
d. to begin enteral support.

b   661 (a)   41. Serum amylase levels are monitored in clients with pancreatitis to
a. establish the presence of lactose intolerance.
b. assess pancreatic function.
c. improve protein status.
d. evaluate the need for drug therapy.

a   661 (k)   42. The characteristics of diet therapy for pancreatitis include all of the following *except*
a. elimination of fat.
b. process from a liquid diet.
c. oral intake may resume after abdominal pain subsides.
d. avoidance of alcohol.

d   659 (a)   43. Health care professionals prescribe enzyme replacement therapy when patients have
a. severe steatorrhea.
b. severe damage to the pancreas.
c. problems with digestion.
d. all of the above

d   661 (a)   44. Mr. Bryant has been put on a fat-restricted diet. Which of the following suggestions can you give him to improve his acceptance of the diet?
a. Make Mr. Bryant aware of the wide variety of fat-free and low-fat products.
b. Provide Mr. Bryant with tips for maintaining high-fat in meals.
c. Advise Mr. Bryant to add MCT gradually.
d. a and c.
e. a, b, and c.

d   660 (k)   45. Which of the following nutrients are affected by the pancreas?
- a. carbohydrates
- b. fat
- c. protein
- d. all of the above

b   660 (k)   46. Pancreatitis is defined as
- a. production of a thick mucus that affects the pancreas.
- b. inflammation of the pancreas.
- c. ulceration along the pancreas.
- d. none of the above

a   661 (a)   47. Patients diagnosed with chronic pancreatitis should be cautioned to avoid
- a. large meals, fatty foods, and alcohol.
- b. red meats, sweets, and complex carbohydrates.
- c. carbohydrates, low-fat dairy products, and coffee.
- d. high-protein foods, food with a high-sucrose content, and caffeine.

For questions 48 and 49: Mrs. Adams is a 48-year-old woman who has the following symptoms: severe abdominal pain, nausea, vomiting, respiratory failure, and reduced blood volume.

c   660 (a)   48. From the information provided, what is Mrs. Adams' diagnosis?
- a. irritable bowel syndrome
- b. liver failure
- c. acute pancreatitis
- d. none of the above

c   661 (a)   49. What dietary treatment could be used for Mrs. Adams?
- a. IV fluids and electrolytes
- b. withholding food
- c. a and b
- d. none of the above

b   661 (k)   50. What is the most frequent cause of chronic pancreatitis?
- a. repeated episodes of acute pancreatitis
- b. alcohol abuse
- c. liver disease
- d. cystic firbrosis

c 661 (a) 51. What additional complication of chronic pancreatitis is a concern for physicians?
- a. dehydration
- b. kidney stones
- c. damage to cells that synthesize insulin and glucogen
- d. nausea

a 661 (k) 52. A hereditary disorder that causes the production of mucus that affects organ function is called
- a. cystic fibrosis
- b. pancreatitis
- c. crohn's disease
- d. none of the above

d 661 (k) 53. What organs can be affected by cystic fibrosis?
- a. pancreas
- b. liver
- c. heart
- d. all of the above

d 662 (a) 54. What are the energy needs of people with cystic fibrosis?
- a. 10 to 15 percent of the RDA
- b. 50 to 75 percent of the RDA
- c. 75 to 85 percent of the RDA
- d. 120 to 150 percent of the RDA

d 662 (k) 55. What information do dietitians use to estimate energy requirements in individuals with cystic fibrosis?
- a. basal metabolic rate
- b. activity level
- c. pulmonary function
- d. all of the above

c 663 (k) 56. An indication for enteral tube feeding a client with cystic fibrosis is
- a. inadequate sodium chloride intake.
- b. the need for water miscible forms of fat soluble vitamins.
- c. weight less than 85-90% of desirable weight for height.
- d. steatorrhea.

b   662 (k)   57. The most appropriate diet therapy for clients with cystic fibrosis is to
a. reduce fat to less than 35 grams per day.
b. supply missing enzymes.
c. limit kcalories to 1200 per day.
d. restrict sodium.

For question 58: Hakeem is a 22-year-old man with Crohn's disease. He is 5'8" and weighs 128 lbs. Upon assessment, he has steatorrhea and reports "having gas and diarrhea" when he consumes milk.

b   663 (a)   58. Based on this data, his diet order should be high-kcalorie, high-protein, and
a. iron restricted.
b. lactose restricted.
c. folate and selenium enriched.
d. no other restriction or enrichment.

c   662 (a)   59. Which of the following conditions results in fat malabsorption but with no need for a severe dietary fat restriction?
a. celiac disease
b. pancreatitis
c. cystic fibrosis
d. crohn's disease

c   663 (a)   60. Advanced malnutrition is indicated below what percentage of weight for patients with cystic fibrosis?
a. 65 %
b. 75 %
c. 85 %
d. 90 %

b   663 (k)   61. Inflammation and ulceration along the GI tract is called
a. irritable bowel syndrome.
b. crohn's disease.
c. pancreatitis.
d. cystic fibrosis.

c   664 (a)   62. Nutritional assessment of a client with Crohn's disease would include all of the following *except*
     a. serum albumin levels.
     b. hematocrit and hemoglobin levels.
     c. serum amylase.
     d. serum iron levels.

b   665 (k)   63. A hereditary disorder that causes a sensitivity to gliadin is called
     a. crohn's disease.
     b. celiac disease.
     c. cystic fibrosis.
     d. pancreatitis.

d   665 (a)   64. For patients with celiac disease, dietitians recommend adapting their diets by
     a. formulating a gluten-restricted diet.
     b. avoiding wheat.
     c. avoiding barley.
     d. all of the above

c   666 (a)   65. An appropriate food for a client with celiac disease is
     a. peanut butter and jelly sandwich.
     b. oatmeal cookies.
     c. applesauce.
     d. cheese and crackers.

a   663 (k)   66. Ulcerative colitis involves which section(s) of the gastrointestinal tract?
     a. large intestine
     b. small intestine
     c. jejunum and rectum
     d. biliary tract

d   664 (k)   67. Diet recommendations for a client with ulcerative colitis may include a
     a. high-fiber diet.
     b. high-protein diet.
     c. high-fat diet.
     d. diet without restrictions.

     For question 68: Mrs. Smith has ulcerative colitis and is scheduled for surgery in two days. Her nutrition status has been deteriorating.

c 664 (a) 68. Which of the following therapies is recommended for nutritional support?
   a. high-kcalorie and high-protein diet
   b. enteral feedings
   c. total parenteral nutrition
   d. clear liquid diet

a 668 (k) 69. Which of the following substances is thought to stimulate adaptation of intestine after a small bowel resection?
   a. glutamine
   b. raffinose
   c. stachyose
   d. oxalate

b 668 (a) 70. Short gut syndrome commonly results in
   a. hyperglycemia.
   b. hypocalcemia.
   c. hypokalemia.
   d. hyperphosphatemia.

b 669 (k) 71. Immediately after intestinal surgery, the primary nutritional effort should be to
   a. increase protein levels.
   b. replace fluids and electrolytes.
   c. provide kcalories.
   d. decrease gas formation.

d 672 (k) 72. Which of the following foods would be the *least* appropriate for a person with diverticulosis?
   a. whole-wheat bread
   b. low-fat milk
   c. raw carrots
   d. strawberries

a 672 (k) 73. Dietary recommendations for a person with diverticulosis include
   a. high-fiber diet.
   b. gluten-restricted diet.
   c. low-fat diet.
   d. diet without restrictions.

a   672 (k)   74. Clients with diverticular disease should
                 a. avoid foods with seeds.
                 b. avoid high-fiber foods.
                 c. restrict fluids.
                 d. increase fiber content quickly.

b   672 (k)   75. What dietary treatment is prescribed to patients suffering with diverticulosis?
                 a. low-fiber diet
                 b. high-fiber diet
                 c. high-fat diet
                 d. high-protein diet

b   669 (k)   76. Procedures that remove the rectum and anus are called
                 a. ileostomy.
                 b. colostomy.
                 c. stoma.
                 d. none of the above

d   671 (k)   77. An ileostomy is characterized by
                 a. formed stool.
                 b. bloody drainage.
                 c. absence of the small intestine.
                 d. loss of fluid and electrolytes.

ESSAY QUESTIONS

1. Discuss the causes of lactose intolerance and explain how calcium and vitamin D deficiencies can develop.

2. Discuss the complications associated with irritable bowel syndrome and how can diet modification be used for treatment.

3. Illustrate the effects of fat malabsorption and describe dietary recommendations used as treatment.

4. Give examples of inflammatory bowel diseases and discuss symptoms and complication and nutrition therapy.

5. What is cystic fibrosis and how is nutrition therapy used to minimize its symptoms?

6. Explain the effects of short-bowel syndrome. What factors affect absorption after small bowel surgery?

Chapter 22
Enteral Formulas

c   682 (k)

1. An enteral formula that is the primary source of all needed nutrients is a(n)
   a. standard formula.
   b. hydrolyzed formula.
   c. complete formula.
   d. isotonic formula.

b   683 (k)

2. Which one of the following formulas is *not* nutritionally complete?
   a. hydrolyzed
   b. modular
   c. protein isolate
   d. polymeric

b   682 (a)

3. A standard formula is to complete proteins as a modular formula is to
   a. broken-down proteins.
   b. single nutrient.
   c. polyunsaturated fat.
   d. saturated fat.

b   682 (k)

4. Standard formulas are used for clients who
   a. require large amounts of kcalories.
   b. are able to digest and absorb nutrients.
   c. are severely malnourished.
   d. require intravenous feedings.

c   682 (k)   5. An example of a protein isolate is
    a. albumin from egg.
    b. casein from milk.
    c. a and b
    d. none of the above

d   682 (k)   6. A characteristic of a hydrolyzed formula is
    a. low in fat.
    b. reduces amount of work needed for digestion.
    c. contains complete protein.
    d. a and b
    e. a, b, and c

d   683 (k)   7. Which of the following is true?
    a. Administering the appropriate modular formulas is very easy.
    b. Enteral formulas can be delivered orally or IV.
    c. Only enteral modules can be used to enhance the concentration of nutrients.
    d. Enteral or intravenous modules can alter formula composition.

d   683 (a)   8. Which of the following solutions provide the *most* energy and nutrients in the *smallest* volume?
    a. 0.5 kcal/ml
    b. 1.0 kcal/ml
    c. 1.5 kcal/ml
    d. 2.0 kcal/ml

a   683 (a)   9. Which of the following formulas has the greatest amount of free water?
    a. 1 kcal/ml
    b. 1.5 kcal/ml
    c. 1.5 kcal/ml, high-protein
    d. 2.0 kcal/ml

e   683 (k)   10. Formulas vary in the amount of
    a. fat.
    b. vitamins and minerals.
    c. carbohydrate.
    d. protein.
    e. all of the above

a   683 (k)

11. Most standard formulas have
    a. low-to-moderate residue content.
    b. high-residue content.
    c. no residue content.
    d. a and b

b   683 (a)

12. For clients suffering from constipation or diarrhea, health care professionals recommend increasing
    a. fat intake.
    b. fiber intake.
    c. vitamin intake.
    d. mineral intake.

d   683 (k)

13. An isotonic formula is
    a. approximately the osmolality of blood serum.
    b. about 300 mOsm/kg.
    c. above the osmolality of blood serum.
    d. a and b
    e. b and c

b   683 (k)

14. A formula with an osmolality above serum is known as a(n)
    a. isotonic formula.
    b. hypertonic formula.
    c. enteral formula.
    d. complete formula.

b   683 (a)

15. Daniel Davis is suffering from abnormal digestion and absorption. The physician orders Daniel to be placed on enteral nutrition. What type of formula would be prescribed?
    a. standard formula
    b. hydrolyzed formula
    c. polymeric formula
    d. modular formula

d   688 (a)

16. When determining nutrient requirements for patients, which of the following should be considered?
    a. medical condition
    b. nutrition status
    c. metabolic rate
    d. all of the above

d   685 (k)   17. Which of the following can be used as an indication for tube feeding?
a. PEM with inadequate oral intake for 5 or more days
b. metabolic stress
c. severe dysphasia
d. all of the above

a   685 (a)   18. What do severe diarrhea and severe acute pancreatitis have in common?
a. contraindications of tube feeding
b. indications of tube feeding
c. both require special formulas
d. Tube feeding is the preferred method for nutrition support.

c   685 (k)   19. The preferred feeding tube placement site for infants is
a. nasoduodenal.
b. nasogastric.
c. orogastric.
d. none of the above

c   686 (k)   20. An opening in the stomach through which a feeding tube can be passed is called a(n)
a. enterostomy.
b. endoscopic jejunostomy.
c. gastrostomy.
d. duodenostomy.

For question 21: Mr. Heiman has multiple sclerosis with dysphagia. He is 5'8" and weighs 127 lbs.

d   686 (a)   21. The most appropriate method of nutrition support for him would be
a. total parenteral nutrition.
b. peripheral parenteral nutrition.
c. liquid supplements.
d. gastrostomy feedings.

d   686 (a)   22. Which of the following is the most appropriate feeding tube site for a 30-year-old man with multiple sclerosis and severe dysphagia?
a. nasogastric.
b. esophagostomy.
c. orogastric.
d. jejunostomy.

For question 23: Mr. Smith is 63 years old with Alzheimer's disease.

c   686 (a)   23. He has an order for a feeding tube because he refuses to eat and is becoming malnourished. Which of the following feeding tubes would be a good choice?
a. nasogastric.
b. nasoduodenal.
c. gastrostomy.
d. transnasal.

d   684 (k)   24. An advantage of enteral nutrition is
a. normal gut function is maintained.
b. costs less than IV.
c. enhanced wound healing during critical illness.
d. all of the above

b   686 (k)   25. A disadvantage of transnasal tube placement is
a. it is not an effective means for tube feeding.
b. the tube can be easily pulled out.
c. the tube is inserted through the nose.
d. the tube can be passed to the jejunum.

a   686 (k)   26. Which of the following feeding sites is appropriate for clients requiring long-term nutrition support?
a. enterostomy
b. nasoentric
c. nasogastric
d. orogastric

c   686 (k)   27. Placement of feeding tubes that may require a surgical procedure is
a. nasogastric.
b. nasojejunal.
c. enterostomy.
d. nasoduodenal.

a   686 (k)   28. Which of the following tube sites has a high risk of aspiration?
a. nasogastric
b. nasoduodenal
c. transnasal
d. jejunostomy

For questions 29 and 30: Mr. Brown is suffering from delayed gastric emptying. Answer the following questions regarding his nutrition support.

b   686 (a)

29. The health care team acknowledges which feeding site to be appropriate for Mr. Brown?
    a. oral feeding
    b. nasoentric feeding
    c. orogastric feeding
    d. intravenous feeding

d   687 (a)

30. Which of the following conditions requires special consideration when determining the feeding tube site for Mr. Brown?
    a. Mr. Brown's cooperation
    b. irritation of the esophagus
    c. long-term tolerance
    d. aspiration pneumonia

c   687 (k)

31. The final location of the feeding tube determines the
    a. size of the tube.
    b. type of formula.
    c. type of feeding.
    d. duration of the feeding.

b   686 (k)

32. Which of the following is less likely to cause regurgitation?
    a. gastric feeding
    b. intestinal feedings
    c. nasogastric feeding
    d. none of the above

b   687 (k)

33. The major disadvantage of intestinal feeding is
    a. loss of control of the pyloric sphincter.
    b. loss of control of stomach emptying.
    c. loss of control of the cardiac sphincter.
    d. delivery of formulas can be initiated early.

b   690 (k)

34. Proper sterile techniques should be used during preparation and delivery of formulas to protect patients from
    a. receiving the wrong formula.
    b. exposure to food-borne illness.
    c. malnutrition.
    d. dehydration.

For question 35: Mr. Seymour is a 56-year-old man with cancer who is 5'8" tall and weighs 130 lbs. His appetite has been poor and he is started on bolus feeding of a 1 kcal/ml formula. Within 24 hours he has increased his weight by 2.5 lbs.

b   692 (a)   35. The appropriate intervention is to
    a. realize he needs more calories.
    b. recognize this represents a likely fluid gain.
    c. change to intermittent feedings.
    d. increase the protein content of his feeding.

For question 36: Tom Teenager is a 15-year-old who is eating some but must also receive enteral feeding for malnutrition associated with Crohn's disease.

b   687 (a)   36. To help Tom carry on normal activities, the health care team might try
    a. bolus feedings.
    b. feeding at night only.
    c. neon colored feeding tube.
    d. all of the above

c   690 (k)   37. Techniques used to prevent the risk of bacterial contamination include all of the following *except*:
    a. flush the feeding tube before and after each use.
    b. change the feeding bags every 8 to 12 hours in an open system.
    c. mix new formula with remaining formula into one bag.
    d. discard open containers of formula not used within 24 hours.

d   691 (a)   38. Intermittent feeding using the gravity drip is the delivery of no more than how much formula over 30 minutes?
    a. 100 ml
    b. 200 ml
    c. 300 ml
    d. 400 ml

b   690 (k)   39. Which of the following statements is true?
a. Open feeding system reduces the risk of bacterial contamination.
b. Enteral formula delivery system ready to be attached to a feeding tube is called a closed feeding system.
c. Formulas in cans, bottles, or powders can all be used in a closed feeding system.
d. none of the above

d   692 (k)   40. Typically, adults require ___ of water daily.
a. 1000 milliliters
b. 1500 milliliters
c. 1750 milliliters
d. 2000 milliliters

b   694 (k)   41. Possible complications of a nutritionally complete tube feeding include all of the following *except*
a. aspiration.
b. hypoproteinemia.
c. dehydration.
d. fluid overload.

For question 42:   Mr. Thomas is receiving an enteral feeding product at 60 cc/hr by continuous drip. At 2:00 p.m. it is time to hang an additional feeding product since there is only 40 cc left in the feeding bag.

b   690 (a)   42. If you decide to continue the feeding, you should
a. pour new feeding into the bag with the remaining 40 cc.
b. let the remaining feeding infuse prior to adding new product.
c. add 20 cc of feeding because your shift ends at 3:00 pm.
d. check your institution's policy regarding hang time.

For question 43: Claire Wilson is an 80-year-old woman on a tube feeding. Upon assessment, her blood pressure is 90/72, serum sodium 146 mEq/l, and a potassium level of 5.6 mEq/l.

d   694 (a)   43. These findings indicate
       a. hypertension.
       b. overhydration.
       c. hyponatremia.
       d. dehydration.

For question 44: Mrs. Arthur is receiving an enteral feeding ready-to-feed formula continuously over 24 hours. She is not on fluid restriction.

c   692 (a)   44. Mrs. Arthur will receive ___ of formula each hour.
       a. 42 ml
       b. 63 ml
       c. 83 ml
       d. none of the above

For question 45: Mr. Simpson is receiving formula intermittently six times a day. He needs 1500 ml in 24 hours.

a   692 (a)   45. How many milliliters of formula is Mr. Simpson receiving at each feeding?
       a. 250
       b. 333
       c. 9000
       d. 12000

For question 46: Mrs. Smith, a client with congestive heart failure, requires 2000 kcal/day. She is receiving a formula with 2 kcal/ml by continuous drip.

b   692 (a)   46. How many milliliters of formula will be given each hour?
       a. 33
       b. 42
       c. 66
       d. 83

c   691 (k)   47. The delivery of up to 300 to 400 ml of formula within 10 minutes is termed
       a. minimal residual.
       b. intermittent feeding.
       c. bolus feeding.
       d. continuous drip.

c   693 (k)

48. Which of the following nursing interventions is appropriate for the delivery of medications through a feeding tube?
    a. Flush feeding tube with water before and after medication.
    b. Give only time release medications through the feeding tube.
    c. Discontinue the tube feeding every hour to enhance drug absorption.
    d. Rinse feeding tube with a solution of meat tenderizer and sterile water before and after medication is administered.

c   695 (k)

49. Daily assessment data to be collected on a client on a feeding tube should include all of the following *except*
    a. intake and output.
    b. body weight.
    c. fat fold measurements.
    d. assessing breath sounds.

c   694 (a)

50. Possible causes of diarrhea in a tube fed client are all of the following *except*
    a. lactose.
    b. bacterial contamination.
    c. opiates.
    d. hypertonic solutions.

c   693 (a)

51. Sarah has been receiving enteral nutrition support for the past 4 days. She has developed diarrhea. What is the most likely culprit?
    a. allergies
    b. dehydration
    c. medication
    d. low-fat formula

a   694 (a)

52. A client who would be the *least* likely to develop diarrhea on a tube feeding is one
    a. with a serum albumin level of 4.0 g/dl.
    b. receiving potassium chloride.
    c. receiving an elixir diluted with sorbitol.
    d. taking magnesium containing antacids.

d   696 (k)   53. Which of the following should be included in medical records regarding tube-feeding?
     a. clients' response to tube insertion
     b. method of delivery
     c. administration schedule
     d. all of the above

     For question 54: Mr. Thomas is receiving an enteral feeding product at 60 cc/hr by continuous drip. At 2:00 p.m., it is time to hang additional feeding product since there are only 40 cc left in the feeding bag.

d   692 (a)   54. When you check the residual you note that there is 50 cc of gastric contents, so you should
     a. stop the feeding and contact the physician.
     b. stop the feeding, irrigate the tube, and then contact the physician.
     c. continue the feeding but decrease the rate to 50 cc/hr.
     d. continue the feeding as ordered.

c   692 (k)   55. In general, gastric residual is considered excessive between
     a. 25 to 50 ml.
     b. 50 to 100 ml.
     c. 100 to 200 ml.
     d. 200 to 300 ml.

b   701 (k)   56. All of the following statements are true *except*
     a. Inborn errors of metabolism are inherited and present at birth.
     b. All inborn errors of metabolism are fatal.
     c. PKU is an inborn error of amino acid metabolism.
     d. Galactosemia is an inborn error of carbohydrate metabolism.

ESSAY QUESTIONS

1. Explain how health care professionals determine the appropriate formula for enteral nutrition.

2. Differentiate between standard formulas, hydrolyzed formulas, complete formulas, and modular formulas. Give examples of situations where these formulas can be used.

3. Describe the various tube sites and provide advantages and disadvantages for each.

4. Explain how diarrhea, hyperglycemia, and constipation can be complications related to tube-feeding. How are these complications corrected?

5. Discuss the complications and medical nutrition therapy associated with PKU.

Chapter 23
Parenteral Nutrition

c   706 (k)

1. Delivery of nutrient solutions directly into the vein is called
   a. standard nutrition.
   b. enteral nutrition.
   c. parenteral nutrition.
   d. tube feeding.

d   707 (k)

2. An IV solution may contain which of the following essential nutrients?
   a. vitamins and minerals
   b. water
   c. fat
   d. all of the above

d   707 (k)

3. Which of the following conditions require special considerations regarding amino acid content of IV solutions?
   a. recovery from stress
   b. liver failure
   c. following intestinal resections
   d. all of the above

a   707 (k)

4. Which of the following forms of glucose is available in IV solutions?
   a. dextrose
   b. fructose
   c. lactose
   d. glucose

1

b   707 (k)   5. How much energy does glucose provide?
- a. 3 kcal/g
- b. 4 kcal/g
- c. 5 kcal/g
- d. 6 kcal/g

a   707 (k)   6. How much energy does dextrose provide?
- a. 3.4 kcal/g
- b. 4.0 kcal/g
- c. 4.4 kcal/g
- d. 5.0 kcal/g

a   707 (k)   7. The protein in a TPN solution is primarily in the form of
- a. amino acids.
- b. protein hydrolysate.
- c. short chain fatty acids.
- d. intact protein.

d   707 (a)   8. A physician writes an order for Mrs. Wilson to receive IV fat twice a week. The purpose of this order is to
- a. provide essential amino acids.
- b. provide nonessential amino acids.
- c. serve as an energy source.
- d. serve as a source of essential fatty acids.

c   707 (k)   9. When fat is administered IV on a daily basis, what is the main objective?
- a. IV fat serves as a concentrated source of essential fatty acids.
- b. IV fat serves as a concentrated source of essential amino acids.
- c. IV fat serves as a concentrated energy source.
- d. all of the above

b   707 (a)   10. A 250 ml bottle of 10% IV fat emulsion provides how much energy?
- a. 200 kcalories
- b. 275 kcalories
- c. 500 kcalories
- d. 550 kcalories

c   707 (a)

11. A 20% IV fat emulsion provides how many kcalories per ml?
   a. 1.0
   b. 1.1
   c. 2.0
   d. 2.1

d   707 (k)

12. Caution should be taken when administering IV lipids to people with which condition?
   a. atherosclerosis
   b. blood coagulation disorders
   c. pancreatitis
   d. all of the above

c   708 (k)

13. The purpose of short term infusion of simple IV solutions is all of the following *except*
   a. maintain acid-base balance.
   b. maintain fluid and electrolyte balance.
   c. provide complete nutritional support.
   d. provide fluid and kcal support.

a   708 (a)

14. Beth has just been placed in recovery following a knee surgery. What intravenous feeding do you expect she will receive during this time?
   a. simple IV solutions
   b. total parenteral nutrition
   c. peripheral parenteral nutrition
   d. no intravenous feeding is required

d   707 (k)

15. The FDA recently issued new specifications for IV multivitamin solutions and added
   a. vitamin C.
   b. vitamin D.
   c. vitamin E.
   d. vitamin K.

For question 16: Joan Sussman is in her second trimester of pregnancy and has experienced hyperemesis gravidarum for 14 days.

d   710 (a)

16. At this point she is a candidate for
   a. peripheral total parenteral nutrition.
   b. central total parenteral nutrition.
   c. peripheral total parenteral nutrition with fat emulsion.
   d. central total parenteral nutrition with fat emulsion.

d   708 (k)   17. Which of the following is an example of a medication that
                            can be added to IV solutions?
                            a. ranitidine
                            b. heparin
                            c. insulin
                            d. all of the above

b   709 (a)   18. How many grams of amino acids would be provided to a
                            client receiving 2,000 ml of a 5% amino acid solution?
                            a. 50 grams
                            b. 100 grams
                            c. 200 grams
                            d. 400 grams

b   709 (a)   19. The amount of kcalories in 3 liters of 5% dextrose
                            solution is
                            a. 150.
                            b. 510.
                            c. 600.
                            d. 660.

c   708 (k)   20. The purpose of an IV of 5% dextrose solution is to
                            a. provide adequate calories.
                            b. decrease the incidence of diarrhea.
                            c. provide fluid.
                            d. prevent aspiration.

b   709 (a)   21. What is the amount of dextrose a person would get if
                            they were receiving 2000 milliliters of 50% dextrose?
                            a. 750 grams
                            b. 1000 grams
                            c. 1250 grams
                            d. none of the above

c   709 (a)   22. Suppose a person is receiving 2000 milliliters of 10%
                            amino acid solution. What is the amount of amino acids?
                            a. 100 grams
                            b. 150 grams
                            c. 200 grams
                            d. 250 grams

d   710 (k)   23. Candidates for PPN are patients
                     a. who are unable to use their GI tracts for long periods.
                     b. who are malnourished.
                     c. who have high nutrients needs.
                     d. all of the above

c   708 (k)   24. Veins that are small in diameter and carry blood from the arms and legs are the
                     a. central veins.
                     b. hepatic veins.
                     c. peripheral veins.
                     d. portal veins.

a   708 (k)   25. Complete nutrient solutions delivered through the central veins provide ___ percent from dextrose.
                     a. 70-85
                     b. 60-75
                     c. 50-65
                     d. 40-55

a   709 (k)   26. A characteristic of PPN is
                     a. IV lipid emulsion provides concentrated source of kcalories.
                     b. dextrose solution provides concentrated source of energy.
                     c. a small volume of fluid is required.
                     d. a and c

a   710 (k)   27. A method of infusing formula into a large-diameter central vein for meeting all nutrient needs is called
                     a. central total parenteral nutrition.
                     b. peripheral parenteral nutrition.
                     c. simple IV solution.
                     d. all of the above

c   708 (k)   28. A typical simple IV solution provides approximately how much energy per day?
                     a. 150 kcalories
                     b. 250 kcalories
                     c. 500 kcalories
                     d. 700 kcalories

b   708 (k)   29. The large-diameter veins are located near the
                        a. extremities.
                        b. heart.
                        c. liver.
                        d. lungs.

d   711 (k)   30. Conditions that may require the need for TPN by central
                        vein include
                        a. GI tract obstructions.
                        b. HIV infection.
                        c. bone marrow transplants.
                        d. all of the above

d   710 (k)   31. A client receiving 3000 kcal per day via parenteral
                        nutrition should
                        a. have it administered via peripheral vein.
                        b. receive dextrose and amino acids only.
                        c. have it administered in bolus form.
                        d. be given nutrition by the central venous route.

d   712 (k)   32. In order to prevent the development of hyperglycemia,
                        what is the recommended maximum amount of
                        carbohydrate in a TPN solution that should be provided
                        daily?
                        a. 4 g/kg body weight
                        b. 5 g/kg body weight
                        c. 6 g/kg body weight
                        d. 7 g/kg body weight

c   713 (a)   33. Which of the following nursing interventions is *not*
                        indicated for a client receiving TPN?
                        a. monitor weights
                        b. maintain input and output records
                        c. speed up the flow rate if the solution gets behind to
                           meet the day's volume
                        d. check blood glucose

                        For question 34: Mr. Rodriguez has been stable on a
                        standard TPN solution for three weeks. During this time
                        his blood glucose has been 150 mg/dl. You check his
                        blood glucose at 10:00 a.m. and it is 240 mg/dl.

d   712 (a)   34. The most likely explanation is
                    a. the dextrose in the TPN solution.
                    b. hypocalcemia.
                    c. refeeding syndrome.
                    d. infection.

                    For question 35: Judy Smith is a 36-year-old who just
                    had bowel resection. She is expected to be NPO for
                    approximately seven days.

b   710 (a)   35. Which of the following would be appropriate nutrition
                    support?
                    a. peripheral total parenteral nutrition
                    b. central total parenteral nutrition
                    c. simple IV solutions with amino acids
                    d. enteral feeding via nasogstric tube

                    For question 36: Susan Taylor is a 59-year-old
                    accountant who sustained multiple abdominal injuries in
                    a motor vehicle accident. She is allergic to sulpha drugs,
                    eggs, and seafood.

b   710 (a)   36. Her nutritional needs will most likely be met by
                    a. peripheral total parenteral nutrition.
                    b. central total parenteral nutrition.
                    c. peripheral total parenteral nutrition with fat emulsions.
                    d. central total parenteral nutrition with fat emulsions.

d   712 (k)   37. An example of catheter or care-related complications
                    associated with intravenous nutrition is
                    a. thrombosis.
                    b. sepsis.
                    c. improperly positioned catheter tip.
                    d. all of the above

a   712 (k)   38. Nutrition-related complications that may develop from
                    intravenous nutrition include all of the following *except*
                    a. hypoammonemia.
                    b. hypoglycemia.
                    c. vitamin and mineral deficiencies.
                    d. dehydration.

e   713 (k)   39. To ensure a patient who is receiving TPN is adapting to the formula, health care professionals monitor
a. electrolyte balance.
b. blood glucose concentration.
c. vital signs.
d. a and b
e. a, b, and c

b   712 (k)   40. Which of the following is correct?
a. The desired volume of TPN solution is immediately provided to the patient.
b. If the administration of solution gets off schedule, the drip rate can be adjusted to the correct hourly infusion rate.
c. After the first 24 hours of starting TPN, infusion rate is decreased by 1 liter a day until the desired volume is being given every 24 hours.
d. None of the above

For questions 41, 42, and 43: The health care team has just ordered Mr. Carter to be put on TPN. He is a 58-year-old man who is suffering from intractable diarrhea.

a   713 (a)   41. Before Mr. Carter starts TPN, what biochemical analysis should be performed?
a. x-ray
b. body mass index
c. calcium balance
d. hand grip strength

d   713 (a)   42. Which of the following should be monitored daily while Mr. Carter is on TPN?
a. input and output
b. body weight
c. catheter site
d. all of the above

c   713 (a)   43. On a weekly basis, the health care team should perform what part of the nutrition care process?
a. analyze assessment data
b. develop a health care plan
c. assess nutrition status
d. implement the nutrition care plan

c   713 (k)   44. The benefits of cyclic infusion of TPN include

                          a. maintenance of high-insulin levels.
                          b. increase in fat stores.
                          c. use of body fat for energy.
                          d. achievement of a negative nitrogen balance.

For question 45: Courtney Troxclair, age three months, has necrotizing enterocolitis. Prior to initiation of TPN, blood tests show:

total protein 7.5 g/dl	hematocrit of 44%
blood urea nitrogen 10 mg/dl	bilirubin 5 mg/dl
blood glucose 80 mg/dl	

c   707 (a)   45. Based on these findings, the TPN solution should contain low levels of

                          a. dextrose.
                          b. amino acids.
                          c. lipids.
                          d. iron.

For question 46: Mary Jones, a 69-year-old diabetic, has been receiving TPN with fat emulsions. She complains of a backache, chills, nausea, and chest pain.

d   712 (a)   46. The *most* likely cause of these symptoms is

                          a. an infection.
                          b. hypoglycemia.
                          c. hyperglycemia.
                          d. a reaction to the fat emulsions.

a   713 (k)   47. Which of the following measurements should be done daily for a client receiving TPN?

                          a. weights
                          b. serum calcium
                          c. serum ammonia
                          d. CBC

For question 48: Sue Watson is receiving 3 liters of a standard TPN solution with 500 m. of a 10% IV lipid emulsion to be hung piggyback three times per week. As the lipid emulsion is being infused for the first time, Ms. Watson becomes chilled and begins wheezing.

d   712 (a)   48. The *most* appropriate intervention is to
- a. continue the TPN and the emulsion as this is a normal and temporary reaction.
- b. continue the TPN and emulsion but call the doctor *stat.*
- c. remove the TPN and the emulsion and notify the doctor when he arrives in 30 minutes.
- d. continue the TPN, remove the emulsion and call the doctor *stat.*

a   712 (k)   49. Reactions to large amounts or rapid administration of IV lipids including chest pains, nausea, palpitations, and cyanosis can be avoided by receiving small amounts of lipid emulsion every
- a. 15 to 30 minutes.
- b. 30 to 60 minutes.
- c. one hour.
- d. Emulsion should be avoided.

c   713 (a)   50. A person on a cyclic parenteral nutrition receives an infusion at a constant rate for
- a. 3 to 6 hours per day.
- b. 6 to 8 hours per day.
- c. 8 to 12 hours per day.
- d. 12 to 14 hours per day.

c   714 (k)   51. Before parenteral nutrition is discontinued, oral intake, tube feeding, or a combination should provide at least what percent of the estimated energy needs?
- a. 50 %
- b. 60 %
- c. 70 %
- d. 80 %

a   713 (a)   52. Which of the following would be the *best* method of delivery of long-term TPN to a 14-year-old?
- a. cyclic infusion
- b. PPN
- c. central TPN
- d. central TPN with lipids five times a week

For question 53: Greg Thomas is a 12-year-old who is being weaned off of TPN. In addition to TPN, Greg is on a soft diet. Greg is 5'2" and weighs 110 lbs. His caloric count reveals he is consuming 1700 kcal/dl.

a   714 (a)   53. Which intervention is appropriate at this time?
a. discontinue TPN
b. oral feeding should be doubled
c. enteral feeding should be considered
d. TPN should be increased to provide an additional 1100 kcal

d   713 (k)   54. When long-term TPN is discontinued, oral feedings are gradually reintroduced because of all of the following reasons *except*
a. intestinal villi may have shrunk.
b. malabsorption may occur.
c. bloating may occur.
d. albumin levels may have dropped.

c   713 (k)   55. An advantage to cyclic parenteral infusion often used in home parenteral programs is
a. a decrease in the cost of the solution.
b. the elimination of the need for a pump.
c. a decrease in the incidence of fatty infiltration of the liver.
d. the ease with which clients can prepare IV solutions.

a   713 (a)   56. Which of the following clients would *not* be a candidate for home cyclic TPN program?
a. an 86-year-old with congestive heart failure
b. a 36-year-old with Crohn's disease
c. a 52-year-old with cancer
d. an 18-year-old with radiation enteritis

a   715 (k)   57. What is the common objective for home enteral and parenteral nutrition tube feedings and TPN in the hospital?
a. to achieve or maintain adequate nutrition status
b. to provide familiar surroundings
c. to allow significant patient participation in treatment
d. to provide constant monitoring by health care professionals

d   716 (k)   58. An example of a condition that utilizes home TPN as a means for maintaining adequate nutrition status is
a. cancer.
b. Crohn's disease.
c. HIV infection.
d. all of the above

c   716 (K)   59. The current average cost of a home parenteral nutrition program is approximately
a. $50,000.
b. $60,000.
c. $70,000.
d. $80,000.

d   722 (k)   60. Which of the following statements is true?
a. JCAHO is an agency responsible for overseeing the accreditation of health care facilities.
b. JCAHO requires health care facilities' nutrition care standards to identify, address, and monitor each client's nutrition requirements.
c. JCAHO requires health care facilities' nutrition care standards to promote coordination and communication across disciplines.
d. all of the above

c   722 (k)   61. A health care delivery system aimed at providing cost-effective health care by coordinating services and limiting access to services is called
a. capitation.
b. HMO.
c. managed care.
d. none of the above

ESSAY QUESTIONS

1. Discuss nutrients that can be administered by vein.

2. Compare simple IV solutions, PPN solutions, and central TPN solutions. Give examples of conditions that would utilize each intravenous feeding method.

3. Discuss possible complications associated with intravenous nutrition and how clients receiving parenteral nutrition are monitored.

4. Describe how PPN and central TPN solutions are started and discontinued. How are they different?

5. Discuss how home enteral and parenteral programs are developed and give examples of candidates who would benefit from such programs.

Chapter 24
Nutrition in Severe Stress

1. Stresses that cause disruption to the body's internal balance that lie beyond its normal and healthy functioning is called
   a. pathological stresses.
   b. severe stresses.
   c. physiological stresses.
   d. none of the above

2. In response to severe stress, the body experiences
   a. hypermetabolism.
   b. increased mobilization into glucose and amino acids.
   c. synthesis of factors to regain homeostasis.
   d. all of the above

3. Metabolic responses observed during stress are mediated by factors that include
   a. immune system responses.
   b. hormonal responses.
   c. inflammatory responses.
   d. all of the above

4. Cytokines are proteins that help regulate ___ responses.
   a. immune system
   b. inflammatory
   c. hormonal
   d. GI tract

d   727 (k)   5. Which of the following is an example of a condition that can lead to severe stress?
a. surgery
b. burns
c. infection
d. all of the above

b   728 (k)   6. Shock is characterized by a sudden drop in
a. blood pressure.
b. blood volume.
c. heart rate.
d. respiratory rate.

b   729 (k)   7. Insulin acts to
a. promote the storage of carbohydrate, lipids, and protein breakdown.
b. promote the storage of carbohydrate, lipids and synthesis of protein.
c. promote the synthesis of protein, and carbohydrate and lipid utilization.
d. promote the storage of lipid, and carbohydrate and protein utilization.

d   729 (k)   8. An example of a counterregulatory hormone that opposes the actions of insulin is
a. cortisol.
b. catecholamines.
c. glucagons.
d. all of the above

c   729 (k)   9. Hypermetabolism generally peaks at ___ days of a stress response.
a. 1 to 2
b. 2 to 3
c. 3 to 4
d. 4 to 5

b   729 (k)   10. The correct order of the stress response phases is
a. acute, adaptive, exhaustion, and recovery.
b. acute, adaptive, recovery, and exhaustion.
c. adaptive, acute, exhaustion, and recovery.
d. adaptive, acute, recovery, and exhaustion.

d   729 (k)   11. To respond to stress, ___ is sacrificed to supply glucose
to amino acids.
a. connective tissue.
b. gut tissue.
c. skeletal muscle.
d. all of the above

d   730 (k)   12. Which of the following hormones promote glucose
production from amino acids during severe stress?
a. aldosterone
b. cortisol
c. catecholamines
d. b and c
e. a, b, and c

b   730 (k)   13. Which of the following hormones promote glycogen
breakdown?
a. catecholamines and cortisol
b. catecholamines and glucagon
c. cortisol and glucagon
d. aldosterone and catecholamines

a   730 (k)   14. Which of the following hormones increase water
retention?
a. antidiuretic hormone
b. aldosterone
c. a and b
d. none of the above

c   728 (k)   15. Sepsis develops when
a. an infection becomes localized in an area.
b. immune factors attack the foreign substances.
c. infectious microorganisms or their by-products invade
the bloodstream.
d. none of the above

b   729 (k)   16. As a result of immune and inflammatory responses to
stress, all of the following changes occur except
a. swelling at the injury site.
b. lower respiratory rate.
c. lower serum iron and zinc concentrations.
d. pain at the injury site.

a   729 (k)   17. The changes that are observed from activation of immune and inflammatory factors during stress are collectively called
    a. systemic inflammatory response syndrome.
    b. stress responses.
    c. immune system responses.
    d. none of the above

c   729 (k)   18. During stress, which of the following physiological responses would be expected?
    a. hypoglycemia
    b. decrease in calorie requirements
    c. negative nitrogen balance
    d. sodium depletion

c   731 (k)   19. Which of the following physiological stressors lowers kcalorie requirements?
    a. elective surgery
    b. infection
    c. negative nitrogen balance
    d. sodium depletion

b   731 (a)   20. What does hypermetabolism, infection, and pressure sores have in common?
    a. they decrease nutrient intake
    b. they increase nutrient needs
    c. they promote excessive nutrient losses
    d. they don't affect nutrition status

d   731 (a)   21. During conditions of fasting, the body responds by
    a. reducing the use of glucose.
    b. producing ketone bodies from energy.
    c. reducing the metabolic rate.
    d. all of the above

e   731 (a)   22. In response to simple fasting, the body
    a. works to conserve its vital proteins.
    b. begins to draw on fat stores to provide ketone bodies.
    c. increases body temperature.
    d. a and c
    e. a and b

d   727 (a)   23. Mr. Smith is a 50-year-old man who sustained multiple broken bones in a car accident. Upon assessment, he is hyperglycemic and edematous. The health care professional should
a. call the physician.
b. suspect undiagnosed diabetes.
c. institute a low-kcalorie, low-sodium diet.
d. recognize these signs are associated with stress.

a   729 (k)   24. The predominant source of endogenous glucose during severe stress is
a. amino acids.
b. glycerol.
c. free-fatty acids.
d. ketones.

b   730 (k)   25. Which of the following systems is among the first to suffer the effects of PEM?
a. skin
b. GI tract
c. kidney
d. cardiac

c   730 (k)   26. An example of an organ that is among the first to be affected by protein degradation is the
a. heart.
b. lungs.
c. GI tract.
d. liver.

b   734 (k)   27. Which of the following are nonessential amino acids?
a. aspartic acid and arginine
b. arginine and glutamine
c. glycine and glutamine
d. alanine and glycine

For questions 28, 29, and 30: Betty is a 45-year-old woman who has recently been involved in an automobile accident. Her injuries include a broken leg and two broken ribs.

d 729 (a) 28. What clinical findings do you expect to find?
      a. hyperglycemia
      b. elevated blood urea nitrogen
      c. increased fluid and sodium retention
      d. all of the above

d 730 (a) 29. In response to her injuries, what hormonal changes do
      you expect Betty will have?
      a. increase in catecholamine excretion
      b. increase in antidiuretic hormone and aldosterone
       release
      c. decrease in cortisol production
      d. a and b
      e. a, b and c

c 727 (k) 30. Inflammatory responses at the injury site would include
      all of the following *except*
      a. slows blood flow.
      b. shrinks diameter of blood vessels.
      c. decreased capillary permeability.
      d. increased flow of immune factors to the site.

a 729 (k) 31. Elevated blood urea nitrogen is attributed to
      a. protein catabolism.
      b. hyperglycemia.
      c. fatty acid catabolism.
      d. all of the above

d 730 (a) 32. During severe stress, the body's protein needs increase
      in order to
      a. produce immune factors.
      b. maintain physical work.
      c. provide inflammatory responses.
      d. a and b
      e. a, b and c

      For question 33: Mr. Watson is a 50-year-old man who
      is 5'10" and weighs 145 lbs. He has lost 25 lbs. over the
      past month and reports "not wanting to eat after his wife
      died." His serum albumin is 4.0 g/dl and his total
      lymphocyte count is normal.

a   730 (a)   33. Which subtype of PEM is suggested by these assessment data?
- a. chronic malnutrition
- b. acute malnutrition
- c. mixed malnutrition
- d. no malnutrition identified

d   731 (k)   34. Which of the following is a possible cause of malnutrition associated with acute stress?
- a. anorexia
- b. hypermetabolism
- c. immobility
- d. all of the above

b   730 (a)   35. Which condition is more likely to require immediate nutrition support for a patient during severe stress?
- a. fasting
- b. PEM
- c. acute malnutrition
- d. none of the above

b   730 (k)   36. Clinical signs of acute malnutrition include
- a. adequate body weight and adequate serum proteins.
- b. adequate fat stores and low serum protein levels.
- c. low body weight and low serum protein.
- d. low body weight and adequate immune function.

b   730 (k)   37. All of the following are characteristics of chronic malnutrition except
- a. depleted fat stores.
- b. low serum protein levels.
- c. underweight.
- d. none of the above

d   730 (k)   38. Nutrition status can be compromised during stress by
- a. PEM.
- b. loss of appetite.
- c. inadequate absorption.
- d. all of the above

e   732 (k)   39. Drugs prescribed in the treatment of severe stress
                        include
                        a. immunosuppressants.
                        b. anti-infective agents.
                        c. analgesics.
                        d. a and b
                        e. a, b, and c

c   730 (a)   40. Health care providers should be aware that giving
                        multiple medications to a person who is severely
                        stressed and malnourished may lead to the development
                        of all of the following *except*
                        a. delayed drug actions.
                        b. drug-nutrient interactions.
                        c. vitamin toxicities.
                        d. all of the above

d   732 (k)   41. The primary purpose of nutrition support for treating
                        stress is to
                        a. maintain immune defenses.
                        b. prevent acute malnutrition.
                        c. preserve organ function.
                        d. all of the above

c   733 (a)   42. The initial task for the health care team for a client under
                        major stress is to
                        a. institute total parenteral nutrition to prevent negative
                           nitrogen balance.
                        b. place a nasogastric tube to begin enteral nutrition
                           supply.
                        c. restore fluid and electrolyte balance.
                        d. calculate calorie needs via indirect calorimetry.

e   733 (k)   43. Which of the following techniques do health
                        care professionals use to monitor fluid needs?
                        a. heart rate
                        b. body temperature
                        c. blood pressure
                        d. b and c
                        e. a, b, and c

b   732 (k)   44. A complication that results when adequate nutrition is reintroduced rapidly is called
     a. refeeding hypotension.
     b. refeeding syndrome.
     c. refeeding hyperglycemia.
     d. refeeding tachycardia.

d   732 (k)   45. Complications that result from refeeding syndrome include
     a. malabsorption and respiratory distress.
     b. translocation and hypermetabolism.
     c. congestive heart failure and convulsions.
     d. a and c
     e. a, b, and c

c   732 (a)   46. Which of the following diets would prevent refeeding syndrome in a client who has PEM?
     a. high-kcalorie, moderate carbohydrate, low-sodium, lactose-free
     b. high-kcalorie, high-protein, moderate-carbohydrate
     c. low-kcalorie, moderate-carbohydrate, low-sodium, lactose-free
     d. low-kcalorie, high-potassium, high-carbohydrate

d   733 (k)   47. Electrolytes normally concentrated in intracellular fluids include
     a. potassium.
     b. phosphorus.
     c. manganese.
     d. a and b
     e. b and c

d   734 (k)   48. Glutamine does which of the following?
     a. maintains immune function
     b. promotes healing of wounds
     c. provides fuel for intestinal cells
     d. all of the above

b   734 (k)   49. The Harris-Benedict equation can be used to
     a. estimate fat expenditure.
     b. estimate basal energy expenditure.
     c. estimate protein requirements.
     d. estimate fat requirements.

b   734 (a)   50. An estimate of the non-protein kcalorie needs of a 70 kg man who has undergone bypass surgery would be
- a. 1525-1700 kcalories.
- b. 1750-2100 kcalories.
- c. 2450-2800 kcalories.
- d. 2950-3175 kcalores.

a   735 (a)   51. How many grams of protein would a 120 lb. woman require after major physiological stress?
- a. 55-82 grams
- b. 82-109 grams
- c. 156-173 grams
- d. 180-240 grams

c   735 (k)   52. Fat intake should be restricted to __ percent for clients with burns.
- a. 5 to 10
- b. 10 to 15
- c. 15 to 20
- d. 20 to 25

b   735 (a)   53. Which of the following leads to an accelerated inflammatory response?
- a. omega-3 fatty acids
- b. omega-6 fatty acids
- c. fish oils
- d. oleic

a   735 (k)   54. Fish oils are rich in
- a. omega-3 fatty acids.
- b. omega-6 fatty acids.
- c. linolenic.
- d. stearic.

d   735 (k)   55. Which of the following stimulates intestinal cells growth and protects the intestine during stress?
- a. growth hormone
- b. insulin-like growth factor
- c. glycogen
- d. a and b
- e. a, b, and c

c   736 (a)   56. Of the following groups of foods, which is *most* appropriate on a clear liquid diet?
a. chicken broth, custard, jello
b. apple juice, lemonade, ice cream
c. coffee, broth, popsicle
d. strained oatmeal, custard, hard candy

d   736 (k)   57. Early feeding following stress does can
a. stimulate intestinal function.
b. minimize hypermetabolism.
c. increase septic complications.
d. a and b
e. a, b, and c

For question 58: Mrs. Cousins is a 56-year-old who had an uncomplicated hip replacement yesterday and complains of severe pain. Her lab work is WNL. She is 5'6" and weighs 145 lbs. She is receiving 5% glucose in NS. Her oral nutrition intake for the last two days has been minimal. Because of sedation, oral intake is anticipated to remain low.

a   736 (a)   58. The most appropriate nutritional intervention for her now would be
a. supplemental formula.
b. high-protein shakes.
c. tube feedings or parenteral nutrition.
d. low-fiber diet.

c   731 (k)   59. Barriers to adequate nutrition during severe stress can include all of the following *except*
a. decreased energy.
b. pain.
c. increased GI motility.
d. anorexia.

For question 60: Jane Smith is a 55-year-old African American woman. She has had an appendectomy and her diet order is "as tolerated". As she is advanced to a full liquid diet, she complains of gas, cramping, bloating, and diarrhea.

c   736 (a)

60. Based on her symptoms, the health care professional should
   a. recommend total parenteral nutrition.
   b. recommend enteral nutrition.
   c. provide a lactose-free full liquid diet.
   d. explain that her stomach will adjust.

For question 61: Jill Merwin is a 21-year-old woman with a history of anorexia nervosa admitted to the intensive care unit with an abdominal gunshot wound. She is 5'2" and weighs 81 lbs. Following resuscitation, her diet order is for a 3500 kcal, high-carbohydrate, high-protein formula to be delivered by vein.

c   732 (a)

61. Jill's most likely response to this diet will be
   a. rapid recovery.
   b. boredom with the type of food.
   c. refeeding syndrome.
   d. constipation.

a   733 (a)

62. For clients who are minimally stressed, clinicians suggest providing ___ to meet protein daily requirements.
   a. 1.0 to 1.5 g protein/ kg bodyweight
   b. 1.5 to 2.0 g protein/ kg bodyweight
   c. 2.0 to 2.5 g protein/ kg bodyweight
   d. 2.5 to 3.0 g protein/ kg bodyweight

d   733 (k)

63. Indirect calorimetry estimates energy output by measuring
   a. the amount of oxygen used.
   b. the amount of carbon dioxide eliminated.
   c. the amount of heat produced.
   d. a and b
   e. b and c

b   733 (a)

64. Which of the following is true?
   a. The greater the stress, the more nitrogen is excreted in the urine, the lower the protein need.
   b. The greater the stress, the more catabolism, the more nitrogen is excreted in the urine.
   c. The milder the stress, the more nitrogen is excreted in the urine, the more catabolism.
   d. The milder the stress, the greater the protein need, the more catabolism.

c   735 (k)   65. Which of the following micronutrients is important for tissue repair?
a. thiamin and riboflavin
b. folic acid and pyridoxine
c. ascorbic acid and zinc
d. iron and magnesium

c   733 (k)   66. During the immediate post-burn period, the treatment of an extensive burn focuses on
a. calculating the protein loss.
b. providing IV dextrose for caloric support.
c. replacing lost fluids and electrolytes.
d. providing supplemental lipids.

c   741 (k)   67. The ability of the GI tracts to protect the body against foreign substances include all of the following *except*
a. intestinal barrier.
b. bacterial flora.
c. high gastric pH.
d. immune system cells.

a   742 (k)   68. All of the following promote changes in bacterial flora that increase bacterial translocation *except*
a. hypetmetabolism.
b. use of antibiotics.
c. decreased GI tract motility.
d. lack of enteral nutrients.

b   742 (k)   69. Malnutrition and inflammatory responses increase the likelihood of translocation by
a. changing the bacterial flora.
b. altering the structure and function of the GI tract barrier.
c. compromising immune factor functions.
d. none of the above

ESSAY QUESTIONS

1. Compare and contrast the metabolic responses to fasting and severe stress.

2. Describe the factors associated with hormonal and metabolic responses to severe stress.

3. Discuss the affect acute stress has on nutrition status and how it alters the body's nutritional needs.

4. Illustrate how PEM can interact with stress response. How is nutrition status further compromised?

5. Darryl recently underwent extensive surgery. He is 30-years-old and is 5'11" and weighs 205 lbs. Using the Harris-Benedict equation, estimate his energy and protein requirements.

6. Give examples of when nutrients are provided to clients following severe stress by oral diets, tube feedings, and parenteral nutrition.

Chapter 25
Nutrition and Diabetes Mellitus

c   746 (k)   1. People with type 1 diabetes need insulin because they
                      a. have become insulin resistant.
                      b. have developed hyperinsulinemia.
                      c. no longer synthesize insulin.
                      d. digest insulin with GI enzymes.

d   746 (k)   2. All of the following conditions are present in diabetic
                      clients with type 2 diabetes *except*
                      a. being over age 45 at onset.
                      b. currently taking insulin.
                      c. being obese.
                      d. no longer producing insulin.

c   746 (k)   3. Which of the following *best* describes clients with
                      type 2 diabetes?
                      a. usually lean
                      b. rapid onset of symptoms
                      c. weight loss needed
                      d. ketosis prone

d   746 (k)   4. Type 2 diabetes generally develops in children and teens
                      who
                      a. are between 10 and 19 years old.
                      b. have a family history of diabetes.
                      c. have a BMI of 27 or greater.
                      d. all of the above

b   746 (k)   5. The hallmark for type 2 diabetes is
                           a. insulin deficiency.
                           b. insulin resistance.
                           c. absence of receptor sites for insulin.
                           d. beta-cell exhaustion.

c   746 (k)   6. Hyperinsulinemia is associated with
                           a. rise in blood glucose, pancreas synthesizes more
                              insulin, and blood insulin decreases.
                           b. decrease in blood glucose, pancreas synthesizes
                              more insulin, and blood insulin increases.
                           c. rise in blood glucose, pancreas synthesizes more
                              insulin, and blood insulin increases.
                           d. decrease in blood glucose, pancreas stops synthesis
                              of insulin, and blood insulin decreases.

a   746 (k)   7. The ability of the body to regulate blood glucose
                           concentration during fasting or metabolic stress is called
                           a. glucose tolerance.
                           b. insulin resistance.
                           c. glucose intolerance.
                           d. insulin response.

b   747 (k)   8. All of the following contribute to weight loss in type 1
                           diabetes *except*
                           a. loss of glucose in the urine.
                           b. polyphagia.
                           c. catabolism of protein.
                           d. loss of ketone bodies in the urine.

b   748 (k)   9. Acetone breath is a symptom of diabetes due to
                           a. insulin resistance.
                           b. ketosis.
                           c. hyperglycemia.
                           d. gangrene.

c   748 (k)   10. Glycosuria usually occurs when blood glucose exceeds
                           a. 140 mg/dl.
                           b. 160 mg/dl.
                           c. 180 mg/dl.
                           d. 200 mg/dl.

d   748 (k)   11. Which of the following is a symptom or complication associated with diabetes?
a. ketoacidosis
b. nephropathy
c. polydipsia
d. all of the above

a   747 (k)   12. Fatigue, increased urination, and acetone breath are symptoms of
a. hyperglycemia.
b. hypoglycemia.
c. macroangiopathies.
d. microangiopathies.

c   748 (k)   13. Hyperglycemic coma can develop when blood glucose is greater than
a. 400 mg/dl.
b. 500 mg/dl.
c. 600 mg/dl.
d. 700 mg/dl.

b   749 (k)   14. Hunger, shakiness, and disorientation are all symptoms of
a. hyperglycemia.
b. hypoglycemia.
c. macroangiopathies.
d. microangiopathies.

c   756 (a)   15. Which of the following foods is considered a meat exchange on a diabetic diet?
a. bacon
b. peanuts
c. ham
d. yogurt

a   756 (a)   16. Which of the following foods is *not* found in the vegetable exchange group?
a. potatoes
b. green beans
c. broccoli
d. tomato juice

b   755 (k)   17. Alcoholic beverages such as rum, gin, and vodka are best substituted for which exchange on a diabetic diet?
a. fruit
b. fat
c. bread
d. milk

c   757 (a)   18. For a diabetic diet, a croissant containing 17 grams of carbohydrate and 30 grams of fat should be counted as
a. 1 bread and 4 fats.
b. 1 fruit and 6 fats.
c. 1 bread and 6 fats.
d. 1 fruit and 4 fats.

For question 19: Mrs. Barclay's physician has prescribed 6U regular insulin and 15U NPH for control of her diabetes. Mrs. Barclay is 5'3", weighs 112 lbs., and is an active woman who plays handball three times per week.

d   755 (a)   19. While preparing her for discharge, the nurse should tell Mrs. Barclay that
a. she does not need to eat extra food for exercise as her diet is designed to cover strenuous activity.
b. she should eat three meals only to cover the action of her insulin.
c. she could miss one injection if she gets too busy.
d. if she drinks alcoholic beverages, she is at risk of hypoglycemia.

c   759 (a)   20. When NPH insulin is administered once daily, before breakfast, hypoglycemic reactions are *most* likely to occur
a. 2 hours after the drug is injected.
b. at midday (before lunch).
c. before the third meal of the day (supper).
d. at bedtime.

a   749 (k)   21. Symptoms of hypoglycemia include
a. confusion and nervousness.
b. increased thirst and polyuria.
c. acetone breath.
d. warm-flushed skin.

b   755 (k)   22. When symptoms of hypoglycemia begin, ___ grams of
carbohydrates should be consumed.
a. 5 to 10
b. 10 to 15
c. 15 to 20
d. 20 to 25

a   755 (a)   23. Which of the following represents an appropriate snack
at the beginning of an episode of hypoglycemia?
a. 4-6 lifesavers
b. 8 oz. orange juice with 1 teaspoon sugar
c. 10 saltine crackers
d. 1 piece of chewing gum

For question 24: While you are making rounds at the
beginning of the evening shift at 4 p.m., Mrs. Davis
complains of feeling dizzy. When taking her pulse, you
note that her hand trembles slightly and feels cool and
moist.

b   749 (a)   24. It is most likely that Mrs. Davis is experiencing
a. a relapse into ketoacidosis.
b. hypoglycemia.
c. respiratory alkalosis from hyperventilation.
d. hyperglycemia.

a   749 (k)   25. Hypoglycemia should be avoided, especially for children
under 7 years old, because it can
a. impair brain development.
b. impair muscle development.
c. impair insulin sensitivity.
d. impair glucose tolerance.

For question 26: A 50-year-old woman with uncontrolled
type 2 diabetes is admitted to the hospital for the
initiation of insulin therapy. She received 25U of NPH
insulin at 8:00 a.m. At 4:00 p.m. she is complaining of a
headache, rapid heart rate, and shakiness.

d   749 (a)   26. The first thing the nurse should do is
a. give her ½ cup of orange juice.
b. call the physician.
c. give her skim milk and two crackers.
d. check her blood sugar.

b 749 (k) 27. The Somogyi effect is *best* described as
       a. rebound hypoglycemia.
       b. rebound hyperglycemia.
       c. dawn phenomenon.
       d. nocturnal hypoglycemia.

a 749 (k) 28. To prevent the Somogyi effect, insulin should gradually be
       a. decreased.
       b. decreased by half.
       c. increased.
       d. increased by half

       For question 29: Mildred Jones is a 28-year-old woman with type 2 diabetes. She is admitted to the hospital for the treatment of the Somogyi effect.

b 749 (a) 29. The health care provider should expect the blood glucose levels for Mildred to
       a. progressively rise from bedtime to the morning hours.
       b. decrease during sleeping hours resulting in hypoglycemia around 3:00 a.m. and rise until dawn.
       c. be normal throughout the sleeping hours and rise suddenly at dawn.
       d. rise at bedtime, be elevated throughout the night, and decrease at dawn.

b 748 (k) 30. All of the following are associated with diabetic ketosis *except*
       a. dehydration.
       b. blood glucose level less than 65 mg/dl.
       c. electrolyte depletion.
       d. labored breathing.

b 748 (a) 31. On the cellular level, diabetic ketoacidosis is a form of
       a. hypertrophy.
       b. starvation.
       c. hypoglycemia.
       d. hyperplasia.

d   749 (a)   32. During an acute illness, clients with type 1 diabetes
should
a. decrease their medications if their appetite is poor.
b. decrease the fluid intake to prevent nausea.
c. drink fluids with sugar if the blood glucose is greater
than 240 mg/dl.
d. monitor urine for ketones.

a   749 (k)   33. Hypoglycemia shares the same symptoms as
a. alcohol intoxication.
b. dehydration.
c. food deprivation.
d. kidney failure.

d   745 (k)   34. A fasting blood glucose level above ___ is classified
as diabetes.
a. 90 mg/dl
b. 100 mg/dl
c. 116 mg/dl
d. 126 mg/dl

d   746 (k)   35. Which of the following are major risk factors for type 2
diabetes?
a. obesity
b. family history
c. high-risk ethnic background
d. all of the above

c   750 (k)   36. Which one of the following characteristics is *not*
associated with syndrome X?
a. insulin resistance
b. hypertension
c. elevated HDL
d. elevated LDL

c   752 (k)   37. Blood glucose is monitored at least ___ times a day
under intensive therapy for diabetes.
a. 1 or 2
b. 2 or 3
c. 3 or 4
d. 4 or 5

For question 38: Mr. Brown is a 65-year-old male who
has suffered two hear attacks last year. He has just
been diagnosed with diabetes.

b   752 (a)   38. Which treatment therapy is appropriate for Mr. Brown?
- a. intensive therapy
- b. traditional therapy
- c. intensive or traditional therapy
- d. Not enough information is given to determine the best therapy for Mr. Brown.

a   753 (k)   39. Which of the following has the greatest effect on blood glucose?
- a. carbohydrate
- b. protein
- c. fat
- d. all have equal effect

c   754 (k)   40. Diet plans for type 1 diabetes should provide __ percent of the total kcalories from carbohydrate.
- a. 20 to 35
- b. 35 to 50
- c. 45 to 60
- d. 60 to 75

d   754 (k)   41. Which of the following are complex carbohydrates?
- a. legumes
- b. fruits
- c. whole-grain breads and cereals
- d. all of the above

b   753 (k)   42. For a diabetic, protein should provide how much of the total kcalories?
- a. 5 to 10 %
- b. 10 to 20 %
- c. 15 to 25 %
- d. 20 to 30 %

d   754 (k)   43. Which of the following can be used as a nutritive sweetener?
- a. fructose
- b. mannitol
- c. sucrose
- d. all of the above

a   754 (a)   44. Mr. Jacobs has high triglycerides. The physician would
                        instruct him to limit dietary fat to less than
                        a. 10% of kcalories.
                        b. 15% of kcalories.
                        c. 20% of kcalories.
                        d. 25% of kcalories.

a   754 (k)   45. All of the following contribute carbohydrates *except*
                        a. olestra.
                        b. sucrose.
                        c. sorbitol.
                        d. xylitol.

c   755 (k)   46. Health care professionals recommend that patients with
                        hypertension and diabetes should restrict sodium to
                        a. 1000 mg or less per day.
                        b. 1500 mg or less per day.
                        c. 2400 mg or less per day.
                        d. 3000 mg or less per day.

b   761 (k)   47. Patients with type 1 diabetes should refrain from
                        vigorous exercise if their blood glucose levels are
                        greater than
                        a. 200 mg/dl.
                        b. 300 mg/dl.
                        c. 350 mg/dl.
                        d. 400 mg/dl.

d   759 (k)   48. An advantage of lispro is
                        a. reduced risk of hypoglycemia.
                        b. reduced after-meal hyperglycemia.
                        c. shorter duration of action.
                        d. all of the above

b   760 (k)   49. Delivery of different types of insulin by injection three or
                        more times a day is called
                        a. advanced diabetes.
                        b. multiple daily injection.
                        c. type 2 diabetes.
                        d. insulin resistance.

a   751 (k)   50. The most commonly used glycated hemoglobin used for
                            screening and monitoring diabetes is
                            a. hemoglobin A_{1c}.
                            b. heme iron.
                            c. heme protein.
                            d. none of the above

b   751 (k)   51. Glycosylated hemoglobin (AIC) can best be described
                            as a(n)
                            a. by-product of fat metabolism.
                            b. reflection of mean blood glucose concentration over
                               two to three months.
                            c. end-product of protein metabolism formed in the liver.
                            d. summary of hemoglobin rates for type I diabetes.

d   745 (k)   52. A hormone that opposes insulin's actions is
                            a. glucagons.
                            b. cortisol.
                            c. catecholamines.
                            d. all of the above

d   762 (k)   53. A hormone that opposes insulin's actions during
                            pregnancy is
                            a. prolactin.
                            b. cortisol.
                            c. progesterone.
                            d. all of the above

b   749 (k)   54. For a diabetic, overdose of insulin, strenuous physical
                            activity, skipped meals, and inadequate intake of food
                            can all result in
                            a. hyperglycemia.
                            b. insulin shock.
                            c. dawn phenomenon.
                            d. rebound hyperglycemia.

c   755 (K)   55. Each of the following food sources provides approximately how much carbohydrate?

2 to 3 tsp honey
4 to 6 oz sweetened soft drink
4 oz orange juice

a. 3 to 4 grams
b. 5 to 7 grams
c. 10 to 15 grams
d. 15 to 20 grams

For question 56: Jane Watson is a 16-year-old with type 1 diabetes. At clinic she reports fasting blood sugars to be within the 100-150 mg/dl range and no postprandial blood glucoses greater than 180 mg/dl. Her glycosylated hemoglobin level is 18%.

c   751 (a)   56. The most likely explanation is
a. chronic hypoglycemia.
b. Somogyi effect.
c. noncompliance.
d. adolescent growth spurt.

For question 57: Mr. Sanchez, a 52-year-old male, is being discharged from the hospital. He participates freely in the discussion during discharge instructions about type 2 diabetes.

c   756 (a)   57. Which statement indicates some understanding of his nutrition plan?
a. "I should avoid dried beans and peas because they have too much starch."
b. "Green peas and green beans are both in the vegetable exchange group."
c. "Sausage won't make my blood sugar go up but it will clog my arteries."
d. "If I don't want to drink 8 oz. of skim milk, I can drink 4 oz. of whole milk instead."

d   752 (k)   58. To promote gradual weight loss, average energy intake should be restricted by
a. 50 to 100 kcalories.
b. 100 to 150 kcalories.
c. 150 to 300 kcalories.
d. 250 to 500 kcalories.

For question 59: Mrs. Lucas is 5'2" tall and weighs 142 lbs. She has been recently diagnosed as having type 2 diabetes.

a   867 (a)   59. The appropriate kcal level for Mrs. Lucas for weight reduction is
a. 940.
b. 1040.
c. 1140.
d. 1240.

For question 60: Hector Martinez is a 70-year-old Hispanic man recently diagnosed with type 2 diabetes. He is having difficulty understanding the exchange system and has limited financial resources.

b   756 (a)   60. Which of the following strategies is *most* likely to help him control his diabetes?
a. emphasis how important it is to follow only the exchange list
b. try an alternate diet approach
c. give him a printed exchange list of traditional Hispanic foods
d. encourage him to join a spa and exercise

For question 61: Mrs. Billings was recently diagnosed with type 2 diabetes. She is 5'8" tall, weighs 200 lbs., 58 years old, and lives a sedentary life style. During the interview, she tells you her lowest weight in her adult life is 160 lbs.

a   752 (a)   61. What is the *most* appropriate kcal level for the management of her diabetes?
a. 1120
b. 1220
c. 1320
d. 1420

For question 62: Mr. Mervin is a 45-year-old man with type 2 diabetes. He is 5'9" and weighs 210 lbs. His diabetes is currently controlled with diet alone.

a   752 (a)   62. Which of the following will help to improve insulin resistance?
a. weight reduction
b. hard candy for hypoglycemic attack
c. antioxidants
d. three meals plus a morning, afternoon, and bedtime snack

b   749 (k)   63. Physiological stress, such as colds and surgery, causes a(n) ___ in blood glucose.
a. decrease
b. increase
c. no change

For question 64: Mrs. Barclay has type 2 diabetes and you are preparing her for discharge. She tells you that she loves red beans and rice and knows that she must eliminate them from her diet because they will elevate her blood glucose level.

a   756 (a)   64. You should explain to her that
a. she can enjoy 1/3 c. beans mixed with 1/3 c. rice in exchange for 2 slices of bread.
b. red beans are eliminated because they are high in complex carbohydrates.
c. red beans are high in water soluble fiber and should be avoided.
d. peas are a better choice than red beans.

For question 65: Mrs. Filbert, age 56, has been diagnosed with type 2 diabetes. During discharge instruction, she makes a number of statements.

c   753 (a)

65. Which one indicates some understanding of her diabetes management?
   a. "If my blood glucose is between 100-180 mg/dl I should not exercise."
   b. "If I eat high-fat foods my blood sugars will be elevated."
   c. "Adding a bedtime snack may prevent nocturnal hypoglycemia."
   d. "Red beans can be exchanged for broccoli on my diet."

For question 66: Mr. Lilly, a 42-year-old male, tells you that he used to take "pills" for his diabetes but is now taking insulin.

d   758 (a)

66. What is the most likely reason that he no longer takes oral antidiabetic agents?
   a. They are only effective in type 1 diabetes.
   b. His body now stimulates enough insulin to meet his needs.
   c. They suppress insulin release.
   d. They were not controlling his blood glucose.

d   756 (k)

67. Drug therapy for type 2 diabetes includes
   a. oral antidiabetic agents.
   b. drugs to stimulate insulin secretion.
   c. insulin and insulin analogs.
   d. all of the above

d   763 (k)

68. Which of the following statements is true?
   a. The most common medical complication of pregnancy is gestational diabetes.
   b. Uncontrolled diabetes in the early stages of pregnancy increases the risk of spontaneous abortions.
   c. Women with gestational diabetes are at high risk of hypotension.
   d. a and b
   e. a, b, and c

e   764 (k)   69. The prenatal care for women who develop gestational
diabetes can include
a. insulin therapy.
b. high-protein intake.
c. reduced carbohydrate intake.
d. a and b
e. a and c

a   763 (k)   70. Women with type 1 diabetes who are attempting to
become pregnant should be aware that uncontrolled
blood glucose can contribute to all of the following
except
a. diabetes in the infant.
b. high-birthweight infant.
c. risk of spontaneous abortion.
d. birth defects.

c   763 (k)   71. The American Diabetes Association recommends that
pregnant women should be screened for diabetes
between ___ weeks of gestation.
a. 10 to 14
b. 19 to 23
c. 24 to 28
d. 30 to 34

b   764 (a)   72. Which of the following treatments is *not* recommended
for pregnant women with diabetes?
a. insulin therapy
b. oral antidiabetic agents
c. physical activity
d. diet modification

c   751 (k)   73. To re-evaluate a diabetic treatment plan, all of the
following information is used except
a. body weight.
b. blood pressure.
c. midarm muscle circumference.
d. blood glucose levels.

For question 74: Jane Smith is a 36-year-old client with
type 1 diabetes who has experienced frequent episodes
of hypoglycemia.

b   751 (a)   74. The most helpful tool for evaluating her management of
                            the disease is
                            a. glycosylated hemoglobin level.
                            b. blood glucose monitoring records.
                            c. triglyceride levels.
                            d. fasting blood sugar level.

ESSAY QUESTIONS

1. Compare and contrast the characteristics of type 1 and type 2 diabetes.

2. Illustrate the metabolic consequences and clinical manifestations of uncontrolled diabetes.

3. Describe strategies for managing conditions of hyperglycemia and hypoglycemia in diabetics and explain why these conditions develop.

4. Describe the techniques health care professionals use to monitor the success of diabetic treatment plans.

5. Discuss how the intakes of protein, carbohydrate, fat, sodium, and alcohol are modified for a diabetic diet and explain why these changes are made.

6. Discuss meal-planning strategies for clients with diabetes mellitus and illustrate how exchange lists and carbohydrate counting are used.

7. Compare and contrast drug therapies used for diabetes and diagram the actions of insulin types.

8. If you were counseling a client who has just been diagnosed with diabetes, what would you say regarding blood glucose control and physical activity?

9. Discuss how diabetes develops as a consequence of pregnancy and what are the treatments used to protect both mother and fetus.

Chapter 26
Nutrition and Disorders of the Heart, Blood Vessels, and Lungs

d   774 (k)

1. Cardiovascular disease usually involves
    a. atherosclerosis.
    b. hypertension.
    c. diabetes.
    d. a and b
    e. a, b, and c

d   774 (k)

2. The aorta carries blood from the heart to the
    a. brain.
    b. kidneys.
    c. lungs.
    d. other major arteries.

a   774 (k)

3. Pulmonary arteries carry ___ blood from the heart to the lungs and pulmonary veins carry ___ blood from the lungs to the heart.
    a. carbon dioxide-rich, oxygen-rich
    b. carbon dioxide-rich, carbon dioxide-rich
    c. oxygen-rich, carbon dioxide-rich
    d. oxygen-rich, oxygen-rich

d   774 (k)

4. The kidneys regulate blood pressure by
    a. hormonal changes.
    b. adjusting blood volume.
    c. altering blood vessel size.
    d. all of the above

c   775 (k)

5. Cholesterol carried on ___ is oxidized and is embedded in artery walls.
   a. chylomicrons
   b. HDL
   c. LDL
   d. VLDL

d   785 (k)

6. If ignored, a consequence of coronary heart disease is
   a. heart attacks.
   b. chronic heart failure.
   c. strokes.
   d. all of the above

b   777 (k)

7. All of the following conditions are modifiable as a risk factor for coronary heart disease *except*
   a. hypertension.
   b. gender.
   c. diabetes mellitus.
   d. high LDL cholesterol.

c   777 (a)

8. Based on the limited data provided, which of the following individuals has the lowest risk for developing CHD?
   a. a 40-year-old man with controlled hypertension
   b. a 50-year-old post-menopausal woman
   c. a 45-year-old woman who is 5'2" and weighs 125 lbs
   d. a 35-year-old woman with a LDL to HDL ratio of 5.0

d   778 (k)

9. Which of the following is included in the standards for CHD risk factors?
   a. being female
   b. body weight 20% less than ideal
   c. HDL greater than 35 mg/dl
   d. LDL cholesterol greater than 160 mg/dl

a   774 (k)

10. Mounds of lipid material and macrophages covered with fibrous connective tissue and embedded in artery walls are
    a. plaques.
    b. platelets.
    c. thrombosis.
    d. embolus.

d   775 (k)   11. All of the following favor plaque development *except*
a. diabetes.
b. elevated LDL.
c. low HDL.
d. low triglycerides.

c   775 (a)   12. High fasting blood glucose is to diabetes as ___ is to atherosclerosis.
a. chylomicrons
b. HDL
c. LDL
d. VLDL

b   775 (k)   13. Which of the following carries cholesterol away from the arteries to the liver?
a. chylomicrons
b. HDL
c. LDL
d. VLDL

d   777 (a)   14. Which of the following significantly affect *other* risk factors associated with CHD?
a. obesity
b. inactivity
c. diabetes
d. a and b
e. a, b, and c

d   775 (k)   15. Sudden tissue death of the heart muscle by blockages of a vessel is
a. acute heart failure.
b. cardiac arrest.
c. MI.
d. all of the above

a   776 (k)   16. When a portion of a clot travels through the blood stream, lodges in a small artery, and causes sudden tissue death it is called a(n)
a. embolism.
b. platelets.
c. aneurysm.
d. thrombus.

b   778 (k)   17. In women, CHD occurs about ___ years later than in men.
a. 5 to 7
b. 10 to 12
c. 15 to 17
d. 20 to 22

d   779 (k)   18. Which of the following ethnic groups is considered at higher risk for CHD?
a. African Americans
b. Asian Americans
c. Native Hawaiians
d. all of the above

c   776 (k)   19. Which of the following is known as the "silent killer?"
a. stroke
b. MI
c. hypertension
d. diabetes

d   776 (k)   20. If left untreated, hypertension can lead to
a. renal failure.
b. a heart attack.
c. a stroke.
d. all of the above

For question 21: Mrs. Thomas had blood work done as ordered by her physician. Her total cholesterol level was 230 mg/dl and HDL was 35 mg/dl.

b   778 (a)   21. Mrs. Thomas' total cholesterol and HDL indicates she is
a. at a desirable level.
b. borderline at risk for CHD.
c. at high risk for CHD.
d. requires more tests.

c   781(k)   22. The dietary guidelines recommend that total fat intake be limited to less than ___ percent of daily kcalories in order to promote a healthy blood cholesterol and lipoprotein profile.
a. 10
b. 20
c. 30
d. 35

b   785 (k)   23. Early dietary interventions after a MI include
    a. low-fat diet.
    b. low-sodium diet.
    c. high-kcalorie diet.
    d. high-fiber diet.

b   783 (k)   24. Dietary guidelines for the management of hypertension emphasize
    a. avoidance of calcium-rich foods.
    b. a diet rich in fresh fruits and vegetables.
    c. 6 oz. wine per day.
    d. avoidance of starchy foods.

d   778 (k)   25. Total cholesterol of 242 mg/dl would be classified as
    a. desirable.
    b. normal.
    c. borderline high.
    d. high.

    For questions 26, 27, and 28: Mr. Johnson is a 60-year-old Caucasian. His has a BMI of 36. His cholesterol measured: LDL 172 mg/dl, HDL 30 mg/dl, and total cholesterol 250 mg/dl.

c   778 (a)   26. From the above information, what is Mr. Johnson's risk of CHD?
    a. very low
    b. moderate
    c. very high
    d. not enough information is provided

c   778 (a)   27. Mr. Johnson's LDL and HDL cholesterol are classified as
    a. low and low.
    b. low and high.
    c. high and low.
    d. high and high.

d   778 (a)   28. What risk factors from the above information place Mr. Johnson at risk of CHD?
    a. LDL and HDL cholesterol
    b. age
    c. obesity
    d. all of the above

b   778 (k)   29. Women younger than ____ tend to exhibit lower LDL cholesterol compared to men the same age.
a. 35 years
b. 45 years
c. 50 years
d. 55 years

d   778 (k)   30. Which of the following puts women at greater risk of CHD?
a. birth control pills
b. hypertension
c. smoking
d. all of the above

For question 31: Mrs. Appleton's physician wants to start her on estrogen replacement therapy, but she does not like medication and is reluctant.

d   778 (a)   31. What could the physician say to encourage Mrs. Appleton to start estrogen replacement therapy?
a. Estrogen replacement therapy reduces CHD risk.
b. Estrogen replacement therapy reduces the risk of osteoporosis.
c. Estrogen replacement therapy alleviates menopausal symptoms.
d. all of the above

For question 32: Mr. Brady is 51 years old and his diastolic blood pressure is 110 mmHg. He has no signs of CHD. The physician places him on dietary therapy to prevent the development of CHD and to control his blood pressure.

b   778 (a)   32. What is his goal for LDL cholesterol?
a. $\leq$ 100 mg/dl
b. < 130 mg/dl
c. $\geq$ 130 mg/dl
d. < 160 mg/dl

b   779 (k)   33. Regular aerobic physical activity
a. lowers HDL.
b. increases HDL.
c. increases LDL.
d. has no effect on cholesterol.

d   791 (k)   34. Medication used to treat cardiovascular disease include
                          a. aspirin.
                          b. antihypertensives.
                          c. diuretics.
                          d. all of the above

c   776 (k)   35. The risk of heart attacks and stroke increase in direct
                          proportion to rising blood pressure when blood pressure
                          is ___ or higher.
                          a. 120 / 80 mmHg
                          b. 130 / 80 mmHg
                          c. 140 / 90 mmHg
                          d. 150 / 90 mmHg

c   778 (k)   36. For adults, normal resting blood pressure averages
                          about
                          a. 100 / 70 mmHg.
                          b. 110 / 80 mmHg.
                          c. 120 / 80 mmHg.
                          d. 120 / 90 mmHg.

c   776 (k)   37. At diastolic pressures of ___ and higher, the risk of
                          heart attacks and strokes increase.
                          a. 120 mmHg
                          b. 130 mmHg
                          c. 140 mmHg
                          d. 150 mmHg

a   776 (k)   38. In atherosclerosis, blood flow to the kidneys
                          a. decreases.
                          b. increases.
                          c. remains unchanged.
                          d. expands.

d   776 (k)   39. Hypertension that goes untreated can cause
                          a. aneurysm.
                          b. heart attacks.
                          c. kidney disease.
                          d. all of the above

c   787 (a)   40. When clients have edema associated with chronic heart
                          failure, physicians usually order
                          a. cholesterol restriction and bile acid sequesterants.
                          b. saturated fat restriction and corticosteriods.
                          c. sodium restriction and diuretics.
                          d. carbohydrate restriction and insulin.

b   779 (k)   41. All of the following are consequences of smoking
                            tobacco *except*
                            a. encourages plaque formation.
                            b. lowers blood pressure.
                            c. deprives the heart of oxygen.
                            d. increases the likelihood of blood clot formation.

                            For question 42: Interventions for post-MI usually
                            include a low-fat, low-kcalorie, salt-restricted diet.

b   786 (a)   42. If a client continues to have pain post-MI you should
                            a. encourage a liquid diet.
                            b. suggest small, frequent feedings.
                            c. restrict sodium even further.
                            d. ask for an order for enteral feedings.

d   783 (a)   43. Which of the following groups of foods are *most*
                            appropriate for a hypertensive client on a low-fat,
                            low-sodium, high-potassium diet?
                            a. macaroni and cheese, carrot and raisin salad, and
                               chocolate layer cake
                            b. fried shrimp, French fries, spinach salad with Italian
                               dressing, and fresh strawberries
                            c. cheese omelet, buttermilk biscuits, and apple pie
                            d. hamburger patty, lettuce and tomato with vinegar and
                               oil, and baked potato with margarine

c   782 (a)   44. Which of the following groups of foods are *most*
                            appropriate for a low-cholesterol, low-saturated fat diet?
                            a. turkey breast, mashed potatoes with gravy, green
                               beans, and coconut pie
                            b. scrambled eggs, toast with jelly, orange juice, and
                               whole milk
                            c. beef tenderloin, wild rice, peas, and angel food cake
                            d. cheeseburger with lettuce and tomato, apple, and
                               chocolate milkshake

                            For question 45: Mr. Bidwell, age 68, has suffered a
                            MI six-weeks ago. On his clinic visit he tells you he has
                            been trying to mange his diet. You ask him to describe a
                            typical dinner.

c   786 (a)   45. Mr. Bidwell probably understands his dietary instructions if he describes a dinner of
- a. baked chicken, macaroni and cheese, green beans and jello.
- b. shrimp creole, rice, salad with blue cheese dressing, and sherbet.
- c. turkey, cranberry sauce, steamed vegetables, and angel food cake.
- d. spare ribs, boiled potato, and coleslaw.

d   780 (k)   46. Which of the following contains fiber that will help reduce blood lipids?
- a. barley
- b. oats
- c. wheat
- d. a and b
- e. a, b, and c

For question 47: Mrs. Gonzales has been placed on a two-gram sodium diet for her hypertension.

c   783 (a)   47. Which of the following statements suggests some understanding of her dietary restriction?
- a. "I will only eat ham twice per week."
- b. "I will use monosodium glutamate (MSG)."
- c. "I will cook with small amounts of salt and add no salt at the table."
- d. "I cannot eat foods seasoned with garlic powder."

b   783 (a)   48. Which of the following meals is lowest in sodium?
- a. pancakes, sausage, and orange juice
- b. chicken breast, baked potato, and spinach
- c. spaghetti with tomato sauce, carrots, and dinner roll
- d. cheeseburger on a bun with lettuce, tomato and ketchup, and milkshake

a   781 (a)   49. Which of the following is the leanest cut of beef?
- a. top sirloin steak
- b. ribeye steak
- c. brisket
- d. hamburger meat

For question 50: Mr. Parks owns a sandwich shop. He has hired you to help him to revise his "lunch specials" to label them "heart healthy". One popular "special" offers a 3 oz. cut of grilled sirloin on a sour dough bun; a salad that includes ½ tomato, lettuce leaf, and ½ avocado.

b   782 (a)   50. Which of the following would be the most effective revision to recommend to Mr. Parks?
a. substitute 3 oz. skinless chicken for sirloin
b. substitute bell pepper for avocado
c. provide a choice of wheat or sour dough bun
d. double the amount of lettuce

d   781 (k)   51. The goals for the American Heart Association diet strategies aim to
a. produce healthy eating patterns.
b. promote a health body weight.
c. control blood pressure at a desirable level.
d. all of the above

d   783 (k)   52. A source of omega-3 fatty acids is
a. fish oil.
b. canola oil.
c. nuts.
d. all of the above

d   789 (a)   53. Dietary interventions for a client in respiratory failure include controlling carbohydrate intake because carbohydrates
a. fuel infections.
b. impair the immune function.
c. decrease oxygenation.
d. generate more carbon dioxide that fat metabolism.

c   789 (a)   54. Overfeeding should be avoided in clients with respiratory failure primarily because
a. albumin levels will decrease.
b. serum cholesterol will increase.
c. CO_2 production will increase.
d. protein energy malnutrition will result.

b   789 (a)   55. Clients who are on ventilators should receive
a. continuous parenteral support.
b. an individualized diet based on indirect calorimetry.
c. a protein restricted diet.
d. a high-potassium diet.

For question 56: Mr. Goldman is a 55-year-old Caucasian who has suffered a MI. His total cholesterol level is 242 mg/dl, LDL 172 mg/dl, HDL 35 mg/dl, and triglycerides 400 mg/dl.

d   786 (a)   56. Which statement by Mr. Goldman suggests some accurate recall of dietary instructions?
   a. "I should drink a glass of wine every day to raise my HDL cholesterol."
   b. "I'm supposed to eat 300 mg of cholesterol/dl."
   c. "I must eliminate red meat from my diet."
   d. "Avoidance of saturated fat is a primary concern."

c   783 (k)   57. Simple sugars cause triglyceride levels to ___ and HDL cholesterol to ___.
   a. decrease, decrease
   b. decrease, increase
   c. increase, decrease
   d. increase, increase

c   787 (a)   58. Prior to feeding someone post-stroke, the health care professional should assess the client for
   a. food intolerance.
   b. salt sensitivity.
   c. dysphagia.
   d. hydration status.

c   787 (a)   59. Dietary interventions for a client with chronic heart failure are aimed at all of the following *except*
   a. reducing the workload of the heart.
   b. preventing fluid overload.
   c. increasing the metabolic rate.
   d. restricting sodium intake.

a   786 (k)   60. The term for PEM associated with chronic heart failure is
   a. cardiac cachexia.
   b. anorexia nervosa.
   c. dyspnea.
   d. tachycardia.

b   787 (a)   61. The major goal of dietary intervention in CHF is to provide
a. extra calories for rapid weight gain.
b. adequate nutrients with limited work for the heart.
c. a decrease in calories and protein.
d. large meals to maximize rest periods for the client.

For question 62: Mr. Kline is a 36-year-old African American with hypertension. He is currently taking a potassium sparing diuretic to help lower his blood pressure.

d   782 (a)   62. Which of the following meals would be most appropriate for Mr. Kline?
a. vegetable soup (canned), ½ c. chocolate pudding, and carrot sticks
b. ham sandwich, potato salad, and frozen yogurt with strawberries
c. cheese sandwich, garden salad, and dried apricots
d. chicken, chief salad, French bread, and an apple

a   784 (k)   63. Moderate consumption of alcohol can reduce the risk of CHD by
a. increasing HDL.
b. deceasing HDL.
c. increasing LDL.
d. decreasing LDL.

For question 64: Mr. Peabody had a stroke seven days ago. Initially he was fed via tube feeding because he had dysphagia. Today the tube has been removed and his diet is advanced.

a   787 (a)   64. Which of the following foods would be the *most* appropriate for Mr. Peabody?
a. pureed carrots
b. cubed meat
c. sliced apple
d. rice

For question 65: Mrs. Green has CHF. She is currently taking the drugs digoxin and furosemide (diuretic) to help control the symptoms. You visit her at home and note she is eating fried chicken, green beans, and a baked potato with sour cream. She is drinking a carbonated cola.

d   787 (a)   65. Mrs. Green's meal contains
                      a. too much fat, sodium, and potassium.
                      b. too much fat, sodium, and calcium.
                      c. too much fat and sodium.
                      d. amounts of fat and minerals require further
                         assessment.

b   783 (k)   66. The effect of diets rich in omega-3 fatty acids is a(n)
                      a. decrease in serum cholesterol.
                      b. decrease in serum triglycerides.
                      c. increase in serum triglycerides.
                      d. tendency to form thrombi.

a   783 (a)   67. A recommendation for clients with hypertension is a low-
                      sodium diet that contains
                      a. high-potassium and high-calcium.
                      b. low-potassium and high-calcium.
                      c. low-potassium and low-calcium.
                      d. high-potassium and low-calcium.

b   785 (a)   68. The purpose of an intravenous infusion immediately after
                      a MI is to
                      a. provide an energy source.
                      b. prevent dehydration.
                      c. provide fuel to the heart muscle.
                      d. prevent a fluid shift.

d   791 (k)   69. Which of the following are prescribed in treating
                      hypertension?
                      a. antihypertensives
                      b. diuretics
                      c. potassium supplements
                      d. all of the above

a   791 (a)   70. A physician placing clients on diuretics to treat
                      hypertension should also be concerned with
                      a. potassium imbalances.
                      b. manganese imbalances.
                      c. phosphorous imbalances.
                      d. B vitamins.

c   786 (k)

71. Which of the following conditions can lead to CHF?
   a. liver disease
   b. diabetes
   c. hypertension
   d. all of the above

b   786 (a)

72. In response to CHF, energy requirements
   a. decrease.
   b. increase.
   c. remain the same.
   d. depend on individual needs.

b   787 (a)

73. Generally, patients with CHF benefit from daily sodium restriction of ___ or less.
   a. 1 gram
   b. 2 grams
   c. 3 grams
   d. 4 grams

d   788 (a)

74. Which of the following are usually restricted after a stroke?
   a. sodium
   b. fat
   c. kcalories
   d. all of the above

b   788 (k)

75. The most frequent cause of acute respiratory failure is
   a. severe allergic reactions.
   b. severe stress.
   c. aspiration pneumonia.
   d. inhalation of toxic gases.

a   789 (k)

76. Indirect calorimetry is used to determine the ratio of ___ produced to ___ consumed.
   a. carbon dioxide, oxygen
   b. oxygen, carbon dioxide
   c. water, oxygen
   d. carbon dioxide, water

b   790 (k)

77. Emphysema and bronchitis are examples of
   a. acute respiratory failure.
   b. chronic obstructive pulmonary disease.
   c. esophogeal deterioration.
   d. none of the above

d   790 (k)   78. Weight loss in patients with COPD can be attributed to
                            a. anorexia.
                            b. elevated energy expenditure.
                            c. repeated infection.
                            d. all of the above

ESSAY QUESTIONS

1. Discuss the risk factors associated with CHD and describe how they can be affected by diet modification.

2. Explain why hypertension is known as the "silent killer."

3. What is the interrelationship between atherosclerosis and hypertension?

4. Provide examples of ways to help clients implement a heart-healthy diet into their lives.

5. Mr. Wilson is a 57-year-old male who just suffered from a heart attack. Describe both his immediate care and long-term therapy.

6. Discuss the nutritional concerns associated with patients with CHF and those who suffered a stroke.

7. Give examples of how nutrition status is compromised due to acute respiratory failure and COPD.

Chapter 27
Nutrition and Renal Diseases

Ans	Page	
b	801 (k)	1. All of the following are functions of the kidneys *except*

Ans **Page**

b   801 (k)   1. All of the following are functions of the kidneys *except*
     a. help maintain fluid, electrolyte, and acid-base balance.
     b. activate vitamin A.
     c. eliminate metabolic waste products.
     d. help regulate blood pressure.

d   801 (k)   2. The most active form of vitamin D is
     a. vitamin D_2.
     b. vitamin D_3.
     c. vitamin D_4.
     d. 1,25-dihydroxy vitamin D.

c   802 (k)   3. Conditions associated with kidney stones include all of the following *except*
     a. fat malabsorption.
     b. gout.
     c. hypothyroidism.
     d. vitamin D toxicity.

d   803 (k)   4. A symptom associated with kidney stones is
     a. frequent urination.
     b. dysuria.
     c. hematuria.
     d. all of the above

d   804 (k)   5. Foods high in oxalate are
a. beets, orange peel, and peanut butter.
b. blueberries, coffee, and legumes.
c. baked potatoes, pepper, and lentil.
d. a and b
e. a, b, and c

e   804 (a)   6. Cathy has been diagnosed with oxalate stones. Her physician instructs her to
a. eat calcium-rich foods.
b. take vitamin C supplements.
c. avoid vitamin C supplements.
d. a and b
e. a and c

d   805 (k)   7. Which of the following can damage the glomerular capillaries?
a. diabetes mellitus
b. hypertension
c. infection
d. all of the above

d   805 (k)   8. Characteristics of nephrotic syndrome include
a. proteinuria.
b. low serum albumin.
c. edema.
d. all of the above

c   805 (k)   9. Nephrotic syndrome in clients with diabetes can be an early sign of
a. hypertension.
b. hypoglycemia.
c. renal failure.
d. hypolipidemia.

a   801 (k)   10. A hormone secreted by the kidneys that stimulates the production of red blood cells is
a. erythropoietin.
b. renin.
c. aldosterone.
d. vasopressin.

c   801 (k)   11. In response to reduced blood flow, the kidneys secrete
                   a. aldosterone.
                   b. erythropoietin.
                   c. renin.
                   d. vasopressin.

b   801 (k)   12. The working units of the kidneys are
                   a. filtrate.
                   b. nephrons.
                   c. tubule.
                   d. glomerulus.

a   807 (k)   13. The normal glomerular filtration rate is ___ for females
                   and ___ for males.
                   a. 120 ml/min, 130 ml/min
                   b. 130 ml/min, 120 ml/min
                   c. 130 ml/min, 140 ml/min
                   d. 140 ml/min, 130 ml/min

d   805 (k)   14. A consequence of nephrotic syndrome is the loss of
                   plasma proteins in the urine, which include
                   a. albumin.
                   b. immunoglobulins.
                   c. vitamin D-binding proteins.
                   d. all of the above

d   806 (a)   15. Daniel is a 10-year-old boy that has just been diagnosed
                   with nephrotic syndrome. Which of the following
                   conditions may develop as a result of his condition?
                   a. beriberri
                   b. pellagra
                   c. anemia
                   d. rickets

a   806 (k)   16. The characteristics of lipids in nephrotic syndrome is
                   a. elevated cholesterol, LDL, and triglycerides.
                   b. elevated cholesterol and lower LDL, triglycerides.
                   c. lower cholesterol, LDL and elevated triglycerides.
                   d. lower cholesterol and elevated LDL, triglycerides.

b   806 (k)   17. Diet, as a treatment for nephrotic syndrome, focuses on
                   a. increasing the fat content in the diet.
                   b. preventing protein malnutrition and edema.
                   c. high-protein diets above the RDA.
                   d. high-sodium intake.

For question 18: Billy Lewis is a 20-year-old man admitted to the hospital with nephrotic syndrome. He is 5'11", 192 lbs. and has edema. His blood values include albumin 1.7 g/dl, K+ 3.3 mEq/L, cholesterol 492 mg/dl, and triglycerides of 680 mg/dl. He is complaining of hunger and wants a snack.

b   806 (a)   18. The most appropriate food choice would be a
    a. sausage biscuit.
    b. grilled chicken sandwich with lettuce and tomato.
    c. peanut butter and crackers.
    d. piece of coconut cream pie.

a   807 (a)   19. Dietary guidelines for a client with nephrotic syndrome restrict all of the following *except*
    a. protein.
    b. fat.
    c. sodium.
    d. all are restricted.

c   807 (a)   20. A high-protein diet for a nephrotic client is contraindicated because
    a. protein foods are usually high in fat.
    b. energy requirements are decreased with nephrotic syndrome.
    c. protein may accelerate nephrotic syndrome.
    d. protein levels in nephrotic syndrome are not altered.

d   806 (k)   21. Diets high in vitamin D and calcium are recommended for children with nephrotic syndrome to prevent
    a. beriberi.
    b. marasmus.
    c. nephrosclerosis.
    d. rickets.

d   807 (k)   22. A client in acute renal failure who is uremic is likely to be
    a. hyperactive.
    b. hypoglycemic.
    c. alert.
    d. anorexic.

c   808 (a)   23. The majority of sodium comes from ___ in a typical diet.
a. salt added at the table
b. salt added during cooking
c. processed foods
d. unprocessed natural foods

b   809 (a)   24. As glomerular filtration decreases in renal failure, so does the tolerance for
a. carbohydrate.
b. protein.
c. fat.
d. vitamins.

a   810 (a)   25. A client in acute renal failure with a potassium level of 6.2 mEq/L will probably require
a. IV dextrose and insulin therapy.
b. IV normal saline with potassium.
c. extra amounts of oral fluids.
d. parenteral glucagon therapy.

c   810 (a)   26. The primary reason for giving TPN with 70% dextrose to clients in acute renal failure is to
a. provide low-kcalories.
b. provide high protein.
c. prevent fluid overload.
d. avoid using lipid emulsions.

c   810 (k)   27. For patients with nephrotic syndrome, recommended daily protein intake is
a. 0.6 g/kg body weight.
b. 0.7 g/kg body weight.
c. 0.8 g/kg body weight.
d. 0.9 g/kg body weight.

d   807 (k)   28. Daily sodium intake should be restricted to about ___ for patients with nephrotic syndrome.
a. 0.5 grams
b. 1.0 grams
c. 1.5 grams
d. 2.0 grams

a   807 (k)   29. A cause of acute renal failure is urinary tract obstruction
                            which is known as
                            a. postrenal.
                            b. prerenal.
                            c. intrarenal.
                            d. azotemia.

a   807 (k)   30. Normal blood urea nitrogen levels are
                            a. 10 to 20 mg/dl.
                            b. 30 to 40 mg/dl.
                            c. 50 to 60 mg/dl.
                            d. 80 to 90 mg/dl.

d   807 (k)   31. Blood urea nitrogen levels of ___ indicate serious
                            abnormal renal function.
                            a. 10 to 20 mg/dl
                            b. 30 to 40 mg/dl
                            c. 50 to 80 mg/dl
                            d. 50 to 150 mg/dl

b   809 (k)   32. Hyperkalemia is when excessive ___ is in the blood.
                            a. calcium
                            b. potassium
                            c. phosphorus
                            d. vitamin D

b   809 (k)   33. The early phase of acute renal failure that is
                            characterized by reductions in urine volume is called the
                            a. diuretic phase.
                            b. oliguric phase.
                            c. hyperkalemic phase.
                            d. recovery phase.

a   809 (a)   34. A patient suffering from acute renal failure is
                            experiencing large fluid and electrolyte losses in the
                            urine. What phase of acute renal failure does this
                            describe?
                            a. diuretic phase
                            b. oliguric phase
                            c. hyperkalemic phase
                            d. recovery phase

For questions 35 and 36: Mrs. Jones is in acute renal failure and has a potassium level of 5.2 mEq/L. Her physician has ordered potassium exchange resin through enemas.

b   810 (a)   35. Additional therapy at this time for Mrs. Jones should be a diet that is
a. high in phosphorus.
b. low in potassium.
c. low in carbohydrates.
d. low in phosphate binders.

c   810 (a)   36. When Mrs. Jones becomes oliguric and receives diuretics, her diet should be
a. higher in potassium.
b. lower in potassium.
c. lower in sodium.
d. higher in protein.

For question 37: Sam Martin is a 9-year-old boy in end stage renal disease. He weighs 35 kg.

c   813 (a)   37. How many kcal does Sam need to promote reasonable growth?
a. 1400
b. 2800
c. 3500
d. 4000

d   807 (k)   38. Which of the following symptoms accompany uremic syndrome?
a. anorexia
b. agitation
c. muscle twitches
d. all of the above

b   809 (k)   39. To meet the energy requirements of a patient with acute renal failure, an estimate of daily nonprotein energy intake should range between
a. 20 to 30 kcal/kg body weight.
b. 30 to 40 kcal/kg body weight.
c. 40 to 50 kcal/kg body weight.
d. 50 to 60 kcal/kg body weight.

b   809 (a)   40. The nonprotein kcalorie needs for a person with acute renal failure who weighs 140 lbs. would be approximately
- a. 1300 to 1900 kcal/day.
- b. 1900 to 2500 kcal/day.
- c. 2500 to 3200 kcal/day.
- d. none of the above

d   810 (a)   41. When prescribing the use of carbohydrate-dense enternal and parenteral nutrition for acute renal failure, physicians are aware it can cause
- a. hyperglycemia.
- b. insulin resistance.
- c. hyperkalemia.
- d. a and b
- e. a, b, and c

b   811 (k)   42. Uremic frost is a symptom of chronic renal failure that affects the
- a. eyes.
- b. skin.
- c. blood.
- d. hair.

c   823 (k)   43. The removal of excess fluids and wastes from the blood using the peritoneum as a semipermeable membrane is called
- a. dialysis.
- b. hemodialysis.
- c. peritoneal dialysis.
- d. none of the above

d   811 (k)   44. In the early stages of chronic renal failure, GFR
- a. falls to 50% of its normal rate.
- b. falls to 60% of its normal rate.
- c. falls to 65% of its normal rate.
- d. falls to 75% of its normal rate.

For questions 45 and 46: A patient is admitted to the hospital who is in the end stage of renal disease.

a   811 (a)   45. What would the health care professionals expect to find regarding the GFR?
a. drop below 20% of normal
b. drop below 40% of normal
c. drop below 50% of normal
d. drop below 75% of normal

a   816 (a)   46. Which of the following are treatment options for this patient?
a. dialysis or kidney transplant
b. diet modification
c. drug therapy
d. enteral nutrition

b   814 (k)   47. Causes of the development of wasting and PEM in renal failures is related to reduced nutrient intake include all of the following *except*
a. protein.
b. phosphorus.
c. calcium.
d. all of the nutrient requirements are higher.

d   812 (K)   48. Excessive nutrient losses in patients with chronic renal failure that contribute to the development of wasting and PEM include
a. dialysis.
b. GI bleeding.
c. malabsorption.
d. all of the above

d   813 (a)   49. As renal insufficiency progresses to en-stage renal disease, requirements for vitamin B_6
a. decreases by 50%.
b. increases by 50%.
c. decreases by 100%.
d. increases by 100%.

c   812 (a)   50. Which of the following is an application of a dietary therapy for clients with chronic renal failure?
a. avoidance of hard candy to prevent dental caries
b. drinking three glasses of milk per day for extra calcium
c. adding extra margarine to toast to increase calories
d. eating spinach to promote elimination of potassium salts

b 809 (a) 51. The fluid allowance for a client with a urine output of 800 ml is
           a. 800 ml.
           b. 1300 ml.
           c. 1800 ml.
           d. 2300 ml.

d 813 (a) 52. Phosphorus levels of 7 mg/dl in chronic renal failure indicate
           a. probable compliance with the diet.
           b. erythropoietin deficiency.
           c. the need to assess fluid status.
           d. the need to assess diet and drug compliance.

d 814 (k) 53. Phosphorus is found in
           a. eggs.
           b. milk products
           c. peanut butter.
           d. all of the above

b 815 (k) 54. Clients with zinc deficiency often exhibit
           a. dysphagia.
           b. dysgeusia.
           c. dyspnea.
           d. dyslipidemia.

a 814 (k) 55. Which of the following medications is used to treat an elevated serum phosphate level during end stage renal disease?
           a. calcium carbonate
           b. glucagon
           c. 50% dextrose solution and insulin
           d. kayexalate

a 809 (k) 56. In the oliguria stage of acute renal failure, urine volume is ___ and fluid needs are ___.
           a. reduced, low
           b. reduced, high
           c. increased, low
           d. increased, high

For question 57: Johanna Klein, a 12-year-old, has chronic renal failure and receives dialysis three times per week. According to her dry weights over the last month, Johanna has lost six lbs.

b 813 (a) 57. What is the most likely explanation for this weight loss?
a. Johanna is responding to the dialysis and is having less edema.
b. Johanna is at risk for growth failure.
c. Johanna is at risk for developing osteodystrophy.
d. Johanna's diet is too low in sodium.

b 822 (a) 58. When Glen Davis, a 46-year-old dialysis client, calls you to report a blood pressure of 160/100 mm Hg, you should
a. refer him to his internist for an antihypertensive agent.
b. ask him when the blood pressure was taken in regards to his dialysis schedule.
c. tell him to further restrict his sodium intake.
d. refer him to his nephrologist for an increase of his diuretic.

d 814 (k) 59. Which of the following foods are considered part of a fluid-restricted diet?
a. soup
b. ice cream
c. liquid medications
d. all of the above

a 814 (k) 60. In the presence of hyperkalemia, daily potassium can be restricted to
a. 1.5 to 3.0 grams.
b. 2.5 to 4.0 grams.
c. 3.5 to 5.0 grams.
d. no restriction is needed.

a 815 (k) 61. Intakes of vitamin C are restricted in patients with chronic renal failure to prevent
a. oxalate stones.
b. scurvy.
c. kidney stones.
d. hypermagnesemia.

b   814 (a)   62. To meet energy needs, a renal diet should be rich in
- a. protein.
- b. complex carbohydrates.
- c. fat.
- d. electrolytes.

For question 63: Mr. Jones has insulin dependent diabetes and end stage renal disease. He becomes hypoglycemic while on dialysis.

c   815 (a)   63. The immediate treatment for Mr. Jones should be 4 oz. of
- a. unsweetened orange juice.
- b. prune juice.
- c. lemon-lime soft drink.
- d. tomato juice.

d   813 (a)   64. Which of the following is an example of a food containing high quality protein?
- a. gelatin
- b. dried beans
- c. peanut butter
- d. fish

d   814 (a)   65. Which of the following fruits is a source of potassium?
- a. grapefruit
- b. cantaloupe
- c. apple
- d. grapes

For questions 66 through 68: John Miller is on dialysis and his current protein allowance is 60 grams.

c   816 (a)   66. After he receives a kidney transplant, the health care professional should expect Mr. Miller's protein intake to be
- a. unchanged.
- b. decreased to 0.5 g/kg of body weight.
- c. increased to 1.0 g/kg of body weight.
- d. unrestricted.

b   816 (a)   67. When Mr. Miller inquires if he should continue to restrict his sodium after transplant, you reply,
  a. "Since your renal function has been restored you do not need to restrict your sodium intake."
  b. "Since you are on immunosuppressants, you need to restrict your sodium level to 3-4 g/day."
  c. "Since you are going to be on diuretics, there is no need to restrict sodium."
  d. "Once you are off the immunosuppressants, you will no longer need to restrict sodium intake."

b   816 (a)   68. Regulation of carbohydrate intake after Mr. Miller's transplant helps to control which immunosuppressant effect?
  a. catabolic effect
  b. glucose intolerance
  c. weight gain
  d. hyperkalemia

c   816 (k)   69. When a client is rejecting a new kidney, his diet therapy will most likely be
  a. unchanged.
  b. changed to a high-potassium diet.
  c. changed to a renal diet.
  d. changed to a high-protein diet.

a   816 (a)   70. Mr. Brown has just received a kidney transplant. His nutrition support would include
  a. high-kcalories and high-protein to limit catabolism.
  b. low-kcalories and low-protein to limit catabolism.
  c. high-fat and high-protein to limit catabolism.
  d. low-fat and low-protein to limit catabolism.

c   802 (k)   71. Conditions associated with kidney stone formation include all of the following except
  a. fat malabsorption.
  b. hyperparathyroidism.
  c. diabetes.
  d. gout.

a   802 (k)   72. An inherited metabolic disorder in which large amounts
                       of the amino acids cystine, lysine, arginine, and ornithine
                       are excreted in the urine is called
                       a. cystinuria.
                       b. hematuria.
                       c. hypercalciuria.
                       d. gout.

b   804 (k)   73. Which of the following is more likely to cause the
                       formation of calcium oxalate stores?
                       a. hypercalciuria
                       b. hyperoxaluria
                       c. hyperthyroidism
                       d. hypocalciuria

b   802 (k)   74. An inherited disorder that results in abnormally high
                       urinary excretions of cystine causes the formation of
                       a. calcium stones.
                       b. cystine stones.
                       c. uric acid stones.
                       d. struvite stones.

ESSAY QUESTIONS

1. A client is diagnosed with kidney stones. What is the appropriate diet therapy
   for her treatment?

2. Explain the nephrotic syndrome and what diet modifications are needed?

3. Compare and contrast the symptoms and consequences associated with
   acute and chronic renal failure.

4. Explain how chronic renal failure can lead to cardiovascular complications.

5. Describe the events leading to the development of bone disease in patients
   with chronic renal failure.

6. Discuss the modifications of phosphorus, calcium, and vitamin D that are
   required for persons with chronic renal failure.

7. Dan, a 34-year-old male, has just undergone a kidney transplant. Discuss
   dietary therapy that will be implemented when he gets out of ICU and explain
   why these modifications are needed.

Chapter 28
Nutrition and Liver Disorders

d   827 (k)   1. The liver synthesizes which of the following?
                        a. albumin
                        b. cholesterol
                        c. lipoproteins
                        d. all of the above

b   827 (k)   2. Which of the following is responsible for returning blood
                        to the heart from the liver?
                        a. hepatic artery
                        b. hepatic vein
                        c. GI tract vein
                        d. portal vein

c   827 (k)   3. The GI tract veins absorb nutrients and transport them to
                        the
                        a. hepatic vein.
                        b. biliary tract.
                        c. portal vein.
                        d. hepatic artery.

a   828 (k)   4. A liver typically weighs
                        a. 3 lbs.
                        b. 4 lbs.
                        c. 5 lbs.
                        d. 6 lbs.

c   828 (k)   5. In liver disease, serum alanine transaminase levels ___ and serum aspartate transaminase levels ___.
a. increase, decrease
b. decrease, increase
c. increase, increase
d. decrease, decrease

a   829 (a)   6. A client with hepatitis who has persistent anorexia and vomiting should be started on
a. parenteral nutrition.
b. enteral nutrition.
c. IV glucose solution.
d. a low protein diet.

d   828 (a)   7. A client with a fatty liver is at risk for
a. heart disease.
b. diabetes.
c. intolerance to sun.
d. cirrhosis.

d   830 (k)   8. Which of the following can cause cirrhosis?
a. CHF
b. infection
c. alcohol abuse
d. all of the above

d   829 (k)   9. Chronic hepatitis can lead to
a. cirrhosis.
b. liver cancer.
c. liver failure.
d. all of the above

e   828 (k)   10. Fat accumulates in the liver by
a. synthesizing too much fat.
b. oxidizing too little fat.
c. taking up too much fat from the blood.
d. releasing too little fat back into the blood.
e. all of the above

d   828 (k)   11. Treatment of fatty liver includes
a. eliminating the cause.
b. a liver transplant.
c. an adequate diet to replenish nutrient stores.
d. a and c
e. a, b, and c

c   829 (k)   12. All of the following are symptoms of hepatitis *except*
a. jaundice.
b. anorexia.
c. kidney failure.
d. nausea.

a   829 (k)   13. The characteristics of yellowing skin and whitening eyes associated with jaundice is cause by the accumulation of ___ in the blood.
a. bilirubin
b. bile
c. triglycerides
d. alkaline phosphatase

c   829 (a)   14. A diet plan for a malnourished person with hepatitis would be
a. low-kcalorie, low-protein diet.
b. high-kcalorie, low-protein diet.
c. high-kcalorie, high-protein diet.
d. not required.

a   830 (k)   15. The most common cause of cirrhosis in the U.S. is
a. alcohol abuse.
b. heart disease.
c. environment toxins.
d. congenital disorders.

c   830 (k)   16. All of the following are metabolic disorders that can cause cirrhosis *except*
a. excessive accumulation of iron.
b. excessive accumulation of copper.
c. excessive accumulation of zinc.
d. excessive accumulation of glycogen.

b   830 (a)   17. Biliary cirrhosis can develop from
a. malnutrition.
b. gallstones that block the flow of bile.
c. failure of the right ventricle.
d. alcohol abuse.

a 830 (k) 18. Cirrhosis that develops with no identifiable cause is
known as
a. idiopathic cirrhosis.
b. Laennec's cirrhosis.
c. nonalcoholic cirrhosis.
d. obstructive cirrhosis.

b 831 (k) 19. In a cirrhotic liver, portal hypertension is the result of
a. increased pressured in the hepatic artery.
b. increased pressure in the portal vein.
c. normal pressure.
d. blood flow through the liver.

c 831 (k) 20. Which of the following findings would be unexpected in a
client with cirrhosis?
a. portal hypertension
b. esophageal varices
c. hypoammonemia
d. ascites

a 831 (k) 21. Normal blood ammonia levels are
a. less than 50 mg/100 ml.
b. greater than 50 mg/100 ml.
c. less than 60 mg/100 ml.
d. greater than 60 mg/100 ml.

b 831 (k) 22. When blood flow through the portal vein is obstructed,
blood travels through smaller vessels around the liver
called
a. ascites.
b. collaterals.
c. bypass.
d. varices.

a 832 (a) 23. For a client with ascites, the nurse should expect a
reduction of dietary
a. sodium.
b. potassium.
c. calcium.
d. magnesium.

d   832 (k)   24. Hepatic encephalopathy is characterized by
a. short-term memory loss.
b. irritability.
c. inability to concentrate.
d. all of the above

a   837 (k)   25. The purpose for limiting animal protein in the diet of
clients with cirrhosis is to decrease their blood levels of
a. ammonia.
b. nitrogen.
c. glucose.
d. cholesterol.

d   832 (k)   26. Ascites worsen from
a. increased aldosterone synthesis.
b. increased blood volume.
c. sodium and water retention.
d. all of the above

d   836 (k)   27. Energy needs for a person with liver disease
range from
a. 95 to 105% of BEE.
b. 105 to 120% of BEE.
c. 120 to 150% of BEE.
d. 120 to 175% of BEE.

b   837 (k)   28. Daily sodium recommendation for a person with liver
disease equals
a. 1 to 2 grams.
b. 2 to 4 grams.
c. 4 to 5 grams.
d. no sodium restrictions

b   837 (a)   29. When signs and symptoms of hepatic encephalopathy
appear, the nurse should anticipate
a. an increase in dietary protein.
b. a restriction of protein intake.
c. the use of agents to slow peristalsis.
d. a reduction of dietary branched-chain amino acids.

c   836 (a)

30. Which of these statements by an adult male with alcoholic cirrhosis of the liver indicates the greatest need for further education?
    a. "I will not eat a 8 oz. steak every night."
    b. "I will eat hard candy and drink soft drinks for extra calories."
    c. "I will limit my drinking to a glass of wine a few times per week."
    d. "I will limit my sodium intake if I develop ascites."

d   837 (a)

31. Which food is highest in aromatic amino acids?
    a. yogurt
    b. whole wheat bread
    c. green beans
    d. hamburger

c   832 (a)

32. Aromatic amino acids may be limited in the diets of clients with hepatic encephalopathy because they
    a. reduce the synthesis of albumin.
    b. elevate bilirubin levels.
    c. may contribute to neurological decline.
    d. cause a false positive on a hemacult test for blood in the stool.

e   833 (k)

33. When brain ammonia is high, the body begins to produce high amounts of
    a. alanine.
    b. glutamine.
    c. ketoglutarate.
    d. a and b
    e. b and c

d   837 (a)

34. Clients in hepatic coma should receive
    a. nothing by mouth.
    b. 100 grams of protein to regenerate albumin levels.
    c. polymeric, high nitrogen enteral products.
    d. protein as dictated by neurological status.

c   838 (k)

35. Supplements of which vitamin decrease prothrombin time?
    a. vitamin A
    b. vitamin D
    c. vitamin K
    d. vitamin E

d   836 (k)   36. An alcoholic patient with advanced liver disease has an
                        increased need for which of the following?
                        a. fats and potassium
                        b. vitamin C and sodium
                        c. protein and simple sugars
                        d. B vitamins and magnesium

b   836 (a)   37. Which of the following is the most appropriate snack for a
                        patient with ascites?
                        a. canned tomato soup
                        b. hard candy
                        c. potato chips
                        d. ham sandwich

                        For question 38: John, a 59-year-old male, is
                        hospitalized with cirrhosis. A family member goes to get
                        a nurse. She tells the nurse John has developed a
                        tremor.

a   833 (a)   38. What would the nurse expect to see when she returns to
                        John's room?
                        a. out-stretched arms and flapping hands
                        b. out-stretched legs and flexing feet
                        c. flapping arms
                        d. twitching head

c   831 (a)   39. Which of the following diet orders would be appropriate
                        for a client with esophageal varices?
                        a. NPO
                        b. high protein
                        c. soft
                        d. clear liquids

c   838 (a)   40. Clients with poor nutrition status and bleeding
                        esophageal varices should be provided with
                        a. duodenal tube feedings.
                        b. a soft diet.
                        c. parenteral nutrition.
                        d. gastrostomy feedings.

d   837 (a)   41. Which nutritional intervention should be encouraged for a client with cirrhosis and steatorrhea?
   a. increasing the intake of polyunsaturated fat
   b. reducing calorie intake by 20%
   c. limiting vitamin B intake per day
   d. limiting fat intake

e   838 (a)   42. Vitamin status that may be affected by liver damage is
   a. B vitamins.
   b. vitamin A.
   c. vitamin D.
   d. vitamin K.
   e. all of the above

a   838 (a)   43. Mineral status that may be altered by liver disease include
   a. calcium, magnesium, and zinc.
   b. magnesium, phosphorus, and copper.
   c. calcium, selenium, and iron.
   d. potassium, zinc, and iron.

b   834 (a)   44. All of the following are associated with increasing nutrient needs in clients with liver disease *except*
   a. ascites.
   b. steatorrhea.
   c. medications.
   d. infection.

d   834 (k)   45. Typical drug therapy used to treat cirrhosis include
   a. antibiotics to limit growth of intestinal bacteria.
   b. laxatives to speed intestinal transit time.
   c. diuretics to reduce fluid retention.
   d. all of the above

c   834 (k)   46. Which of the following is converted to SAMe?
   a. methylene
   b. methotrexate
   c. methionine
   d. menadione

b   837 (k)   47. In conditions where cirrhosis is present with no signs of impending coma, protein intake should be
   a. 0.5 to 1.0 g/kg body weight.
   b. 1.0 to1.5 g/kg body weight.
   c. 1.5 to 2.0 g/kg body weight.
   d. 2.0 to 2.5 g/kg body weight.

a   833 (k)   48. The aromatic amino acids are
   a. phenylalanine and tyrosine.
   b. leucine and isoleucine.
   c. alanine and glycine.
   d. lysine and cysteine.

c   833 (k)   49. The branched-chain amino acids include
   a. phenylalanine, tyrosine, and isoleucine.
   b. lysine, valine, and tyrosine.
   c. leucine, valine, and lysine.
   d. glycine, leucine, and cysteine.

d   837 (a)   50. The benefit of diets high in plant foods for people suffering from liver disease is
   a. speeding up intestinal transit time.
   b. reducing time available for absorption of ammonia.
   c. fewer ammonia-forming constituents.
   d. all of the above

c   837 (a)   51. Health care professionals utilize which method to assess fluid balance
   a. body weight.
   b. abdominal girth.
   c. a and b
   d. none of the above

b   837 (k)   52. The *best* indicator that liver function is improving in a client with cirrhosis is
   a. rapid weight gain.
   b. sudden weight loss.
   c. increased abdominal girth.
   d. arm anthropometrics.

c   838 (a)   **53.** An example of nutrition support for clients suffering with bleeding esophageal varices is
   a. simple IV solutions to maintain fluid/electrolyte balances.
   b. parenteral nutrition.
   c. a and b
   d. none of the above

c   831 (a)   **54.** Normal values for serum albumin are
   a. 1.5 to 2.5 g/100 ml.
   b. 3.5 to 5.0 g/100 ml.
   c. 5.0 to 6.0 g/100 ml.
   d. none of the above

d   831 (a)   **55.** During liver disease albumin levels ___ and ammonia levels ___.
   a. increase, increase
   b. increase, decrease
   c. decrease, decrease
   d. decrease, increase

a   836 (a)   **56.** During hospitalization, alcoholics need
   a. extra kcalories.
   b. low-sodium diet.
   c. intravenous alcohol.
   d. extra fat.

d   831 (k)   **57.** A physical sign of altered liver function is
   a. ascites.
   b. edema.
   c. jaundice.
   d. all of the above

a   837 (a)   **58.** If ascites have developed, recommendations for daily fluid intake is
   a. 1.0 to 1.5 liters.
   b. 1.5 to 2.0 liters.
   c. 2.0 to 2.5 liters.
   d. none of the above

d   844 (k)   **59.** A complication that can develop due to gallstones is
   a. cholangitis.
   b. cholecystitis.
   c. choledocholithiasis.
   d. all of the above

c   845 (a)   60. Which of the following is the *least* likely at to develop gallstones?
- a. a woman with diabetes
- b. a woman taking birth control pills
- c. a 35-year-old man who is inactive
- d. a 60-year-old man with poor appetite

ESSAY QUESTIONS

1. Explain the nutritional concerns associated with fatty liver and hepatitis and the related treatments.

2. Describe the consequences of cirrhosis and explain how it leads to portal hypertension, esophageal varices, ascites, elevated blood ammonia levels, and hepatic coma.

3. Develop a diet for a client with cirrhosis, including protein, carbohydrate, fat, and sodium intakes.

4. Explain the importance of adequate nutrition support for patients before and following a liver transplant.

Chapter 29
Nutrition, Cancer, and HIV Infection

Ans	Page		
c	848 (k)	1.	The name of the cancer that arises from the blood-forming cells of bone marrow is called a. carcinomas. b. gliomas. c. leukemias. d. melanomas.
a	848 (k)	2.	Melanoma is a type of cancer that arises from a. pigmented skin cells. b. lymph tissues. c. epithelial tissues. d. glandular tissues.

For question 3: Mr. Nelson asks you what he can do to prevent cancer.

| a | 851 (a) | 3. | You should recommend that he do all of the following *except*
a. avoid all food additives.
b. avoid excess kcalories and fat.
c. limit salt consumption.
d. eat a variety of foods, especially fruits and vegetables. |

1

c   850 (k)   4. Which of the following cancers is *not* influenced by dietary habits?
a. colorectal
b. stomach
c. lung
d. prostrate

b   850 (k)   5. Research suggests that reducing the consumption of which food may reduce the risk colorectal and breast cancers?
a. fresh fruits
b. dietary fat
c. fiber
d. simple sugar

b   848 (k)   6. A new growth of tissue that forms an abnormal mass with no function is a
a. aalignancy.
b. tumor.
c. benign mass.
d. metastasite.

d   849 (k)   7. Which of the following are factors that influence the development of cancer?
a. immune system
b. environment
c. genetics
d. all of the above

d   849 (k)   8. Exposure to which of the following is associated with causing cancer?
a. air pollution
b. smoking tobacco
c. sunlight
d. all of the above

b   849 (a)   9. Due to the effects aging has on the immune system, the incidence of cancer ____ with age.
a. decreases
b. increases
c. decreases by two
b. increases by two

b   850 (k)

10. Which of the following cancer sites is associated with high intake of saturated fat?
    a. cervical
    b. prostrate
    c. liver
    d. stomach

d   850 (k)

11. All of the following cancer sites are associated with high intakes of alcohol *except*
    a. esophagus.
    b. liver.
    c. breast.
    d. pancreas.

b   850 (k)

12. Evidence of a protective effect from prostrate, breast, and stomach cancer is adequate intake of
    a. meat.
    b. fruits and vegetables.
    c. unsaturated fat.
    d. protein.

e   850 (k)

13. Which of the following is a carcinogen present in food or beverages?
    a. nitrosamines
    b. linoleic acid
    c. urethane
    d. a and b
    e. a and c

a   851 (k)

14. Antipromoters of cancer include all of the following *except*
    a. alcohol.
    b. antioxidants.
    c. cruciferous vegetables.
    d. dietary fiber.

a   850 (k)

15. Carcinogens are ___ of cancer.
    a. initiators
    b. promoters
    c. antipromoters
    d. none of the above

c   851 (k)   16. The main reason cruciferous vegetables are considered cancer antipromoters is because they
         a. are high in fiber.
         b. are low in fat.
         c. contain phytochemicals.
         d. support the immune system.

b   851 (k)   17. Dietary fiber is considered a cancer antipromoter because it
         a. activates enzymes capable of destroying carcinogens.
         b. increases the rate of peristalsis.
         c. contains tryptophan.
         d. decreases the risk of obesity.

c   851 (k)   18. Based on the American Institute for Cancer Research, all of the following are recommended for reducing the risk of cancer *except*
         a. limit weight gain during adulthood to less than 11 pounds.
         b. avoid alcohol consumption.
         c. limit daily consumption of meat to less than 3 ounces.
         d. avoid tobacco use.

d   852 (k)   19. Which of the following is a characteristic of cancer cachexia syndrome?
         a. malnutrition
         b. wasting syndrome
         c. anorexia
         d. all of the above

d   853 (k)   20. An example of therapy used in the treatment of cancer is
         a. chemotherapy.
         b. bone marrow transplant.
         c. radiation.
         d. all of the above

b   853 (k)   21. Methotrexate, medication used for chemotherapy, resembles
         a. iron.
         b. folate.
         c. vitamin K.
         d. selenium.

c   853 (k)   22. Radiation enteritis is inflammation and scarring of the
___ cells.
a. skin
b. epithelial
c. intestinal
d. beta

For question 23: Bill Freeman, a 36-year-old man, was recently diagnosed with cancer.

c   855 (a)   23. Which of his statements suggest some understanding of the role of nutrition in cancer?
a. "Eating a diet rich in fruits and vegetables can cure cancer."
b. "Omitting alcohol from my diet will prevent spreading."
c. "A well-balanced diet will help me to keep my strength up."
d. "A low-fat diet is the best diet to maintain my health."

d   852 (a)   24. The mechanism by which cancer cachexia syndrome develops is
a. altered metabolism.
b. cytokines.
c. dysphagia.
d. a and b
e. a, b, and c

b   853 (k)   25. Nutrient losses observed in cancer patients are due to all of the following *except*
a. inadequate digestion.
b. inadequate nutrient intake.
c. malabsorption.
d. vomiting.

a   853 (k)   26. In cancer, nutrient needs are elevated due to all of the following *except*
a. malabsorption.
b. hypermetabolism.
c. insulin resistance.
d. nutrient deficiencies.

a   853 (a)   27. Cancer induced causes of anorexia include all of the following *except*
      a. lowered metabolic rate.
      b. pain.
      c. early satiety.
      d. psychological stress.

a   852 (k)   28. The major precipitating event in the cancer cachexia syndrome is
      a. anorexia.
      b. malnutrition.
      c. wasting syndrome.
      d. hypermetabolism.

c   856 (k)   29. Which of the following conditions does diet therapy play only a supportive role?
      a. heart disease
      b. diabetes
      c. cancer
      d. renal disease

d   854 (k)   30. Radiation and chemotherapy are both associated with all of the following *except*
      a. reduced nutrient intake.
      b. altered metabolism.
      c. increased nutrient losses.
      d. reduced nutrient losses.

c   853 (k)   31. Bone marrow transplants can be used as a treatment of all of the following *except*
      a. leukemia.
      b. lymphomas.
      c. pancreatic cancer.
      d. breast cancer.

a   854 (k)   32. Destruction of healthy donor cells by the immune system is known as
      a. tissue rejection.
      b. radiation therapy.
      c. chemotherapy.
      d. bone marrow transplant.

a   855 (a)   33. Of the following surgeries, diabetes mellitus is a possible side effect of
a. pancreatic resection.
b. esophageal resection.
c. gastric resection.
d. intestinal resection.

a   855 (k)   34. Malabsorption of ___ is associated with gastric resection.
a. vitamin B_{12}
b. vitamin C
c. niacin
d. zinc

d   855 (a)   35. A careful drug history, including complementary therapies and diet supplements, is taken when a client has HIV infection or cancer for all of the following reasons *except*
a. use of alternative therapies are common.
b. use of alternative therapies may impair nutrition status.
c. use of alternative therapies may contribute to drug-nutrient interactions.
d. use of some alternative therapies is illegal.

For question 36: Sarah has been fighting leukemia. At her last doctors visit, she complained of having no appetite, feeling weak and tired, and she had lost five more pounds.

d   857 (a)   36. Sarah would benefit *most* from
a. dietary supplements.
b. TPN.
c. tube feeding.
d. b or c

For questions 37 and 38: Tommy has been undergoing chemotherapy treatments for the past month. Health care providers have noticed that he is leaving food on his plate and appears to look thinner. Additionally, Tommy has been experiencing several episodes of nausea and vomiting.

d 858 (a) 37. What is a good suggestion that could be used to encourage Tommy to eat?
    a. recommend smaller, more frequent meals
    b. recommend not eating at least two-hours before treatments
    c. encourage Tommy to eat jello, broths, and popsicles
    d. all of the above

b 858 (a) 38. Which of the following is a strategy to control nausea and vomiting?
    a. recommend adding sauces and seasonings to meats
    b. recommend small, frequent meals
    c. suggest foods that are easy to prepare and eat
    d. encourage Tommy to try new foods and experiment with herbs and spices

b 858 (a) 39. The best dietary intervention for a cancer patient experiencing a metallic taste is to
    a. serve meat very warm.
    b. use poultry, fish, or eggs for protein.
    c. avoid all foods containing protein.
    d. provide mouth care after meals.

c 856 (k) 40. A typical diet therapy for cancer patients with problems maintaining weight includes providing
    a. 50% of basal energy expenditure.
    b. 100% of basal energy expenditure.
    c. 150% of basal energy expenditure.
    d. 200% of basal energy expenditure.

b 855 (a) 41. One of the goals of nutrition support for a person with cancer is to
    a. reverse cachexia.
    b. limit the loss of lean body mass.
    c. increase metabolism.
    d. regenerate lean body mass.

a 856 (k) 42. Dietary modifications that should be taken into consideration in regard to cancer of the liver include
    a. protein-, sodium-, and fluid-restriction.
    b. protein- and electrolyte-restriction.
    c. protein- and fat-restriction.
    d. none of the above

c   856 (k)

43. Which of the following cancer sites may require tube feeding or TPN and fat- and lactose-restricted diet treatment?
    a. kidneys
    b. pancreas
    c. intestine
    d. brain

c   856 (a)

44. The rationale for providing a high-kcalorie, high-protein, and high-calcium diet to a bone marrow recipient is that this diet
    a. prevents potassium loss.
    b. prevents steatorrhea.
    c. counteracts protein and calcium loss.
    d. helps support the immune system.

d   857 (a)

45. The most appropriate form of nutrition support for immunosuppressed, anorexic bone marrow transplant patients is
    a. oral supplements.
    b. enteral feedings.
    c. peripheral IVs of fluids and electrolytes.
    d. TPN.

a   857 (a)

46. The rationale for adding glutamine to the TPN solution for bone marrow recipients is that glutamine
    a. helps prevent bacterial translocation.
    b. reduces the need for insulin.
    c. prevents stetorrhea.
    d. improves nutrient absorption.

a   859 (k)

47. The severe complications associated with the end stage of HIV infection are referred to as
    a. acquired immune deficiency syndrome.
    b. human immunodeficiency virus.
    c. opportunistic infection.
    d. all of the above

d   859 (k)

48. Which of the following is a strategy to prevent HIV transmission?
    a. the use of a latex condom and a spermicidal agent
    b. avoid contact with contaminated needles
    c. avoid unprotected sexual contact with others
    d. all of the above

b   859 (k)   49. Once a person is infected, approximately how many weeks does it take before laboratory tests can detect the presence of the HIV virus?
a. 3 to 5 weeks
b. 6 to 12 weeks
c. 12 to 14 weeks
d. immediately after contact

b   861 (k)   50. On average, how many years does it take for HIV infection to progress to AIDS?
a. 5 years
b. 10 years
c. 15 years
d. 20 years

c   860 (k)   51. To prevent food-borne illness, cold foods should be kept at a temperature of
a. 20° F or less.
b. 30° F or less.
c. 40° F or less.
d. 50° F or less.

b   860 (k)   52. To prevent food-borne illness, hot foods should be kept at a temperature of at least
a. 160° F.
b. 140° F.
c. 130° F.
d. 120° F.

a   861 (k)   53. The cells essential for immune function that are affected by HIV infection are
a. CD4+ T-cells.
b. red blood cells.
c. pigmented skin cells.
d. hemoglobin.

d   861 (k)   54. An early symptom of HIV infection is
a. diarrhea.
b. night sweats.
c. skin rashes.
d. all of the above

d   862 (k)   55. Which of the following are causes of anorexia in patients
                            with HIV infection?
                            a. dementia
                            b. depression
                            c. herpes virus
                            d. all of the above

b   862 (k)   56. All of the following contribute to reduced food intake
                            which leads to wasting in HIV infection *except*
                            a. cancer.
                            b. diarrhea.
                            c. medical treatments.
                            d. infection.

b   862 (k)   57. Wasting associated with HIV infection can be attributed
                            to all of the following *except*
                            a. reduced food intake.
                            b. excessive nutrient losses.
                            c. altered metabolism.
                            d. cancer.

a   862 (k)   58. Lipodystrophy associated with HIV infection is the
                            accumulation of fat
                            a. around the abdominal area.
                            b. in the face.
                            c. in the extremities.
                            d. none of the above

d   862 (k)   59. Which of the following is a characteristic of AIDS-
                            defining illness?
                            a. bacterial pneumonia
                            b. cancer
                            c. wasting
                            d. all of the above

b   862 (k)   60. Central body fat as a consequence of HIV infection is
                            associated with all of the following *except*
                            a. insulin resistance.
                            b. hypolipidemia.
                            c. cardiovascular disease.
                            d. diabetes.

c   863 (k)   61. A type of cancer common to people with HIV infection is
a. adenomas.
b. gliomas.
c. Kaposi's sarcoma.
d. thrush.

b   863 (k)   62. HIV enteropathies are
a. bacterial and parasitic alterations associated with HIV infection.
b. diarrhea and malabsorption associated with HIV infection having no known cause.
c. viral and protozoan manifestations associated with HIV infection.
d. none of the above

c   862 (k)   63. Thrush interferes with dietary intake for all of the following reasons *except*
a. altered taste sensations.
b. pain.
c. impaired fat absorption.
d. reduced saliva.

b   863 (a)   64. The major nutritional problems seen in clients with HIV infection are
a. dysgeusia and dyspepsia.
b. diarrhea and malabsorption.
c. weight gain and iron deficiency anemia.
d. dyspnea and gastroesophageal reflux.

d   863 (k)   65. A treatment for HIV infection is drug therapy that includes
a. protease inhibitors.
b. nonnucleoside reverse transcriptase inhibitors.
c. nucleoside reverse transcriptase inhibitors.
d. all of the above

d   864 (K)   66. An anabolic agent given to clients with HIV infection is
a. megestrol acetate.
h growth hormone.
testosterone.
b and c
a, b, and c

a   859 (k)   67. Nutrition support can be most effective for treating
patients with HIV infection during the
a. early stage.
b. presence of opportunistic infection.
c. presence of cancer.
d. end stage.

d   865 (a)   68. Daniel, 28-year-old male, has just been diagnosed with
HIV infection. Nutrition education for Daniel should
include
a. providing a high-kcalorie, high-protein diet to restore
weight.
b. suggestions for alleviating anorexia.
c. proper food preparation techniques.
d. all of the above

c   865 (a)   69. Daily protein recommendations for clients with HIV
infection should be
a. 0.5 to 1.0 gram/kg body weight.
b. 1.0 to 1.5 grams/kg body weight.
c. 1.5 to 2.0 grams/kg body weight.
d. 2.0 to 2.5 grams/kg body weight.

For question 70: Terry Pike is a 28-year-old with HIV
infection. Recently he has been experiencing severe
diarrhea. Terry's physician has identified that he has an
infection in the large intestines.

a   865 (a)   70. All of the following dietary modifications would be
appropriate for Terry *except*
a. a diet high in water insoluble fiber.
b. a low-residue diet.
c. caffeine restrictions.
d. low-fat diet.

b   860 (a)   71. In order to decrease the occurrence of food-borne
infections in people with HIV infection, you should
encourage them to
a. buy only organic produce.
b. wash produce thoroughly.
c. eat only canned produce.
d. microwave all produce prior to eating it.

c   866 (a)   **72.** Clients with HIV infection who develop severe gastrointestinal infections with intractable diarrhea may benefit *most* from
    a. regular oral diet.
    b. tube feeding.
    c. TPN.
    d. none of the above

d   867 (a)   **73.** In a client with AIDS receiving TPN solutions, all of information is useful for nutrition status assessment *except*
    a. diarrhea.
    b. fluid intake.
    c. depression.
    d. total lymphocyte counts.

a   861 (a)   **74.** Which of the following tools is *least* helpful for assessing the nutritional status of a client with AIDS?
    a. triceps skinfold thickness
    b. 24-hour food record
    c. serum albumin
    d. change in weight

ESSAY QUESTIONS

1. Illustrate the proposed causes of cancer development.

2. Explain the dietary factors that may influence the development and prevention of cancer.

3. Compare and contrast the mechanism and consequences of cancer treatment.

4. Explain the role nutrition therapy plays in the treatment of cancer.

5. Describe factors that can affect nutrient intake, nutrient losses, and metabolism in clients with HIV infection.

6. Explain how wasting observed during HIV infection is similar to that seen in cancer clients.

7. Discuss how proper nutrition can affect the course of the HIV infection.

8. Gayle, a 30-year-old female, has HIV infection. Explain why she should be concerned about food-borne illnesses and how she can minimize exposure.